LPN/LVN Student Handbook

Nancy J. Brown, RN, MSN
Director, Practical Nursing Program
San Juan Basin Technical School
Cortez, Colorado

Sandra M. Boyd, RN, MS
Assistant Professor of Nursing
Lamar University
Beaumont, Texas

B. Gayle Twiname, PhD, RN
Associate Professor of Nursing (Retired)
Lamar University
Beaumont, Texas

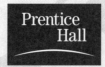

Prentice
Hall

Upper Saddle River, New Jersey 07458

Library of Congress Cataloging-in-Publication Data
Brown, Nancy J. (Nancy Jo), RN.
   LPN/LVN student nurse handbook / Nancy J.
   Brown, B. Gayle Twiname, Sandra M. Boyd.
     p. cm.
   Includes index.
   ISBN 0-13-094182-4 (alk. paper)
   1. Practical nursing—Handbooks, manuals, etc.
2. Practical nursing—Study and teaching—Handbooks,
manuals, etc.
   I. Twiname, B. Gayle. II. Boyd, Sandra M. III. Title.
   [DNLM: 1. Nursing, Practical—Handbooks.
WY 49 B879L 2003]

RT62.B698 2003
610.73'06'93—dc21   2002022478

Publisher: Julie Levin Alexander
Executive Editor: Maura Connor
Executive Assistant: Regina Bruno
Executive Editor: Barbara Krawiec
Editorial Assistant: Sheba Jalaluddin
Development Editor: Maureen Muncaster
Director of Manufacturing and Production: Bruce Johnson
Managing Editor: Patrick Walsh
Production Editor: Linda Begley, Rainbow Graphics
Production Liason: Mary C. Treacy
Manufacturing Manager: Ilene Sanford
Manufacturing Buyer: Pat Brown
Senior Marketing Manager: Nicole Benson
Creative Director: Cheryl Asherman
Senior Design Coordinator: Maria Guglielmo-Walsh
Product Information Manager: Rachele Strober
Cover Design: Joseph DePinho
Interior Design: Donna Wickes
Media Managing Editor: Amy Peltier
Media Project Manager: Stephen Hartner
Printing and Binding: RR Donnelley and Sons
Cover Printer: Phoenix Color

Pearson Education LTD.
Pearson Education Australia PTY, Limited
Pearson Education Singapore, Pte. Ltd
Pearson Education North Asia Ltd
Pearson Education Canada, Ltd.
Pearson Educación de Mexico, S.A. de C.V.
Pearson Education—Japan
Pearson Education Malaysia, Pte. Ltd
Pearson Education, Upper Saddle River, NJ

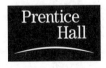

10 9 8 7 6 5 4 3 2 1
ISBN 0-13-094182-4

Contents

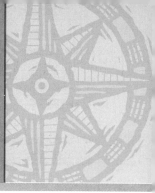

Preface

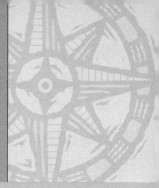

PURPOSE OF THE HANDBOOK

You have probably just finished reading the title of this book and are wondering: "What is this *student handbook*?" The short answer is that it is a book to keep on hand—to keep with you. The long answer is that it is a text specifically designed to help you learn the essential elements of topics that are central to your successful functioning as a professional practical or vocational nurse.

Nursing is a challenging profession. There is a lot of new information to remember and apply. Used in combination with other texts, this handbook will help you keep feelings of being frustrated and overwhelmed to a minimum. Because the core concepts and essential issues are presented concisely, and many valuable learning tools (most of which you will not find in your other textbooks) are included, this text will be a dependable companion throughout your nursing education and beyond.

Perhaps the best way to describe the potential usefulness of this text is to think of it as a map that will help get you to your destination safely, without getting lost. In order to understand or remember what is most essential regarding a particular topic, you can consult this "map," and take the most direct route.

The authors wish you success in your nursing career. Enjoy the journey!

FEATURES

Ask Yourself This component of the text presents questions for you to answer before and after reading the text. Your responses are recorded right in the text in the spaces provided. Through the process of zeroing in on what you already know (questions at the beginning) and what you still need to know or reinforce (questions at the end), you will be able to individualize your learning in accordance with your own learning style. In addition, this exercise in self-examination will help you to develop better analytical and retention skills.

Cyberlinks Included in this component of the text are Web sites that will provide the opportunity for you to engage in interactive exercises that tickle your curiosity and are fun and informative. For example, relating to the topic entitled *Stress,* you can evaluate your own stress level by completing the questionnaire and activities on the Web site. In addition, at www.LPNresources.com or www.LVNresources.com you can explore any topic as expansively as you desire by connecting to the Web links listed.

Core Concepts and Essential Skills   Concepts and skills central to your professional practice as an LPN/LVN are designated by icons and are presented in an easy-to-read and -remember format.

A Case in Point   Each topic is accompanied by an example representing an integration of related material. Through the reading of these examples (cases), the material comes to life. Your learning of the topic is reinforced because the case prompts you to personalize the information.

Flash/Study Card Cyberlink   At the end of each topic discussion, the opportunity is provided to make your own flash cards. Using flash cards is a proven strategy in improving your recall. Flash cards enable you to check and sort: checking to see if you know the answer to the question posed; sorting what you know from what you don't know. The capacity to make flash cards using the CD-ROM allows you to make cards for any topic or course.

Mapping Concepts Word Bank   Concept mapping is another proven technique to help you retain information that can be used with this or any text. This technique, which is explained in detail in the Study Skills section of the text and on the CD-ROM with your textbook, provides you with a concrete, visual learning tool. The format of concept mapping is similar to how the brain formats knowledge for storage. Important general concepts are placed in boxes or specifically identified in some manner, and then linked to specific concepts. Concept Mapping acts as a summary and puts the information in capsule form. It is easy and quick. Once you know how to do it, you will find numerous applications beyond your studies.

ADDITIONAL FEATURES

Study Skills Section   A comprehensive discussion of ways to study and recall what you have learned. Highlights are: assessing learning style, test-taking skills, using faculty and the computer as resources, and time management.

Behavioral Competencies Section   Concepts and skills related to communication, documentation, patient teaching, and the nursing process are among the topics discussed.

Core Issues Section   Universal health care issues are discussed, with essential skills related to each topic emphasized. Among the issues targeted are: stress, pain, ageism, sexuality, spirituality, and death and dying.

Clinical Competencies Core concepts and essential skills are included for topics ranging from drug calculation and infection control to electrolytes and IV infusion. All of the many competencies are LPN/LVN specific.

Advance Skills Section In addition to providing helpful information relating to passing the NCLEX-PN examination, advance skills pertaining to leadership and management are also included.

ACKNOWLEDGMENTS

The authors would like to thank the many individuals who have been instrumental in the development and production of this handbook. We are especially appreciative of the production and editorial staff of Prentice Hall:

Barbara Krawiec for her endless support, encouragement, and faith in this whole project

Michael Sirinides and Sheba Jalaluddin for encouragement and attention to details

Mary Ann Frew for her creativity and development ideas

Maureen Muncaster for her tireless energy and resolve

Nicole Benson for her marketing know-how

Mary Treacy for her part in the final birth of the book

We also appreciate the efforts of those staff members of Rainbow Graphics for crafting the book into the finished product:

Linda Begley and Rhonda Peters, the senders and receivers of numerous emails, for their perseverance, patience, and understanding

And lastly, we would like to acknowledge the practical/vocational nursing students for whom this book is written.

We learn so much from those we teach!

The Authors

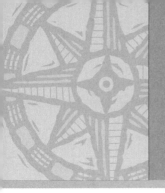

Concept Maps and Flash Cards

As educators and authors of this text, we recognize that every student who enters an LPN/LVN program wants to successfully complete the program and, subsequently, begin his or her career.

Completing the program requires learning an amazing amount of information, not just for the sake of passing tests, but for the sake of integrating and transforming the content of all the courses into the knowledge and skill base required to competently function as an LPN/LVN. We recognize also that some students are better equipped for learning than other students. It is our goal to help equalize the chances for success for all students who have the will and interest to pursue a career in health care.

Various learning tools included in each chapter accompany the presentation of core concepts and essential skills in this text. Two of these tools are special features of this text: concept mapping and flash cards.

CONCEPT MAPS

Concept mapping is a visual learning tool that is intended to help you summarize the chapter and make learning meaningful. They can be utilized in all your courses. The technique used to formulate a concept map is an extremely valuable exercise because connections (memory links) are made in the way the brain is known to store information. When making a concept map, concepts are placed within boxes and linked to one another by lines. The general, more inclusive concepts are at the top; the more specific, less inclusive are lower on the map and linked to the general concepts by drawing connecting lines.

What is unique about concept mapping is that there is no one right way to construct it. How you, the student, can best link concepts is what will help you to learn. At the end of each chapter, some starter words are suggested (Concept Map Word Bank). However, you may want to use others or use some and not all of the words provided. The point is to concretize the key points in the chapter and understand how they are interrelated.

The steps in constructing a concept map are as follows:

1. Choose words that represent general concepts presented in the chapter. Headings can be helpful in pinpointing major ideas, but should not be limiting. One well-constructed map may not contain words in the headings for that chapter. Another map for the same chapter may contain words identical to the headings. Place the key idea or word in a box at the top. The map could contain many or few boxes.

2. Choose words that represent specific concepts presented in the chapter. Place these in boxes situated below the general concept boxes.

3. Link the boxes together by drawing a line from one to the other to connect them. Words or phrases that designate the relationship between the general and specific concepts may be written on the connecting lines. It may not be necessary to write connecting words or phrases on the lines. Remember, there are many ways to link concepts. Much of the value in using this tool comes from examining your own map and revising it until it clearly represents connections you understand. The more mapping you do, the more creative you will become, and the easier it will be to arrange the boxes in a meaningful way. A CD-ROM is provided with this text which enables you to make your own concept maps.

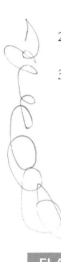

FLASH CARDS

The use of flash cards to learn key concepts, ideas, or terms is a form of a check-and-sort system. Flash cards are a useful strategy in trying to find out what you know and what you don't know. You then target what you still need to study and learn. Flash cards can also be used as a drill—you repeat the checking, sorting what you don't know from what you know as many times as you need to retain the information.

A CD-ROM is provided with this text, which enables you to make your own flash cards. You can also make your own flash cards using 3 x 5 index cards. Write the question or term on one side and the answer or meaning on the other.

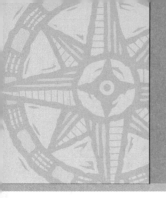

Reviewers

Cheryl A. Brown, RN, M.Ed
Hillsborough County Voc/Tech
    Center
Tarpon Springs, FL

Candace Gioia, RN, BSN, CNOR
Department Chair
Pinellas Technical Education Center
Clearwater, FL

Teresa Jo Grooms, RN, BSN
Southern State Community College
Hillsboro, OH

Geneva Lamm, RN, MSN
Chairperson
Ivy Tech State College
Columbus, IN

Brenda Miller, BSN
LPN Faculty
Central Kentucky Technical College
Lexington, KY

Diane Neville, RN
Instructor
American Career College
Los Angeles, CA

**Diane L. Okeson, RN, MN, ARNP-
    CNS**
Dean of Nursing and Allied Health
Pratt Community College
Pratt, KS

Betty Owen, RN
LPN Professor
Southern Arkansas Community
    College
Eldorado, AR

Mary Lou Roux, RN, BS
Program Coordinator
Fulton Montgomery Community
    College
Johnstown, NY

Nettie Seale, RN, M.Ed
LPN Instructor
Kiamichi Technical Center
Stigler, OK

Raedean Windish, RN, BSN, MS
LPN Instructor
CASPN
Springfield, IL

About the Authors

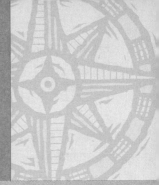

NANCY J. BROWN, RN, MSN

Nancy Brown received her Bachelor of Science in Nursing from the University of Missouri and a Master of Science in Nursing from the University of Colorado. She has been actively involved in teaching practical nursing for the past 10 years. Other teaching experience includes staff development positions in long term care and state institutions for 9 years, where she worked closely with LPNs in practice. Nancy had been involved in nursing administration as a Director of Nursing prior to going into nursing education. She received the "Teacher of the Year" award in 1998 from San Juan Basin Technical School where she currently teaches. In addition to teaching practical nursing, Nancy also coordinates and teaches within the Certified Nursing Assistant program. She is very active in her church and is known as one of the "puppet people" by those who don't remember her name!

SANDRA BOYD, RN, MS

Although officially retired, Sandy continues to teach part time at Lamar University. Her most recent teaching experience has been developing and conducting a web-based, undergraduate nursing research course. Sandy obtained her BSN from Wayne State University in Detroit and her MS in Adult Education from the University of Houston. Her long nursing career has included service in the United States Air Force Nurse Corps and the Veterans Administration. In addition to Michigan, nursing has taken Sandy to Ohio, California, and Texas. Her activities have included staff nursing, nursing administration, and nursing education positions at many levels such as staff development, hospital-based RN programs, BSN, and LVN programs. She has served as program director for two LVN programs in Texas. In addition, Sandy started CEN (Continuing Education for Nurses), a business that provided continuing education programs specifically to meet the needs of LVNs in Texas. She is a member of Sigma Theta Tau International and Phi Kappa Phi. To many she is known as the "chicken lady" since for the past 20 years, she has raised chickens and always has an abundant supply of "yard eggs" which she shares with one and all.

B. GAYLE TWINAME, PhD, RN

Gayle is a retired associate professor of nursing. Gayle has a Ph.D. in Nursing Research from Texas Woman's University; and an M.S.N. in Adult Psychiatric/Mental Health Nursing from the Medical College of Georgia. She worked in a number of different areas of nursing including: Oncology, ER, NICU, IV Therapy, Psychiatric/Mental Health, Consulting, and Nursing Education. She has published a number of articles in refereed journals and is a member of Sigma Theta Tau International and Mensa. Gayle also has a master's degree in counseling and was certified as an individual and group psychotherapist as well as a clinical nurse specialist in adult psychiatric/mental health nursing. Gayle's life and career changed significantly 11 years ago when she was diagnosed with multiple sclerosis. Accepting the challenges that significant life changes can bring, she is now more focused on staying well. Gayle enjoys writing, spending time with friends, computing, kayaking, and learning new skills within the scope of her limitations.

MAPPING FOR YOUR SUCCESS

A. LEARNING SKILLS

FEATURES INTRODUCTION: CONCEPT MAPPING AND FLASH CARDS

1. Recognizing Your Learning Style
2. Time Management
3. Study and Test-Taking Skills
4. Writing a Paper

B. USING RESOURCES EFFECTIVELY

5. Printed Resources
6. Computers
7. Consumer Groups and Health Information

C. SPECIAL PERFORMANCE ISSUES

8. Legal Considerations
9. Risk Management

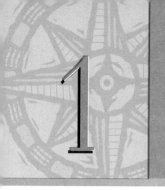

Recognizing Your Learning Style

 ASK YOURSELF

1. What do you think *learning style* means?

   _____

   _____

2. How do you think you learn best: are there any study techniques that you
   use that helps you retain the information studied; are there ways in which
   material is presented that helps you to retain it?

   _____

   _____

 CYBERLINKS

Interactive Want to be an A+ student? Knowing your learning style will help.
www.howtolearn.com/personal.html helps you evaluate your own learning
style and provides you with information of how to get higher grades.

Supplemental www.LPNresources.com can help enhance your learning by
leading you to discover other links with more information about the topic
that you are studying.

The concept of learning style refers to an individual's particular set of study
habits that produce the best results. Recognizing how *you* learn best will provide you
with a compass that will enable you to successfully map your success. You can then
develop study techniques that will best suit your needs. Understanding the differences in learning styles will also help you to effectively teach patients.

ESSENTIAL SKILLS **LEARNING STYLE ASSESSMENT**

There are numerous tests available which help to identify your learning style. Your
school learning center or counselor will have access to these. Many of these tests
analyze your answers to questions about your current study habits, work ethic and

personality traits. The information gathered from these sources provides you with an evaluation of how you learn best. Your nursing school might even have given you an admission test, which had a section on learning styles. Those results should have been shared with you. If you have not taken a test to determine how you learn best and one is available, schedule an appointment with the counselor as soon as possible. The Internet also has learning-style tests available online that you might consider.

| CORE CONCEPTS | **TYPES OF LEARNING STYLES** ——————

Although there are many ways of characterizing learning styles, most experts recognize visual, auditory, or tactile as being the most common. In this chapter, we will explore each of these, and, hopefully, you can recognize the seeds of your own style in one or more of them. Remember that most people are a combination of these styles, although usually one of these styles is dominant.

Visual Learners   Visual learners are lookers. They learn best when the instructor uses videos, overheads, or computer-generated "power point" presentations. Their learning is also enhanced by the use of the blackboard or posters. They need to actually see things to understand them. They are extensive note takers in class. If this is your predominant style, completing your reading assignments, reviewing your notes, and drawing diagrams and charts will all help you to learn better, regardless of the type of content being presented. Making *flash cards* and *mapping concepts* are forms of visual learning described on pages viii–ix. Students who draw connections representing their understanding of a patient's disease condition to how it affects the rest of the body know the pathophysiology of disease better than those who just write out an explanation of the condition in their notes. *The vast majority of students are visual learners.*

Auditory Learners   Auditory learners are listeners. They are better able to retain information if they tape record lectures rather than take notes. Students who are auditory learners also seem to learn material better if they read the reading assignments aloud, or tape record themselves reading aloud for the purpose of listening to the tape as often as they desire. Being able to play back the tape helps the auditory learner feel secure about having caught all that was said. Repeatedly playing back the tape, for them, reinforces learning. Having lectures on tape, however, can be a useful learning tool for anyone who does a lot of driving. Because some schools have a policy regarding the taping of lectures, check with your instructor before bringing a tape recorder to class. Some schools or instructors will require that you sign a paper regarding the purpose of tape recording in which you promise to use the recording for studying only. One drawback of this learning style is that other noises and conversations readily distract the student. Auditory learners may have to use earplugs during testing to eliminate any noise that would cause them to lose their focus. At our school, earplugs are available in the learning center for student use. *Auditory learners comprise the second largest group of learners.*

Tactile Learners   Touching is used by tactile learners to retain information. These learners require an opportunity to practice what they have learned before they fully understand it. If you are a tactile learner, you will want to practice your nursing skills as often as you can both in the laboratory and at home. It is helpful to have someone else watch you practice skills, such as another student, who can make comments and suggestions regarding your technique. Tactile learners benefit the most by their clinical experiences in which they can actually see patients with

A CASE IN
POINT

Cindy entered the licensed practical nurse/ licensed vocational nurse (LPN/LVN) program just one month ago. She shares with several of her classmates that she is overwhelmed. So many classes, term papers, and assignments are boggling to her. The worst part, she confesses, is that she isn't able to remember much of what she learns. She knows she is anxious, but she thinks that some of the teachers talk too fast and she can't take the notes as quickly as she needs to in order to get all the information written. One of the students who is listening to Cindy recognizes the problem and tells Cindy that she too is the kind of learner who has trouble taking notes and needs to listen more than once to information in order to understand and retain it. She suggests that, like herself, Cindy bring a tape recorder to the classes in which she is having the most difficulty. Since the instructors all encourage students to use whatever means they can to learn the concepts and skills required, Cindy purchases a tape recorder. Fast forwarding to a few months before Cindy graduates from her program, she is proud of her accomplishments. She has learned the lesson that awareness achieved by asking yourself questions about who you are and what your thoughts and feelings are, and then understanding and accepting them, provides the very best map for success.

certain disease conditions and perform the appropriate nursing care. Interactive computer programs are also especially beneficial for the tactile learner.

Instructors are aware that they will have students possessing a variety of learning styles in the same class. Most instructors utilize different teaching techniques to meet the needs of all of the students. However, just as students have different learning styles, teachers become comfortable with certain teaching styles. If you are having difficulty learning due to the instructor's teaching style, find a tactful way of letting her or him know about your particular needs. The role of the instructor is to teach, and the role of the student is to learn. The style of one should in some way be compatible with the style of the other, so that learning occurs effectively.

ASK YOURSELF

1. Are you clear about your own style of learning? After reading this discussion, how would you characterize your learning style?

   _____

   _____

2. Are there any obstacles in the way of your learning in the manner best for you? If so, what are they? What steps will you take to remove or diminish the impact of these obstacles?

   _____

   _____

 CYBERLINKS: FLASH CARDS

Use the CD-ROM that accompanies your textbook to discover how to make flash cards for reviewing and retaining what you have learned.

 CONCEPT MAP WORD BANK

Learning Styles

Purpose

Assessment

Types

Refer to Concept Maps and Flash Cards on pages viii–ix for an explanation of how to create and use concept maps. In addition, the CD-ROM guides you through the construction of concept maps by providing a more detailed introduction, more illustrations of examples, and key steps to follow in designing your own maps.

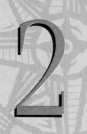

Time Management

 ASK YOURSELF

1. Are you always in a rush, pressed for time, and cramming a lot into a little space of time? Or do you seldom feel rushed, and plan your time wisely?

   _____

   _____

2. Referring to the above question, what do you think are the reasons why you manage time the way you do?

   _____

   _____

 CYBERLINKS

Interactive Never have enough time to do what needs to be done? Check out **www.mindtools.com/page5.html**, scroll down to specific time management tools and learn how to make realistic time estimates and prioritize lists, and much more.

Supplemental **www.LPNresources** can help enhance your learning by leading you to discover other links with more information about the topic that you are studying.

Have you ever played the party game where you had to see how many crackers you could stuff into your mouth, chew as much as you could, and then be the first person to whistle without choking or spitting on someone? Do you ever feel like your life is like that? Sometimes, we cram so many things into our day that we cannot completely comprehend it all; we may "chew" a little but we never really digest it. When we become so frustrated with all we have to do, we feel as if we are choking on our responsibilities, and we may actually snap at other people (although, hopefully, we are not spitting on them). We forget that the goal is to be able to whistle . . . or sing . . . or laugh! If you are feeling that way, a good dose of time management skills should help to lighten your load.

Although this chapter does not propose to have all the answers to help you, we hope it will offer some advice that you can use. We call it the POP plan of time management. POP stands for: Plan, Organize, and Prioritize. The POP plan is discussed again in this text in Chapter 35. Our inclusion of the principles of time management here in this section of the text is to help you to find effective ways of managing time, which is for students, many with work and family responsibilities, an obstacle the size of Mount Everest. Now, besides having family, work, and other responsibilities filling up your day, you are expected to attend classes, attend clinicals, practice skills, work on class presentations, write reports and nursing care plans, study, and get good grades.

While we are personalizing this discussion of time management, its principles can be applied to any situation: home, school, or in a clinical setting.

ESSENTIAL SKILLS   MANAGING YOUR TIME AT HOME

Planning   Planning is the equivalent of gathering your assessment data on your patients in nursing school. You need to see the whole picture before you can begin to see what problems there are and how you can work on them.

- Make a list of all of the things you do at home. It might include paying the bills, cleaning, laundry, car repairs and maintenance, cooking, taking out the trash, and so on. You get the idea. It's kind of like your home job description.
- Have your family and friends who are closely involved in your life make a list as well if this will impact your organization of time.
- Sit down with family and friends, compare lists, and discuss them. They may come up with things you forgot or did not realize you were doing.
- Now, add things to the list that will be necessary during the school year. Your list is getting very long, but do not panic, because we are not finished.

Organizing   This piece of the process is to take the information you have gathered in your planning time and see how it can be organized.

- Are there any things on your list that someone else is also doing? Do you share the job of bill paying, for instance? Could the other person take over the job totally?
- Do you have things that you could combine? When we asked a nursing class one year to come up with time-saving hints for the rest of the class, we had one creative student who said she cleaned her bathroom while she was sitting on the toilet!
- Is everything on your list absolutely necessary? Could someone else do it? Sometimes, we want so much to be the perfect mother, perfect wife or girlfriend, perfect daughter that we forget that we are human and cannot do it all. Do not be afraid to give up some things on your list.

- Learn to delegate. As a nurse, you will have to do that as well. First, ask what other support people can do to help out. If people volunteer to assume certain duties, they are more likely to follow through than if you assign them without any input. Once they have volunteered, delegate that job to them.
- Do you have obvious time wasters? The telephone, Internet, and television are great devices, but how much time do you spend with them?
- Get your home organized; let go of the clutter. That will really save on cleaning time.
- Now, your list should begin to be more manageable.

Prioritizing   Now, you are ready to sort out your list as to which is the most important thing for you to accomplish.

- Look at your list of duties or goals realistically, and decide which are the more important issues for you. These are the things you want to spend the most time on.
- Once you have prioritized, look at the things that are at the bottom of your list. Can any of those be eliminated? Remember, these are the things that you are going to devote the least amount of time to.
- In addition to looking at what is important to you, you also need to look at things that have a time element attached to them. Decide if there are things you need to do right away, such as paying bills by a certain deadline before your electricity is cut off. That would give that task high priority.

An important aspect of time management is having the support and cooperation of those around you. If the significant people in your life are not willing to make some sacrifices and change the way things have always been done, it will be very difficult for you to plan and manage your time wisely at home.

Besides looking at the routine tasks at home, do not forget to add fun things to your list such as exercise, going out to eat or to the movies, going to your child's school play or athletic event, or going to church. In other words, do not just concentrate on being a student. Plan for all elements of your life. You may even construct a weekly calendar and place it on the refrigerator with events of the week penciled in. These should include all activities of the week, not just classes.

ESSENTIAL SKILLS	MANAGING YOUR TIME AT SCHOOL

Every school should give you a calendar at the beginning of the year telling you what classes you have when, when the school holidays are, and so on. You should also have a course syllabus for each course you are taking. The course syllabus should give you your reading assignments as well as the dates for all of the exams. You will need a day planner or organizer, so you can lay everything out in one place.

Planning   You need to plan ahead for each class, so that you are not doing assignments at the last minute. Remember, you should be spending 3 hours outside of class in study and preparation for every hour you spend in class. That is a whopping chunk of your time.

- Get a day planner or organizer.
- Write down on your planner when your classes meet, when assignments are due, what chapters to read by when, and when the school holidays are.
- Always keep your day planner with you, in case there are changes in assignments or test dates. Sometimes, we teachers do make mistakes or miscalculate and have to change things!
- Plan on the times that you will be studying to allow for the other pieces of your life. Write them in on your home calendar as well, so the family or roommates know what to expect.

Organizing   For school, this is kind of a combined step with planning. If you know what your assignments are and when they are due and if you know your test dates, you can organize your time around preparation to meet your deadlines. Do not make the mistake of waiting until the night before an assignment is due to work on it. Do not wait until the night before an exam to begin to study. These actions just do not work. Your assignment will not be a quality paper, and your cramming may help for the test, but what about afterwards? Retention of the material is not good. Where you will need it most is in patient care, not on an exam.

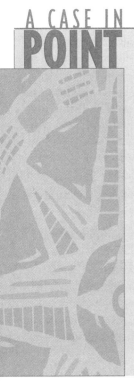

A CASE IN POINT

Toni is a single parent, with two children, ages 7 and 4. She obtained a school loan in order to further her education and become an LPN/LVN. While she is happy with her career choice, she is constantly distracted. When she is at home, she is thinking about school responsibilities. When she is at school, she is thinking about her children and their needs. There doesn't seem to be any "down" time to read a non-textbook or even a newspaper. Getting good grades is a challenge. Amazingly, with all she has on her plate, she is averaging a B in all her courses. Still, homework and laundry pile up. Meals are sometimes inadequate and rushed or consist of fast food. Toni's 4 year old misses her while he is in day care and she is at school. She wonders if things couldn't be easier if she could just get a grip. She decides to evaluate her use of time in all the areas of her life.

Prioritizing This is easy with school assignments. Just ask yourself:

- Which is due first?
- Which will take the longest to do?

The two questions stated above should help you prioritize what needs to be done and when.

Our students have suggested a way of using time effectively at home, which influences the effective use of time at school. The advice given is this: Have everything ready for school the night before. Make sure your car has gas in it. Know where your car keys are. Make sure the books you need and your assignments are in your backpack or book bag. Put them in a visible place, so you are not looking for anything in the morning. Lay out the clothes you are going to wear. Pack your lunch (and your children's if needed), so you just have to pick it up.

| ESSENTIAL SKILLS | **MANAGING YOUR TIME AT CLINICALS** |

Planning The planning for clinicals actually begins before your clinical day.

- Know where your clinical assignment is located. Obtain directions if it is an unfamiliar place.
- Know what your instructor's expectations are for your performance. Are you expected to visit the clinical site the day before and gather patient data? Do you need drugs cards for all of the medications you will be giving? Are you supposed to have a nursing care plan when you arrive for the clinical?
- If your school provides you with a form to document patient data, be sure you take it when you review your patient's chart. This will guide you on collecting enough patient data to prepare you for the nursing care you will be expected to give.
- Prepare for your clinical by reviewing the patient's medical condition in your textbook; look up her or his drugs; review lab results and what they mean; review any nursing skills you might be asked to perform; if there is a special diet, review that as well.
- Know what you are supposed to wear, and make sure it is clean.

Organizing If you have visited the health care facility ahead of time and gathered your patient data, it is much easier to get organized.

- A nursing care plan will help you to organize your nursing care as well as your day.
- Note the times your patient or patients have medications or treatments ordered. Does your patient go to a rehabilitation unit, such as physical therapy? Is your patient scheduled for surgery or a diagnostic procedure?
- Prepare a schedule for yourself, especially if you are caring for more than one patient, so that nursing interventions are done timely (see Figure 2-1).

Figure 2-1 A Sample Schedule of Patient Care

Patient Name	Room Number	0600	0700	0800	0900	1000	1100	1200
John Smith	205B		Meds.	Drssg. Chg.		P.T.		Meds.
Barbara Jones	207A	BG Chem.	Meds.		O.T.		Meds.	
Bobby Ore	208A	Preop	Surg.				Return	

Prioritizing If you are caring for more than one patient, you need to assess the conditions of all shortly after you arrive at clinical and get report. This will often help you to see what immediate needs the patients have and what you need to do first.

- If patients have special procedures that have certain times attached, that also helps you to prioritize. For example, if your patient is due at physical therapy by 8:30 A.M., you know that you need to get his personal care done early and make sure his medications and treatments have been done prior to going to physical therapy.
- If one of your patients has an immediate need such as an obvious breathing problem or an incontinent stool, you would want to manage this before moving on to other nursing interventions. You need to identify those signs or symptoms that need to be communicated to the primary nurse or your clinical instructor immediately.

There are more suggestions for time management in the clinical setting in Chapter 35. There is even a time management exercise for you to do if assuming the role of a charge nurse.

Time management requires a lot of planning, organizing, and prioritizing in your home life, school, and clinical. It will save you a lot of frustration in the long run if you are able to manage your time well. See what works for you and what does not. If your management plan is not working, you need to be flexible enough to go back and revise it so that it does. It is worth the creative effort as the rewards are many.

STOP ASK YOURSELF

1. What is problematic in your life regarding *how much time you have versus how much time you need* in order to attend to your particular set of responsibilities and circumstances?

2. Referring to the above question and the information in this chapter, what do you think you can do to alleviate the time crunches you feel?

_____

_____

 CYBERLINKS: FLASH CARDS

Check to see how much you now remember by making your own flash cards. Use the CD-ROM that accompanies your textbook to discover how to make flash cards for reviewing and retaining what you have learned.

 CONCEPT MAP WORD BANK

Time Management

Description

Principles

At home

At school

At clinicals

Refer to Concept Maps and Flash Cards on pages viii–ix for an explanation of how to create and use concept maps. In addition, the CD-ROM guides you through the construction of concept maps by providing a more detailed introduction, more illustrations of examples, and key steps to follow in designing your own maps.

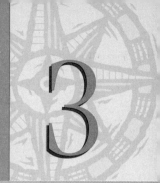

Study and Test-Taking Skills

3

ASK YOURSELF

1. What study methods or tools have you found to be most effective?

   _____

   _____

2. What types of tests (multiple choice, true–false, essay, timed) do you find most difficult?

   _____

   _____

CYBERLINKS

Interactive Did you know that a poorly designed work/study environment could cause musculoskeletal injuries? You can take a test to see if you are at risk:

> www.medbroadcast.com Scroll down to the "Menulist" and click on "Ergonomics." You will learn to set up an optimal workstation, take a stretch break, and the best postures for typing and using a mouse.

Supplemental www.LPNresources.com can help enhance your learning by leading you to discover other links with more information about the topic you are studying.

Studying and test taking are not new to you. We know that you have been doing both for quite awhile. Studying and test taking in nursing school may be more difficult, but not any different from what you have already experienced. Therefore, you probably already know what works or doesn't work for you. Do you study better in groups or on your own? Do you do better outlining assigned readings or just highlighting them or both? Whatever you prefer, find a system that works for you and stick with it!

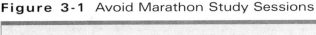

ESSENTIAL SKILLS   **FINDING A SYSTEM THAT WORKS**

The best way to find a system that works for you is trial and error. Here are some ideas that might speed the process along.

1. Most people prefer a *designated study place.* Some people prefer to study in absolute quiet. Others find that background noise or music actually increases their concentration. Be sure that you have adequate lighting, comfortable seating, and all of the supplies that you need to avoid frequent interruptions. Many of our students who are mothers sit down and do their studies along with their children. They find it makes for great "together time."

2. *Avoid marathon study sessions.* It is essential that you take breaks, get up, walk around, and stretch (Figure 3-1). You need to keep your blood moving, and you need to give your mind a break. It is much easier to study for shorter intervals, and it will probably increase your understanding. If you study consistently from the beginning of the course to the end, and review prior content, you shouldn't have to resort to marathon studying or cramming for exams.

Figure 3-1 Avoid Marathon Study Sessions

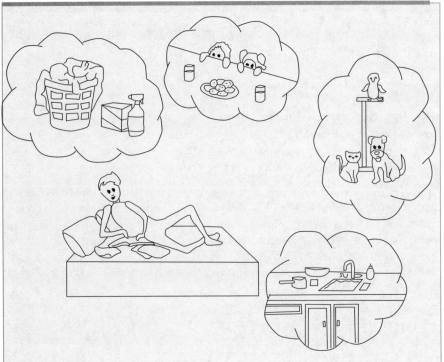

3. *Focus on what you are reading.*
   - If you are worried about something, take the time to deal with it, or put it in the back of your mind until you take a break.
   - If you have to, write down the things that distract you from your studying.
   - Sometimes, the "I forgot to . . ." pops into your mind. Keep a list of these things so you can move on and get back to your reading.
   - If you have a major personal problem that is interfering with your studying, you may need to seek outside help.

Students who try to cover up major difficulties often end up failing courses because of them. Find someone you can talk with and, if you are comfortable, let your faculty know. Nursing faculty has dealt with many a problem, and may know what resources are available to help you. If you are not comfortable with the faculty, seek out a friend, counselor, family member, minister, priest, rabbi, or family physician. Many schools have counselors who would be available to help you sort out your difficulties. The information you give them is confidential and will not be shared with your nursing instructors unless you give permission. Find someone that you trust and get help. Is it worth potentially destroying your career to keep your silence?

| CORE CONCEPTS | **PREPARATION FOR LECTURES** |

Nursing courses build on one another. You can't isolate and forget material from one or more courses. For example, if you hated anatomy and physiology, you can't throw your notes away and never think about it again. Why? Because anatomy and physiology is found in nearly all practical/vocational courses; so once it is over, you can't forget the material. If you don't believe a course or certain course material is important to your education, you will tend to forget the material. It is vital for you to remember that all of your courses are important building blocks to graduation. Units within a course also build on one another. We had students get angry with us, because they had learned their math conversion tables for the conversion exam and couldn't believe they were expected to have retained that information for the next math exam!

| ESSENTIAL SKILLS | **CLASS PREPARATION** |

1. *Have the right tools.*
   - *Notebook.* We suggest to our students to have a loose-leaf notebook for each class. Spiral notebooks don't allow for the insertion of your course syllabus and any handouts the teacher might give you. Loose-leaf notebooks also allow you to put in clear plastic sleeves to hold any study cards you might have made.
   - *Pencils or pens.* Have more than one pencil, and have it sharpened before class.
   - *Textbook.* Bring the textbook for the class. Often, the instructor will draw your attention to important graphs, photos, or tables that you would want to remember.

- *Highlighter.* If the instructor points out important statements or definitions in your textbook, you will want to highlight these to emphasize their importance.

2. *Attend all classes.* Most of us have our own way of taking notes in class. Some of us highlight, draw pictures, or scribble in the margins. No one will take notes the way that you do! We also learn through all of our senses. When you get notes from others, you lose a great deal in the interpretation. You will also spend a lot of time trying to decipher someone else's notes. If you have an emergency, ask someone you trust to tape record the class and tell you what they remember from class. Use their notes only as a backup. Much is learned simply from participating in a class discussion that may not be included in anyone's notes.

3. *If possible, sit in the front of the classroom.* Students who sit up front tend to follow the lectures better and pay attention more. The back of the room usually attracts students who want to be distracting. It is difficult to take adequate notes when the student next to you is providing details about his or her latest "hot date."

4. *Be prepared for class.* It is important to read the required reading prior to class. When you have done the reading, you will be able to concentrate more on what the instructor is saying, and you will be able to ask intelligent questions to clarify anything you didn't understand. Before actually reading, read the chapter title, headings, and key words if they are given. Look up words you don't know to make your reading proceed more smoothly. Look at charts, graphs, tables, and photos. Sometimes, it helps to read the first paragraph and then the last to give you an idea about the content of the reading (Meltzer & Palau, 1997, pp. 14, 15). Some students find it helpful to underline and some to highlight. Others actually take notes on the reading. They may outline the chapter. They may divide their notepaper in half, take notes from the reading on one half of the paper and notes from the lecture on the other half, comparing the information. That way, if there is any disagreement between what the textbook said and what the instructor said, you can have it explained at the time. Doing something, anything, with the reading makes it more memorable than simply reading.

5. *If you are having trouble hearing or seeing the board, overheads, or videos, inform your instructor.* Don't let pride stand in the way of your doing well in school. We had a student who failed two courses one year, because he sat in the back of the room and did not tell anyone he had impaired hearing. When he returned the following year, he confessed the problem. We always made sure he sat up front, and the school provided him with a device to amplify the teacher's voice, enabling him to successfully pass the program. We have had others with impaired vision who did not want to get glasses. If you think you might have a hearing or visual problem, report it right away. Many schools have the resources to test your hearing or vision or can refer you to someone who can. Schools must make reason-

able accommodations to ensure that your impairment does not stand in the way of your success in the school.

6. *Actively listen.* Be aware of what things are distracting to you, and concentrate your focus on the instructor. If students around you are talking and interfering with your learning, ask them to be quiet. If you are not comfortable doing that, then bring the distraction to the attention of your instructor. Believe it or not, sometimes instructors are unaware of those irritating little side conversations and need someone to let them know about the disruption they are causing. Getting enough rest the night before class also helps you pay attention. There's nothing worse than dozing off in class and missing a half page worth of notes.

7. *Take good lecture notes.* The students who do the best in classes are usually those who know how to take good notes. Don't try to write down everything the instructor says. We appreciate students who think every word we say is important, but having every "a," "an," and "the" down in your notes is unnecessary. Write down important concepts, and try to put them in your own words. Learn your medical abbreviations early, and use them when taking notes. Make up your own abbreviations for commonly used words rather than writing every word out. Having done your reading ahead of time also helps when taking notes, as you won't have to constantly ask the instructor to spell or repeat so many words or phrases. If you have difficulty keeping up with note taking, bring a tape recorder and record the lecture. You can take it home and replay the lecture as often as you need to. Remember, though, there are some instructors who will not allow you to use a tape recorder.

8. *During class, be alert for clues to questions that might appear on exams. As you listen to lecture, listen for words like:*
   - "The most important part of . . ."
   - "This would make a good test item."
   - "The main thing to remember is . . ."
   - "To repeat . . ."
   - "The major emphasis is . . ."

9. *Review and edit your notes within 24 hours of writing them.* Be sure to make any corrections or add any important information that you can recall.
   - It may help to recopy your notes in an outline fashion while it is still fresh on your mind.
   - Highlight any major concepts, and note any areas that you might have missed or for which you need clarification.
   - Read your text again to see if it can provide the answers to your questions.
   - If you are unable to fill in the blanks or clarify the content, check with your instructor to get the correct information.
   - Remember that relying on other students does not always provide accurate information!
   - If you and your instructor have modems, you may be able to e-mail your questions. We require our students to have access to e-mail, so that they

may direct questions to us and we may answer them timely. This prevents a lot of calls and last-minute struggling to understand a difficult concept before an exam.

- If e-mail is not available, check for your instructor's office hours, or call the instructor with your questions.

CORE CONCEPTS	TESTING

Testing is a part of all education programs. Most nursing programs use teacher-made exams that are similar to the *National Council Licensure Examination for Practical Nurses (NCLEX-PN)* test that you will take upon graduation to be eligible for your nursing license. The NCLEX-PN is made up of multiple-choice questions, so most likely you will have a great deal of experience with multiple-choice questions during your nursing education.

Before Exams

1. *Plan ahead.* Look at your syllabus or course description to know when exams are scheduled and what material will be on each one. Spend time each day on the material.
2. *Find out what type of exam you will be taking.* Is it multiple-choice, matching, fill-in-the-blank, or essay questions? Find out the expected number of items and approximate length of time allotted for the test.
3. *Clarify any content that you don't understand if you haven't already done so.*
4. *Know your instructor!* Is this the first exam that you have had from this instructor? If so, you may be at a disadvantage. Sometimes, it takes a first test to understand what an instructor expects. It can help you to determine what the instructor focuses on. The focus may vary from instructor to instructor, as they are all individuals. Does this instructor:
   - Focus on details or on general concepts?
   - Focus on the textbook or lectures?
   - Rely heavily on outside reading assignments or audiovisuals?
   - Use a combination of all of the above?

   Sometimes, only time will tell. It is best to be as prepared as possible for the first exam and use it as a learning experience!
5. *Continue to review the material that will be on the exam.*
   - Remember that studying for an exam begins as soon as new content is introduced following the previous exam. If you learn better by discussion, try becoming involved in a study group; if you learn better alone, set up a certain time each day that will be your study time.
   - As each new area of content is introduced, review previous material first and then focus on the new content. For example, if the first area of content is anxiety, go over your notes and read the text and any other material. If the

next area of content to be introduced is mood disorders, you need to go back and review anxiety and then add information about mood and so on.

- You should never need to cram for an exam, because you will be ready. This is also a great way to avoid the disasters of feeling ill or having a family emergency the night before an exam. These things do happen and students who have saved up to cram the night before will end up failing an exam.

6. *Be sure to get a good night's sleep the night before the exam.* Do not rely on medication to help you sleep, as it can interfere with your sleep cycles. If you have been studying on a regular basis, you should need only to review the material, not cram. A good night's sleep will give you the energy you need for the exam!

The Day of the Exam

1. *Eat a meal before the exam.*
   - If you have class from 8 A.M. to 11:30 A.M. and an exam at 11:45 A.M., eat a good breakfast and then eat a snack high in complex carbohydrates, not simple sugars, prior to the exam!
   - If you rely on sugar, remember that you will hit a low sometime during the exam!
   - Eating the right foods has been shown to increase test performance!

2. *Plan ahead so that you leave yourself plenty of time to get to the exam without the added stress of being fearful that you will be late.*
   - Be sure that you have gas in your car and air in the tires.
   - Be sure that you leave time for the little things that can keep you from getting to the exam on time.
   - Don't allow too much time, though, because it will give you additional time to worry if you are a worrier.

3. *Do not rely on drugs to either stimulate you or relax you prior to the exam.* Medications can have side effects or untoward effects that can interfere with your concentration. Don't forget that caffeine is a drug. A little may help energize you and help you concentrate, but a lot will have the opposite effect.

4. *If possible, go to the classroom where you'll have the exam and sit down.* Do not sit around and compare notes or questions with other students at the last second. This may serve to make you more nervous and less confident. All questions you had should have been cleared up by the instructor prior to the exam.

5. *It is important that you maintain some anxiety.* Anxiety tends to improve performance as long as it is controlled and minimized. We can remember playing a relaxation tape for students who had problems with test anxiety. The relaxation tape was so good that several of the students fell asleep! The students were so relaxed that they actually did worse on the exam because they had so little anxiety.

6. *Be sure that you follow the directions on the exam and from the faculty.*
   - Check to be sure that you have all of the pages on the exam in the correct order.
   - Be sure that all of the pages are legible and that you have the correct number of test items.
   - No matter how carefully an instructor checks over an exam before copying it, corrections may need to be made before you begin. Listen for them. Ask for clarifications if there is something you don't understand.

7. *Be sure to fill in the Scantron or computerized test form accurately.*
   - Answer all of the questions to the best of your ability; if two answers seem correct, choose the more obvious one; if no answers seem correct, choose the one that is most nearly correct.
   - Be certain that you have not left a blank on the answer sheet and that all questions correspond to the number on the form. We have had students leave out an entire page of an exam because they were not paying attention to the numbering.
   - If you will be using formulas during the exam, write them on a corner of the test if allowed. The same applies if you have acronyms that have helped you to study; write them in the corner.
   - Leave the tough questions until last. Make a star by them, and come back to them. Sometimes, a later question in the test will give you a good idea as to what a previous answer might be. Learn to look for related questions.
   - Don't read into the question information that isn't there. We have had students miss questions because they added information based on an experience they had had in their clinicals. Do not add to or subtract from the instructor's intention.
   - Erase all stray marks completely. The Scantron machine will often count the erasure instead of the answer you intended if the erasure is not complete.
   - Make sure your name is on the test!

8. *Be careful when changing answers.*
   - Students invariably want to know if they should change answers on an exam.
   - For the most part, we find that students tend to change answers from right to wrong. But, we have had the occasional student who actually does better by changing answers.
   - You know yourself best. Keep track of the answers you have changed and compare them at test review.
   - Did you improve your score or not? If you didn't, then make a rule for yourself that you will not change answers on the next exam.

9. *Do not cheat.*
   - It does you no good, and it will affect your patients in the long run.

- Do not let other students cheat off of you, for the same reasons. I can recall one of my nursing instructors asking me to think about this scenario. She told me to close my eyes and imagine that I had just awakened in the recovery room after major surgery. Then she said to imagine that the student cheating off me was the one providing my nursing care. Would you be comfortable with this student taking care of you? Think about waking up with that student holding your life in his or her hands. If the student cheated his or her way through school, he or she does not know much.
- Most schools have a process for making faculty aware of cheaters. It will benefit all of those involved if you report cheating and other unethical behavior.
- Once students graduate, they don't leave their lack of ethics behind and often jeopardize patients as a result. It is our opinion that a student who would cheat on an exam is the same student who would make a medication error and not tell anyone or chart a treatment as having been done when it wasn't.
- Most nursing programs have a policy related to cheating that usually involves dismissal from the program. Don't take the chance of ruining your career before it actually begins.
- Do not do anything during a test that would give others the perception that you are cheating. Keep your eyes on your own paper at all times.

10. *Beware of the post-exam autopsy.*
    - This is similar to the pre-exam "did you study X, Y, Z," but focuses on questions that were on the exam.
    - The autopsy usually begins with "What answer did you get for that question about . . . ?"
    - Students tend to form groups and as individuals begin to compare notes.
    - Invariably, some will walk away "knowing" that they have "failed" the exam.
    - Rarely does a student feel better following the exam autopsy.
    - Whether or not you choose to participate is your choice, but we would recommend that you head for home or your next class, or treat yourself to something fun!
    - The post-exam autopsy is different from the test review, which, in many schools, occurs immediately after the exam when you can learn the most. This is led by the instructor who gave the exam. In most cases, the instructor will not argue the answers of questions with you during this review, but if you feel strongly about one or more of the questions, see the instructor during a break or after class. It's especially important if you can show a textbook that agrees with your point of view.

ESSENTIAL SKILLS ── **TYPES OF EXAMS** ──────────

There are two main types of testing you might face: objective tests and essay tests. The objective tests include those that contain multiple-choice, short-answer, matching or true–false questions. Most schools use multiple-choice exams or some combination of the above. As stated earlier, multiple-choice questions prepare the student for the NCLEX-PN exam. Essay exams are rarely used in practical/vocational nursing programs. However, we may require our students to construct a nursing care plan based on a case study to be part of their exam. This is a definite test of application of knowledge.

Anatomy of a Multiple-Choice Item   Multiple-choice questions consist of a *stem* and usually four or more *distracters,* or choices.

> The chapter you are reading is about: (Stem)
> a. pathophysiology
> b. pharmacology
> c. anatomy
> d. studying and testing
> } (Distracters)

How to Take a Multiple-Choice Exam   The most recommended way to take the test is to read the entire item, including the stem and all of the distracters. However, some students find it beneficial to cover the distracters, read the stem, and select an answer even before looking at the choices. Then if the choice you mentally selected is present as a distracter, it is probably the correct answer. Most students can choose two distracters that are wrong—which gives them a 50% chance of getting the answer right. Examples of the described distracters are indicated by an asterisk. There are all kinds of tips for doing well on a multiple-choice test. We have given several examples below. We're not sure how reliable they are, but here are some we have heard.

1. The longest distracter is usually the answer.
   One of the primary contributors to heart disease is:
   a. exercise
   b. eating a high-fat diet* (correct answer)
   c. weight loss
   d. vitamin intake
2. If two distracters have the same terms or mostly the same terms, then one of them is probably the answer.
   Skin cancer is most often caused by:
   a. a diet high in vitamin D
   b. long-term sun exposure*
   c. unprotected sun exposure* (correct answer)
   d. swimming
3. If you have no idea what the answer is, choose b or c.

4. If the item lists more than one thing in each distracter, be sure to read the whole list. Avoid choosing answers if any one of the listed items is incorrect.
   In basic life support, ABC stands for?
   a. airway, bleeding, circulation[*]
   b. anatomy, biology, chemistry
   c. airway, breathing, circulation (correct answer)
   d. anxiety, bleeding, circulation[*]

5. Be wary of items that state "always," "never," or any other absolutes.
   When confronting a hostile patient, the nurse would:
   a. speak softly (correct answer)
   b. yell loudly to get the patient's attention
   c. always call for help[*]
   d. start screaming loudly

6. Make sure you are reading the words "not" or "except."
   All of the following symptoms can occur with a stroke except:
   a. Headache
   b. One-sided weakness
   c. Chest pain (correct answer)
   d. Loss of ability to speak or swallow

As you progress through your nursing courses, you will probably find that the test items tend to get harder over time. This occurs because the instructors are trying to help you apply what you have learned in a variety of settings. Most test questions will reflect leveling. This means that they will be more difficult. Instructors are looking for the following skills:

1. *Knowing.* These items ask you to regurgitate what you have learned. A bit like a parrot, they expect you to repeat back what you have heard. For example: What does ABC stand for in basic life support? If you have memorized ABC, you can state airway, breathing, circulation.

2. *Comprehension.* These items ask you to repeat something that you have learned, only in a different way. For example, if you have been told that stress is the major cause of automobile accidents, your instructor may ask a question about two people involved in an automobile accident. The instructor may want to know what is the probability that the accident was stress related. Your answer would be the highest possible number since you were told that stress is the major cause of automobile accidents (therefore, the highest percentage).

3. *Application.* These items ask you to put material you have learned into new situations. For example, you drive up to the scene of a car accident and find that there are two injured people. One is having difficulty breathing and the other is bleeding from a superficial cut on her right knee. Which of these patients would you take care of first? Remember your ABCs and prioritize! You would care for the person having problems breathing first and then the person who is bleeding.

True–False Questions   The general rule with true–false questions is that the longer statements are the ones most likely to be true. There are also more likely to be more true statements. As with multiple choice, the questions containing absolutes like "always" and "never" are more likely to be false. Break the statement down into parts; if one part is false, then the whole statement is false. On these types of questions, your first response is usually correct.

Matching   Check with the instructor to see if answers may be used more than once. Do the more obvious and easier matches first.

Short-Answer or Fill-ins   Although you will be having mostly multiple-choice exams, you may be given a short-answer question as part of the test. In short-answer questions, put down as much information as you have. The more you have down, the more likely you are to receive all or partial credit. Look for clues in the rest of the exam. Make an educated guess on all questions; don't leave anything blank unless wrong answers count against you. If you are taking a test with fill-ins, look at the length of the blank. That often indicates the length of the word. Also, make sure your answer fits in grammatically with the rest of the sentence.

Essay Questions   Essay questions are a great way to determine what a student knows about a particular subject, but they are extremely difficult to grade because it is hard for the faculty to be objective. The primary thing to remember about essay questions is that you need to read and answer what is asked. Many times, students read part of the question and start writing an answer without digesting the whole question. It is helpful if you underline the verb in the question. For example, if the question asks you to describe how you would decide which patients would need to be seen first in a physician's office, be sure to detail how you would make that decision. On the other hand, if it asks you to list the steps taken by an office nurse to prioritize his or her day, then be able to list those steps. After reading and understanding the question and what it is asking, some students choose to do a quick outline to organize their thoughts. Other students prefer to just start writing.

- Do whatever works for you.
- Be sure that you answer in complete sentences using correct spelling and grammar.
- Be sure to be as objective as possible unless the question specifically asks for your opinion about something.
- Be concise in your answer, but include as much information as possible.
- Beware of running on or throwing in as many words as you think the teacher wants to see. (As nursing faculty, we are very good at determining when a student does not really know an answer and is just filling up a page with words.)
- If you have no idea what the question is asking, see if your instructor can provide you with more detail or clarify it for you (some will and some will not).

- If you are not sure of an answer, write down anything that you think relates to the question, because you may get partial credit. Many times, essay questions have a high point value, so it is better to get partial credit than none.

CORE CONCEPTS | **TEST ANXIETY**

Unfortunately, some students experience test anxiety in any testing situation, and it is vital for these students to learn to deal with this disabling anxiety. Most test anxiety results from negative childhood messages that are incorporated into the subconscious. According to Erwin & Dinwiddie (1983), there are several types of unconscious messages that lead to test anxiety.

Unconscious Messages that Create Anxiety

1. *You are stupid, a dummy, or not very smart.*
   - Basically, the student who heard this message believes that he or she will never do anything right.
   - This message sets the student up for failure by creating a no-win situation.
   - During study time, the student thinks, "Why bother? I can't pass the test anyway."
   - Studying becomes a hopeless endeavor, and the student does not do well on the exam, which reinforces the message that he or she is "stupid, a dummy, and not very smart."
2. *Be perfect.*
   - Students who have been told that they have to be perfect force themselves to achieve all A's because their parents focused only on A grades.
   - If the child had five A's and one B, he or she was punished for receiving the B rather than congratulated for the A's achieved.
   - This student studies so compulsively that he or she often neglects other needs.
   - The student is often so worried about not achieving perfection that he or she tends to be easily distracted during testing.
   - If the student doesn't know the answer to one question, the panic tends to snowball and the student believes that he or she will fail the exam.
3. *You are phenomenal.*
   - This child has been told over and over again how bright, intelligent, and amazing he or she is.
   - This child grows up to believe that he or she has to live up to others' expectations.
   - Unfortunately, it is impossible to live up to such high expectations all the time.

- The student begins to have doubts and believes that other people will discover that he or she is not as perfect as others believed him or her to be.
- This sets the student up for failure since he or she feels like an impostor most of the time.

If you believe that you have test anxiety that is interfering with your ability to take and pass exams, please seek help. It is possible to change these messages, and many techniques have been found to be useful in controlling test anxiety. Most schools have a testing or counseling center that can help you learn to control your anxiety levels.

If you do panic during an exam, stop the exam at that point and close your eyes. Breathe slowly and deeply. Visualize a safe, peaceful place. We often tell students to find that safe, peaceful place prior to the exam so they can go right to it. Use positive self-talk. Tell yourself that you can do this. Then open your eyes and return to the exam. Answer easy questions first to bolster your self-confidence.

Some studies have found that eating some form of ginger prior to an exam helps to relieve test anxiety. This could be in the form of ginger tea or gingersnaps. It can't hurt, and it might be refreshing.

Learning how to take exams is an essential component of nursing school. The more exams you take and the more information you have, the more you will succeed. Remember that test taking is a learning experience too. Do the best that you can do, and remember that you are more than your grades. Ten years from now, you won't remember what you made on that fundamentals exam! You'll just know that you are a practical/vocational nurse who successfully completed your nursing program.

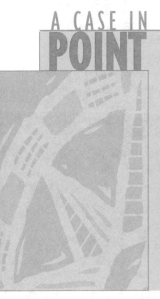

A CASE IN POINT

Brad, an LPN, thinks maybe he stays up too late the night before a test because the morning of the test, he feels foggy and not too sharp. He has been unhappy about the grades he has been getting. He discusses this with his study group. One of the other students asks him why he stays up so late. She thinks it is better to get a good night's sleep. Brad explains that he has to cram. Another student suggests that maybe he study a little each day instead of cramming. From talking to the others in his group, Brad recognizes he has poor study and test-taking habits and decides to go to the counselor for help.

ASK YOURSELF

1. Having read this chapter and taking into account your strengths and weaknesses, what new study methods are you resolved to use?

---

2. Referring back to your response to Ask Yourself question #2 at the beginning of the chapter, how will you apply the information presented to make test taking less difficult?

 CYBERLINKS: FLASH CARDS

Check to see what you now remember by making your own flash cards. Use the CD-ROM that accompanies your textbook to discover how to make flash cards for reviewing and retaining what you have learned.

 CONCEPT MAP WORD BANK

STUDY SKILLS
Personal assessment
Class preparation

TESTING
Preparation before
Preparation day of test

TYPES OF EXAMS
Suggested Methods

TEST ANXIETY
Unconscious messages

Refer to Concept Maps and Flash Cards on pages viii–ix for an explanation of how to create and use concept maps. In addition, the CD-ROM guides you through the construction of concept maps by providing a more detailed introduction, more illustrations of examples, and key steps to follow in designing your own maps.

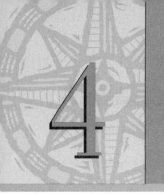

Writing a Paper

4

 ASK YOURSELF

1. What do you like and what do you dislike about writing papers?

2. What resources do you usually consult to help you write a good paper?

 CYBERLINKS

Interactive Is writing a paper your least favorite academic activity? Visit www.ipl.org to learn how to not only write a paper, but to write an A+ paper. Scroll down to "Reference Center" and then click on "A+ Research and Writing."

Supplemental www.LPNresources.com can help enhance your learning by leading you to discover other links with more information about the topic that you are studying.

Nursing responsibilities include communicating in writing as well as speaking. As unfair as it may seem, sometimes judgment of your intelligence is based on the level of your ability to use the English language. The purpose of this chapter is to help you express yourself well on paper.

As a practical/vocational nursing student, you will be asked to write different types of papers on a multitude of topics. You might be asked to write papers on certain diseases or specific changes occurring within the nursing profession. A paper entitled "If I Had Only Six Months to Live" is an example of an informal paper that does not require research but instead requires that you be able to express your own personal thoughts on paper. Papers on a current topic in pharmacology or new uses of technology within the nursing profession are examples of formal papers, which require research.

ESSENTIAL SKILLS **GUIDELINES FOR WRITING PAPERS**

Whatever the topic, remember that the writing of any paper requires preparation. It is vital that you begin preparations for writing the paper long before the paper's due date. It is also essential that you follow the general basics of good writing.

1. *Consider the following when choosing a topic.*
   - Be wary of choosing a topic that is one of the instructor's favorites or one that he or she has written a book about or has done research on; your ideas most likely will be scrutinized closely because of the topic.
   - Don't choose controversial topics that the instructor might be emotionally involved in, unless it is a debate or pro-and-con paper.
   - Be cautious of topics about which you can find little information.
   - On the other hand, be cautious of topics that have too much information available. It is important to narrow the focus or you will never be able to find it all and you will have to wade through tons of material.

2. *Be certain that you find out what style the papers are to be written in.* Most nursing schools use American Psychological Association (APA) format for formal papers.
   - Purchase the APA manual, or go to the library and read the important sections that relate to citations and references.
   - Be sure that you can access the manual easily or that someone you know has a copy for those crisis times when you will need to refer to it. Believe us, it is worth the money to buy a copy for peace of mind, ease of access, and the points that you will earn because you are following the format correctly.
   - Another way to obtain the APA format is through the Internet. Just typing in "APA format" in a search engine will bring you to a number of sites that will give you the format for citing of written materials, such as books and journals, as well as the citing of electronic references off the World Wide Web itself.

3. *Be certain that you obtain the specific criteria from your instructor.*
   - Most courses will have the paper criteria included in your course syllabus. Read all of the criteria first. Make sure you understand when the paper is due, how long it is supposed to be, and how many references are required.
   - Clarify any questions you might have immediately.
   - Don't wait until you are at the library gathering information or at home typing.
   - If certain parts of the paper have a higher point value, then those should be the areas to which you devote the most time and energy.
   - Be careful to distribute your time wisely.
   - It makes no sense to write five pages of a paper on a section worth 10 points and one page on a section worth 50 points.

4. *Gather your resources together.*
   - Will you be using the Internet or a modem to connect to the library computer to complete your search of the literature?
   - Will you need to go to the library in person?
   - Be sure to keep some type of card system that provides detailed notes of each source you plan to use.
   - Refer to your APA manual (or the format your school is using) to determine what is needed in the citations and references.
   - Most style manuals require that you at least keep track of the author(s), title, journal or publisher, and date published. The process of writing down this information will save you many hassles when you can't find a reference, the year is illegible on your copy of the article, or the journal name is not listed on the article.
   - When you proofread your paper, double-check all of your references to see if they are accurate.
   - If you are using Internet references, keep copies of all of your resources. (We require that our students turn in all copies of Internet references with their papers.)

5. *After doing sufficient research, it should be possible for you to construct an outline.*
   - Having an outline helps you to organize the data you have collected.
   - If you do not have an outline, you might find yourself overwhelmed with the amount of information you have. It does not all have to go into your paper!
   - Think of a paper as if you were planning a great vacation. Your focus, or topic, is your destination, and your outline is your road map. You will have a smoother journey if your route has been planned out.

6. *The paper should have a definite beginning or an introduction explaining what your paper is about.*
   - You might even state in your first paragraph what types of information you will be presenting throughout the entire paper.
   - Then follow the guidelines you set up for yourself in that first paragraph.

7. *The paper should have a definite conclusion.*
   - You may want to restate what you covered in the paper.
   - Summarize your findings.
   - If it is allowed, state how you feel about the paper and your summary. Sometimes your opinion is inappropriate in a formal paper, and sometimes it is acceptable. Find out how your instructor feels about this.

8. *If it is at all possible, do not reinvent the wheel.*
   - If it is allowed in your school, you might be able to use the same topic more than once with a possible variation.
   - Save all of your notes.
   - It saves you a lot of time when research for one paper provides a basis for another.

How is this possible? Think of a topic that you are really interested in. An example might be eating disorders. Ways that you could adapt this topic to several different courses include the following:

- Eating disorders in adolescence for pediatric nursing
- Eating disorders during pregnancy for obstetrics
- Drug treatment for eating disorders in pharmacology
- Nutrition and eating disorders for nutrition class
- Treatment of eating disorders for psychiatric nursing
- The relationship between eating disorders in young women and their participation in group sports for research

Of course, one drawback to this approach is that you will probably never want to read or write anything about the chosen topic again! So, be sure that when you choose a topic you really like it or at least want to know a lot more about it!

9. *Make a hard copy of your paper for your file, and save it on a disk as well.*

ESSENTIAL SKILLS | **SPELLING, GRAMMAR, AND PUNCTUATION**

No matter how much research you have done and how much time and energy you have devoted to your paper, you can still lose points for poor spelling, grammar, and punctuation. We know this is nursing, not English composition, but in order to express yourself well, you must be able to use the correct spelling, grammar, and punctuation.

1. *Spelling*
   - If you are using a computer to type your paper, be sure and use the spell-check.
   - However, do not rely totally on your spell-check. You may be using a correctly spelled wrong word. The computer does not know the difference between "to," "two," and "too." You must also proofread your paper, and have someone else proofread it as well.

2. *Grammar*
   - Be sure you use complete sentences. This is a sentence that contains a subject and a verb. A sentence fragment is just a string of words that is missing one or the other of these.
   - It is inappropriate to use abbreviations in a paper. It might be faster and easier to write "approx." than "approximately," but it is not acceptable in a paper.
   - Remember that the language of a paper may be more formal than if you were talking.
   - Do not use a preposition to end a sentence. Prepositions are words such as "to," "of," and "from."
   - If you have a sentence that fills up an entire paragraph, it is too long and needs to be broken down into two or more shorter sentences.

3. *Punctuation.*

- Everyone should know that you place periods after statements and question marks after questions. It is the other punctuation marks that give us the most trouble.
- Colons are used after the greeting in a business letter and before giving a list of items or points you want to cover.
- A semicolon is used to separate two parts of a sentence in which you don't want to break the thought. An example would be: "The nursing student excelled in her fundamentals class; however, she flunked math."
- Commas have many uses. They are needed to separate a series of three or more items or thoughts. They are used after an introductory phrase. An example would be, "Although she was very tired, the nursing student continued to work on her paper." Commas are also used when two clauses are joined by a conjunction such as "but," "because," "or," or "and" if both of the clauses could stand alone. An example would be, "The nursing student fell asleep in class, because he stayed up all night to study."

ESSENTIAL SKILLS   GUIDELINES FOR PREPARING THE FINAL COPY

Always proofread and check your paper before submitting it. Some instructors will actually give you the opportunity to turn your paper in early to enable the instructor to scan and make suggestions. If this is the policy with your instructor, take advantage of it!

When checking a paper, be sure of the following:

- You have the correct paper. It has your name and the correct course information on it. It has a cover page if one is required.
- It has the correct number of pages.
- The pages are in the correct order.
- The lettering is dark enough to read and consistently clear.
- There are no additional or unwanted lines, streaks, or other distracting marks from printers or copiers.
- The bibliography or reference page is attached to the paper.

Writing papers can be fun and challenging. Do remember that computers require a certain amount of special handling. This includes the printer as well. We had a student whose paper was completed on time, but her printer would not print. She brought her disk to school to print, and the school computer could not read the disk. By the time she got the problem straightened out, the paper was one day late. Important facts to keep in mind are to back up all of your work, proofread your paper, and have someone else read it as well. Be sure everything is in order before handing in your paper.

You may not be writing formal papers after you become an LPN/LVN, but you will need to be able to express yourself well to maintain your credibility as a competent, efficient nurse. Use your time in school wisely to develop your own writing style. Learn as you write. It is not only the mastery of the content of your paper that is important but the mastery of your use of words!

CORE CONCEPTS	**PAPER ETHICS**

Invariably, there are some students who try to beat the system and cheat either by copying someone else's paper or getting another student to write a paper for them. Important cautions:

- Do your own work!
- Do not plagiarize! Plagiarism is the use of someone else's words or ideas written as if they were your own. If you are using a direct quote from another source, place the words in quotation marks, and cite the source within the body of your paper as well as on your reference page. You need to cite your reference even if you have reworded another author's ideas. *Many schools will give you a "0" for your assignment, or dismiss you from your nursing program if you are found to have plagiarized the material in your paper!*
- Put everything in your own words!
- Document your work from accepted sources!
- Do not do someone else's work for them!

Unfortunately, student nurses tend to be "caretakers." They are often "helpers" and feel that they are "needed" when others seek them out for help with papers. There is nothing wrong with sharing information or resources, but when you are doing more work than the person you are helping, you are allowing yourself to be used! You are not doing the person a favor; you are hindering his or her learning!

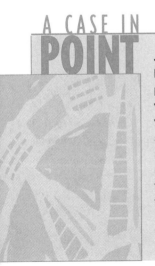

A CASE IN POINT

Joan is Suzie's best friend in the program. Suzie has a paper due and is not confident about her paper-writing skills. She asks Joan to help her write the paper. Joan has a paper of her own to write but wants to help her friend in any way she can. The paper is due in three weeks. About six days before the paper is due and Joan has no time to spare, Suzie asks Joan for help. Joan wants Suzie to name the time and place. Suzie tells Joan that she will give her the topic and the research she gathered but that Joan can write Suzie's paper anytime before the due date.

At some point in your career you will find yourself in the position of being asked to help a fellow student with paperwork or with some other matter perhaps in the clinical setting. Be sure that your help is really needed and that you are not doing someone else's work for them. Nurses who depend on others to always do for them will also cut corners in other ways. They may short change patients on their medications, or rely on others to chart for them. The possibilities are frightening!

 ASK YOURSELF ───────────────────────────────────────

1. Referring to the guidelines for writing papers (pages 29–31), how will you use this information to generally improve your paper writing?

   _____

   _____

2. What additional resources, if any, do you need to acquire to help you to write the best papers?

   _____

   _____

 CYBERLINKS: FLASH CARDS ───────────────────────────

Check to see what you now remember by making your own flash cards. Use the CD-ROM that accompanies your textbook to discover how to make flash cards for reviewing and retaining what you have learned.

 CONCEPT MAP WORD BANK ─────────────────────────────

WRITING PAPERS
Preparation
Topic Selection
Proofreading

Refer to Concept Maps and Flash Cards on pages viii–ix for an explanation of how to create and use concept maps. In addition, the CD-ROM guides you through the construction of concept maps providing a more detailed introduction, more illustrations of examples, and key steps to follow in designing your own maps.

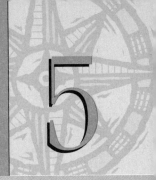

Printed Resources

ASK YOURSELF

1. Which of your current textbooks do you like best and least?

_____

_____

2. Do you read your textbooks before or after class or both? What is the motivation for your choice?

_____

_____

CYBERLINKS

<u>Interactive</u> If, after reading your textbook, you have some unanswered questions, visit **www.ipl.org** and obtain the answer. Scroll down to "Reference Center" and click on "Ask a Reference Question."

<u>Supplemental</u> **www.LPNresources.com** can help enhance your learning by leading you to discover other links with more information about the topic that you are studying.

You will have many resources available to you as you progress through nursing school. Important resources you will most often use are textbooks and journal articles. The appropriate utilization of these resources is key to successful learning.

CORE CONCEPTS | **TEXTBOOKS**

It is essential that you purchase all the required textbooks for your program. To save money, you may buy used, older editions from previous graduates. Keep in mind that the information in these editions is dated, and you may need to go to the library or to current classmates for more recent information.

There are a few other concerns regarding textbooks of which you need to be aware. Most students believe that information given in textbooks is always reliable.

We have had students point out that information in a text sometimes conflicts with what we have said in class. It is for this reason that you should note the following points:

1. Texts are not infallible—many contain errors.
   - If your instructor says one thing and you read something else in your textbook, be sure to ask for clarification.
   - A good way to clarify a conflict is to ask your instructor, "If you ask a question on the test, which answer should I give?"
   - Be as specific as you can possibly be when asking a question.

2. Be wary of information in a text that contradicts common sense.
   - If you are studying dosages and calculations and you read that $4 \times 15 = 45$, or if you read that a major cause of heart disease is eating too many vegetables, you will know that there is an error.
   - If there is one major error, chances are there are several more.
   - Be sure to point out any errors you discover to your instructor.
   - Be careful! Many students overlook an obvious error because they naturally believe that textbooks are perfect.

3. Texts are often out of date.
   - New information is learned on a daily basis, and some areas of technology change minute to minute.
   - Texts are written over a period of a year or two, and in production for another year or more.
   - When reading about areas that are in constant flux such as AIDS, drug development, and others, you will need to rely on more up-to-date sources.

4. Texts reflect the beliefs and biases of the writer or writers.
   - Your instructor may or may not agree with the writer's experience and conclusions. Sometimes, the textbook will say "A." Your instructor will say, "I think B."
   - Be sure that you clarify which response is desired in a testing situation.

In many nursing courses, you will be looking for information that is not in your textbooks.

The following are reference sources that should help you locate more information with minimal frustration.

- *Librarian:* This individual can be of immense help. We highly recommend that you take a trip to the library of your school or of the hospital where you will be doing your clinicals and meet the reference staff. They will not do the work for you, but they can help you use your library time wisely! Just remember, some hospital librarians will not be able to assist you unless you are actually in their facility doing a clinical.
- *Medical dictionary:* Although most of your textbooks have some medical terminology, we strongly recommend that your personal library contain a

recent medical dictionary. Nursing often involves the use of a language we call "medicalese," and you will need your dictionary to help with translations. A good medical dictionary also gives a concise picture of pathophysiology of most disease conditions.

- *Diagnostic tests and implications text:* If your school does not require such a textbook, this is a good resource aid to have. Although most medical–surgical texts will cover some of this information, it is more completely covered and more easily found in a text specifically related to diagnostic tests and their implications for nursing. It certainly helps when you are working on nursing care plans and trying to make sense of the patient's lab reports!
- *Cumulative Index to Nursing and Allied Health Literature (CINAHL):* This is one of the most often used multidisciplinary databases. It includes nursing literature as well as 15 to 20 allied health fields. You can access CINAHL by the hard-copy version as well as by CD-ROM and online at the library.
- *Morbidity and Mortality Weekly Report (MMWR):* This is an excellent source when you are searching for information focused on communicable disease issues, as it is a weekly publication of the Centers for Disease Control and Prevention (CDC). This can be found online at http://www.cdc.gov/.
- *World Wide Web:* Due to the broad range of information available and widespread use of personal computers, computer usage, resources available online, and cautions concerning usage will be more fully covered in Section VI. This is a resource that should be utilized by every nursing student.

CORE CONCEPTS | **JOURNAL ARTICLES**

One of the best ways to supplement information found in textbooks is to read journal articles. Journal articles are often referenced at the end of each chapter in many textbooks. These referenced journal articles may be especially helpful in learning more about the content within a specified chapter.

Knowing the type of journal to research is also very important as there are over 100 American nursing journals. Contents vary from journals with a broad range of topics, such as the *American Journal of Nursing,* to those with a narrow focus such as the *Journal of Intravenous Nursing.*

Journal articles are usually more timely than textbooks, but information may still be 6 months to 1 year old or more at publication. Articles may also contain errors. A majority of the information contained in texts and journals is accurate; however, you need to remain on alert.

In addition, unless the data introduced in the article contains a report of an independent, objective research study or studies, the information contained in the article might also be the opinion of the author or what he or she found true in his or her practice.

Be wary of articles or research that is supported by major companies with a vested interest in the information presented in the article. For example, one of authors of this textbook read that eating a vegetarian diet can be detrimental to your health. Interestingly, a member of a beef producers' organization wrote this article. Another example is: An article may suggest that drug A is better than drug B, but if the pharmaceutical company that makes drug A paid for the research, then the credibility of the article is in question! Locating journal articles related to specific topics can be facilitated by researching the Cumulative Index (CINAHL mentioned above). However, you may need to use interlibrary loan services to receive a hard copy.

Remember, it may take 10 to 14 days for the article to arrive at your library, so plan ahead. Some journals are available online, such as those found with http://www.nursingcenter.com. You might be able to actually download an article and print it on your personal computer. There are similar cautions concerning journal articles as there are with textbooks.

You are no doubt going to find that your main reference sources in school will be your textbooks. These have been selected by faculty who believe that the adopted book will do the best job of presenting the course material. However, there are still going to be information gaps in any text. This chapter has presented some basic references, which we believe will help you fill in the gaps.

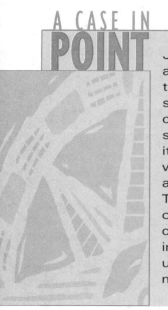

A CASE IN POINT

Julie, a practical nursing student, was confused about a concept that was presented one way in the text and another by the teacher. Another student agreed that the two sources offered conflicting views. They decided they had better study the information as the teacher presented it. When they were tested on the material, they were both surprised to see that they had answered the related questions incorrectly. They approached the teacher and asked which of the two sources (teacher or textbook) was correct. The teacher replied that the information in the text was correct and that she was unaware that she had presented the same material incorrectly.

ASK YOURSELF

1. What resources are available to you, in your library or from another source, to supplement textbook information?

   _____

   _____

2. What guidelines have your teachers given (same or different guidelines) regarding how far back in time (years) that journal information is relevant?

   _____

   _____

 CYBERLINKS: FLASH CARDS

Check to see what you remember by making your own flash cards. Use the CD-ROM that accompanies your textbook to discover how to make flash cards for reviewing and retaining what you have learned.

 CONCEPT MAP WORD BANK

TEXTBOOKS

JOURNALS

Refer to Concept Maps and Flash Cards on pages viii–ix for an explanation of how to create and use concept maps. In addition, the CD-ROM guides you through the construction of concept maps by providing a more detailed introduction, more illustrations of examples, and key steps to follow in designing your own maps.

6 Computers

 ASK YOURSELF

1. What do you most like about using a computer?

   _____

   _____

2. What do you most dislike about using the computer?

   _____

   _____

 CYBERLINKS

<u>Interactive</u> Racking your brain because you can't solve a computer problem? Get fast, free tech help through e-mail at **www.ipl.org** Scroll down to "Reference Center," then click on "Computers and Internet Resources," and then to "ePeople Helpdesk Online."

<u>Supplemental</u> **www.LPNresources.com** can help enhance your learning by leading you to discover other links with more information about the topic you are studying.

Regardless of your level of comfort using the computer, becoming successful in nursing requires that you have basic computer skills. Many individuals use the computer in their leisure for personal communication or for surfing the net. Health care facilities, however, have found the computer to be indispensable in completing a variety of tasks required in their day-to-day operations. Accessing patient records and inputting patient information is now accomplished using the computer.

As a student, you may also find the computer to be essential to your education. Your instructors will likely assign papers to be written containing information you have researched and typed on the computer. You may have interactive CD-ROM educational programs, which you will be required to master. Even your NCLEX-PN board exam will be on the computer. Needless to say, if it has not already been, the computer will now become a routine part of your life.

ESSENTIAL SKILLS | **PREPARING TO USE THE COMPUTER**

You may decide not to invest in your own computer and printer. Most nursing pro-grams have computer labs available for student use for either research on the Internet or for typing and printing papers. However, you can get a reasonably inex-pensive computer to use at home and not worry about access on your campus. Even color printers have become very affordable.

Whether or not you will be using your own computer, be sure that you choose a word processing software program that is capable of doing all the work you will need throughout the nursing program. If your school uses a specific type of software and you will be using their computers, be sure that the same software is available in all the places where you plan on working. There is nothing worse than being forced to use the library computers because the nursing department is closed, and finding out that the library uses an entirely different software program! Be sure that you familiarize yourself with the software program. It is helpful to have a book about the program that you can use. Either the software book itself or books from the *Idiot's Guide* or *Dummies* series will be useful. Most common computer programs have several books available for you to look through. Find one that you can live with. If you are not that skillful with computers, find yourself a computer trouble-shooter in case of emergencies. Trust us, emergencies do happen. If you decide to use the school's computer, we recommend the following:

1. Find out if you can connect to any or all of the school computers by modem.
   - Can you download data from other places?
   - Be certain that your data is protected by a password and that you don't share it with others!

   We once had a student report that one of her friends had destroyed her paper because her friend was failing the class and wanted her to fail too. (These kinds of incidents do not often happen, but once is enough.)

2. If your nursing program does not include a computer class in your curriculum, take advantage of any short computer courses that are offered on campus.
   - Most schools have free or reduced-fee sessions to help students learn a variety of software programs.
   - Some schools might have an abbreviated 1- to 2-session class; others may have a longer 10-session class.
   - These sessions can help you get started and provide lots of information in the way of handouts and tips.
   - An added plus of taking a course is that you have contact with someone who may help you find the computer person you may need as a future resource.

3. Take a day or two to find out how the various computers on campus are used.
   - You need to check for signup sheets, busiest hours, and what software programs are available. If the business department also uses the computer

lab for regular classes, find out the times that the lab is open for the use
of other students.

- Jot down notes to keep with you so that you can refer back to them during the crisis times when your favorite computer is taken! One problem
is that throughout the semester, students frequently end up with similar
course deadlines. This can cause long lines at most campus computers.
- Be sure that you prepare for a time when you will not be able to use the
computer. Be flexible!
- Allow for busy hours and downtime in your planning.

ESSENTIAL SKILLS   **GUIDELINES FOR TROUBLE-SHOOTING
COMPUTER PROBLEMS**

While it is true that computers are a godsend for most of us, they are not without
their drawbacks. Mistakes often occur when you are first learning to use a computer
to write papers. Even seasoned, computer-literate students can run into problems
with campus computers. We wanted to share some of the problems that we have
encountered during our years of teaching, and present possible solutions.

- If you are planning to use a library or school computer, be sure that you
check for viruses before loading any diskettes on to your own—or anyone
else's—PC. Multiple-use computers frequently carry viruses that are capable of destroying all of your information and stored data.
- To access the school computers, you may need to work at odd hours or on
weekends. Be certain that you allow enough time to complete papers so that
one day of downtime will not disrupt your schedule. *Plan ahead!* A number of students have run into problems when a school computer was down
or there was an unexpected power failure. A lot of students may have papers
due around the same time. If you have to schedule times, make sure that
you will be able to complete your work on time. Always remember to back
up your work on a diskette before leaving the computer.
- Be sure to save your work after every couple of paragraphs or, if your computer program has an AutoSave, set it for at least every page. If you need to,
consider setting a timer for every 20 to 30 minutes to help you get into the
habit of saving your work; otherwise, you could be wasting precious time.
Be certain to back up your work at the middle and end of every work session. Even if you have saved your work on the hard drive, you still need to
save it on a diskette. We would recommend a double backup such as two
separate diskettes, a diskette and a tape, or a diskette and a zip drive—anything to ensure that you have a copy in at least two places. We recommend
also that you print a hard copy at the end of each work session. By having
a hard copy, you can read your material and make any necessary changes
before your next work session (Figure 6-1).
- If using a home computer, be sure that your printer has toner in it and is

Figure 6-1 Back Up All Data Several Times

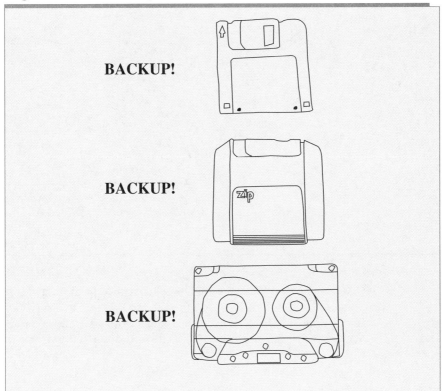

BACKUP!

BACKUP!

BACKUP!

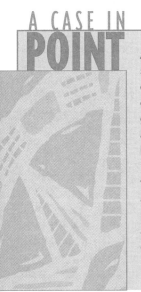

A CASE IN POINT

A student's helpful husband decided to load some new software on the family computer the day before her research paper was due. Not only did he delete the word processing software program that her paper was saved on, but she was also unable to retrieve information from her backup diskette. She came to class the next morning totally distraught with nothing to show for an entire semester of work. The school had a policy regarding point deductions for late papers so she lost some points. If she had had a hard copy to turn in, even if it wasn't a final copy, she may not have lost as many points (Figure 6-2).

Figure 6-2 Be Sure to Make a Hard Copy of Your Drafts

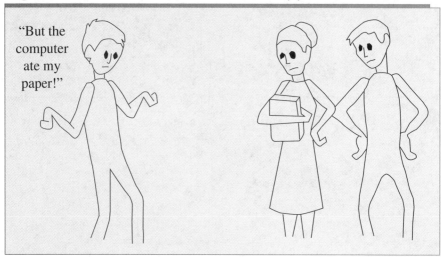

"But the computer ate my paper!"

in good working order. We had a student who went to print her paper at home, only to find out she was out of toner. When she came to school, with her paper on a diskette, none of the school printers would accept it. This resulted in her paper being a day late, because she did not prepare ahead.

CORE CONCEPTS | **NURSING INFORMATICS** ────────

To help ensure your success as an LPN/LVN, it is necessary to introduce nursing *informatics,* a new term related to the use of computers. Nursing informatics refers to a specialty area of nursing that combines the sciences of computers, nursing, and communication to provide the best nursing care possible. Although you are a nursing student and not an informatics specialist, you will still be required to be computer literate within the clinical setting. Hospitals and nursing homes have purchased user-friendly computer systems to provide better overall patient care.

All lab work, x-rays, and the like should be accessible much more quickly through the computer. Nurses can construct individual care plans for patients on the computer, download patient information, check physicians' orders, and input patient information. Many hospitals are already using handheld computers, or palm pilots, to record patient information right at the bedside. Communication between departments and between staff members is also accomplished via the computer instead of the telephone or handwritten memos. Some hospital computer programs even allow you to print off patient education materials to send home with your patient or allow you to research health topics right from the nurses' station computers. The field of computer technology is growing daily, and to be an efficient practical/vocational nurse in today's world, you must grow with it. Who knows? You might choose nursing informatics as your specialty field sometime in the future and be the nurse designing the computer programs that health care facilities are rapidly purchasing!

 ASK YOURSELF

1. What computer skills do you think you still need to acquire?

_____

_____

2. Referring to your response to the above question, how and when do you plan to acquire these skills?

_____

_____

 CYBERLINKS: FLASH CARDS

Check to see what you now remember by making your own flash cards. Use the CD-ROM that accompanies your textbook to discover how to make flash cards for reviewing and retaining what you have learned.

 CONCEPT MAP WORD BANK

COMPUTERS
Using the computer
Solving problems

Refer to Concept Maps and Flash Cards on pages viii–ix for an explanation of how to create and use concept maps. In addition, the CD-ROM guides you through the construction of concept maps by providing a more detailed introduction, more illustrations of examples, and key steps to follow in designing your own maps.

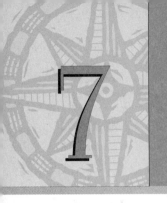

7

Consumer Groups and Health Information

1. Have you used the computer for the purpose of researching a topic? How successful were you in finding the information that you wanted?

   _____

   _____

2. What, if any, are your frustrations in using search engines?

   _____

   _____

 CYBERLINKS

Interactive Find any group or information on any topic at www.ipl.org. Go to Reference Center on menu, then Associates on the Net, then to Health and Medical Science and click on "Consumer Groups." There are many interesting possibilities on this site. For instance, you can obtain a response to your inquiry about problems related to wearing contact lens. The sky is the limit at this site.

Supplemental www.LPNresources.com can help enhance your learning by leading you to discover other links with more information about the topic you are studying.

The previous chapter contained information regarding the use of the computers in the health care profession. This chapter will deal with accessing information on the computer from the World Wide Web.

Many years ago, health professionals knew a great deal of information and shared very little of it with their patients. Most consumers accepted that the doctor was supposed to know everything, and the general public was to follow the doctor's recommendations. Today, with the advent of new technology and the Internet, patients frequently know as much as or more about their health conditions than their physicians and other health care professionals. Nurses can no longer be assured that they know more than the patient does. Consumers are questioning their treatment protocols, and nurses are expected to have some answers.

CORE CONCEPTS	**THE INTERNET AND NURSING**

To keep abreast of the information, health care professionals must stay current in their profession and knowledge base. It is important for nurses to be informed and to be able to provide consumers with knowledgeable feedback regarding all aspects of their health care. One of the primary ways to stay ahead is to use the information offered on the Internet via the World Wide Web (WWW).

To make use of the Internet, one must have a computer, a modem (allows your computer to communicate via telephone lines), and some type of online service (America Online, CompuServe, Prodigy) or Internet service provider (ISP) (Strauch, 1997). (Check your telephone book for local service providers.) You will also need some type of software to connect with and view the various Web sites. Most online service providers and ISPs will provide you with the necessary software free of charge, or you may wish to purchase a Web browser such as Netscape Navigator or Microsoft Explorer. Antiviral software is recommended so that you will not pick up viruses when you download files to your personal computer.

After you have connected your service and can access online information, you will need to learn how to access various Web sites. Typing in a Web address or uniform resource locator (URL) will allow you to access Web sites (Figure 7-1). It is extremely important that you type in addresses exactly as they appear. Some Web addresses are very long but you must type them character by character (Levine & Young, 1994). An example of a URL or Web address might be http://www.person nell/groups.brs.net/479832/bcusc.org. The following are actual URL addresses of some health-oriented Web sites:

- http://www.rheumatology.org
- http://www.nimh.nig.org

ESSENTIAL SKILLS	**SEARCH ENGINES**

Most Web sites or Web pages allow you to travel from one site to another via links. A link is usually highlighted in a color that is different from the main text of the page. By clicking on the highlighted area, you can travel to that Web page or Web site and continue your search. To assist you in your search for information on the WWW it is important to locate either a Web directory or search engine (Strauch, 1998). These two items allow you to search the WWW for the desired information (Figure 7-2). One way to think of this is to consider looking for a specific book in a huge library. It would be possible, but it might take a long time. On the other hand, if you had some type of computerized card file, you could easily cross-reference and find the desired book. A Web directory or search engine is similar. It can wade through the mass of WWW information to find what you are looking for.

Figure 7-1 Connection from Home Computer to a Web Site

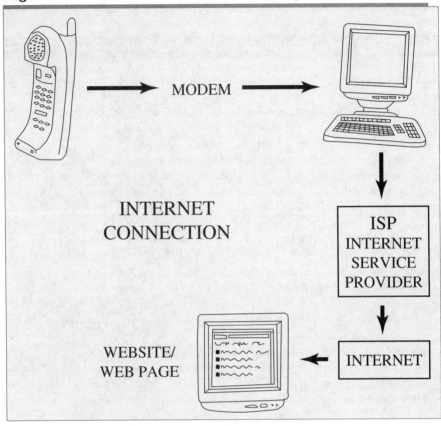

Figure 7-2 Yahoo! Search Engine

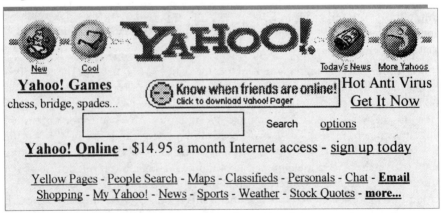

Source: Reproduced with permission of Yahoo! Inc. © 2000 by Yahoo! Inc. YAHOO! and the YAHOO! logo are trademarks of Yahoo! Inc.

When using a search engine, you type in the words that you are looking for in the search blank. For example, if you were interested in learning more about hospice care, you would type in the word *hospice*. After a few seconds, the search engine will tell you how many Web sites matched your query. Depending on what search engine you choose, you may have 10 matches (hits) or you may have 10,000. Be aware that the search engine is retrieving all the Web sites that use the word *hospice*. Many of the search engines list the better-matched sites first with a numerical value such as 98% (Figure 7-3). If you searched more than one word, it will also tell you that the site matched 1 of 2 terms, or 2 of 2 terms. You can scroll down the list of sites and find the ones that you are interested in. As you look through the sites, note their URL addresses. For example, look at the list in Figure 7-3. Do you recognize any of the URL addresses? The first match at 85% is from a .edu or educational facility; however, you will note that it is primarily a list of books and papers. The second site at 81% is also from the same URL but deals with other information. The third site at 80% has to do with the national MS 150, which is a bike race to raise money to fight the disease. The fourth URL is from the National MS Society (note the .org).

When using a search engine, it is important to note what its capabilities are. For example, Yahoo! is a general search engine that searches by category and is good for basic searches. However, you may miss some important information. If you request a search through Yahoo! and yield little results, Yahoo! will direct you to AltaVista, which provides a more detailed search. The number of hits that you get through AltaVista might be overwhelming to you. Lycos is helpful when you want to do a more detailed search, although they have recently added some categories for a more basic search (Strauch, 1998).

Although search engines can assist you with finding the information you need, it is important to note that no search engine will provide you with all of the possible Web pages on a particular topic. As a matter of fact, recent research has found that even the best search engine will index only about 40% of all Web pages (Beaumont Enterprise, 1998). Steve Lawrence and C. Lee Giles of the NEC Research Institute (1998) found that due to the vast amount of information on the Web, even the most sophisticated search engines have a difficult time sorting through it. The main problem is that hundreds of Web pages are added daily to the approximate 325 million Web pages that already exist. Lawrence and Giles found that HotBot covers about 34% of existing pages and AltaVista covered about 28%. Lawrence and Giles found that using five search engines on one topic produced three times as much information as just using one search engine (Beaumont Enterprise, 1998).

Because of this problem, mega-search engines have been developed that will research a variety of search engines for you. Two of these are Metacrawler (www.metacrawler.com) and Dogpile (www.dogpile.com). A newer one of these is called Mamma (www.mamma.com) advertised as the "mother of all search engines." Since it is worthwhile to use two or three search engines, try the mega-search engines first to find the best possible answers to your question. If this is too overwhelming to you, go ahead and use a variety of individual search engines first and then try one of the mega-search engines. Compare your results to see which

Figure 7-3 Search Engine Results Showing Number of Terms and Percentages

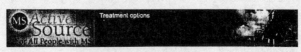

Enter words below and click Search.

Multiple sclerosis   **Search**

Home | Search Options | Help

Search Results for "Multiple sclerosis"

Web Sites   Web Pages   Related News

RECOMMENDED SITES
- **National Multiple Sclerosis Society** - Official site
- **Multiple Sclerosis Chats** - Find scheduled chats and discuss with others
- **Multiple Sclerosis** - Symptoms, conditions, treatments, resources and info

SPONSORED LINKS
The search results below are provided by a third party and are not necessarily endorsed by AOL
- **MSActiveSource.com**

- **The Raj Natural Health Center**
- **Hyperbaric Therapy Multiple Sclerosis**

MATCHING SITES   (1 - 10 of 1349)   next >>
Show Me: AOL and the Web | AOL Only | Most Popular Sites
Results from the WorldWideWeb may contain objectionable material that AOL doesn't endorse.

The National Multiple Sclerosis Society
    Dedicated to ending the devastating effects of multiple sclerosis.
    http://www.nmss.org
    Show me more like this

Rotorua & District Multiple Sclerosis Society
    With information on Multiple Sclerosis, Field Officer services, activities, and links.
    http://www.cole.gen.nz/MS
    Show me more like this

MSOhio Online Multiple Sclerosis Support Group
    MSOhio is sponsored by the Northeast Ohio Chapter of the National Multiple Sclerosis Society. MSOhio offers weekly online support chats, an "E-mail Pal Program" and has an extensive "Links" page. The Cleveland Clinic has linked directly to the MSOhio site.
    http://www.msohio.org
    Show me more like this

Multiple Sclerosis, University of Chicago Medical Center
    Information on multiple sclerosis for patients, physicians, medical students, and health care professionals. Information on clinical trials for newer treatments.
    http://ucneurology.uchicago.edu/Neurological_Disorders/...
    Show me more like this

Doctor's Guide to Multiple Sclerosis
    The latest medical news and information for patients or friends/parents of patients diagnosed with Multiple Sclerosis.
    http://www.pslgroup.com/MS.HTM
    Show me more like this

Multiple Sclerosis (MS) Support
    Infosci's Information about Multiple Sclerosis is available from this Server

SEARCH HERE:

amazon.com.

- **MULTIPLE SCL...**
- **Buy Books Here**
- **SEARCH AMAZON!**

Search books:
MULTIPLE SCL...

BARNES&NOBLE

RELATED HOT SEARCHES
- multiple sclerosis symptoms
- symptoms of multiple sclerosis
- national multiple sclerosis society
- stiff neck in multiple sclerosis
- multiple sclerosis society

Figure 7-3 Search Engine Results Showing Number of Terms and Percentages (Continued)

AOL Search: Search Results for "Multiple sclerosis"   Page 2 of 2

http://www.infosci.org
Show me more like this

Healthology Multiple Sclerosis Focus
A comprehensive resource for patients and families living with multiple sclerosis.
http://www.healthology.com/focus_index.asp?f=m_sclerosi...
Show me more like this

Help for Multiple Sclerosis
A Scientifically Safe, Patented, and Natural Non-Drug Alternative for Multiple Sclerosis.
http://naturalessentials.com/ms.htm
Show me more like this

Multiple Sclerosis - Suite101.com
Unique, starting-point website in a banner-free community. Offers monthly discussions, articles, and links to reputable web sites that inform, enlighten, and support those seeking reliable information on MS.
http://www.suite101.com/welcome.cfm/multiple_sclerosis
Show me more like this

National Multiple Sclerosis Society, Delaware Chapter
A one stop information source for people with Multiple Sclerosis and those that support them.
http://skyconsulting.com/mssdel
Show me more like this

<u>Next 15 Sites (of 1349) for Multiple sclerosis >></u>

MATCHING CATEGORIES   (1 - 5 of 67) next >>
1. Health > Conditions and Diseases > Neurological Disorders > Demyelinating Diseases > **Multiple Sclerosis**
2. Regional > Oceania > New Zealand > Health > Conditions and Diseases > **Multiple Sclerosis**
3. Regional > North America > United States > Delaware > Health > Conditions and Diseases > **Multiple Sclerosis**
4. Health > Conditions and Diseases > Neurological Disorders > Demyelinating Diseases > Multiple Sclerosis > **Support Groups**
5. Health > Conditions and Diseases > Neurological Disorders > Demyelinating Diseases > Multiple Sclerosis > **Associations**

Search Again for "Multiple sclerosis" Using These Search Services:
Picture Search Preview • News Search • Web Search • Personal Home Pages • Message Boards
Newsgroups • Health • Kids Only

Additional Search Resources:
People • ClassifiedPlus • Movies • White Pages
Yellow Pages • International Directories

Enter words below and click Search.
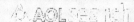
Multiple sclerosis   **Search**
Home | Search Options | Help

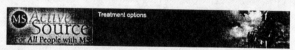

provides you with the best information. You may get some overlapping Web pages or links with your individual searches, but your search will be much more thorough. It is also recommended that when searching for medical information you consider a search engine that searches only health or medical information. Although search engines are not 100% thorough, they are still better than the alternative of trying to sift through Web information on your own.

If you want to search for health information, you might choose to use Health A to Z or Achoo. As you become more familiar with the Internet and the various search engines, you will probably find one or two that you rely on for most of your searching. Also note that most search engines offer advanced searches that can help you streamline your search even further. There are a number of search engines and Web sites listed at the end of this chapter. For a more extensive listing of health-related sites, the book *Nurse's Guide to the Internet* by Leslie Nicoll is now available. This author is the editor-in-chief of *Computers in Nursing*, a journal devoted to the use of computers in health care.

Every once in awhile you will run into problems when attempting to search using a search engine. Before you give up, consider the following:

- If your search ended up with few results, consider trying a different term. For example, if you are searching for information on hyperlipidemia, you may need to use the word *cholesterol* to get started.
- If your search ended up with too many results, consider narrowing it. For example, if you searched for medications, you might need to search for heart medications or diabetes medications.
- Be sure that you spell the search terms correctly.
- If you are searching for diabetes treatments, it helps to write the search as diabetes *and* treatments, this way, the search will include both terms together, not just one and then the other.

CORE CONCEPTS   **OTHER SEARCH OPTIONS** ————————————

Ask Jeeves   This service helps you search by asking a question rather than searching for specific terms. All you do is type in your question (Figure 7-4). You will then be shown similar questions with "go to" buttons leading to the answer (Strauch, 1998). For example, we asked Jeeves, "What are the symptoms of diabetes?" Follow-up questions are found in Figure 7-5. We think that Jeeves did an excellent job of answering this question. It also helped provide a number of sites for further investigation. Be sure to remember Jeeves when you are doing all of that homework! Ask Jeeves is located at **http://www.askjeeves.com.**

Robots   Robots (spider search engines) are similar to search engines in that they allow you to sort through vast amounts of data on a subject that you specify. Robots are able to individualize responses after you identify the information that you want. Robots are able to deliver information that is the most relevant to you, whereas

Figure 7-4 Questions for an Ask Jeeves Search

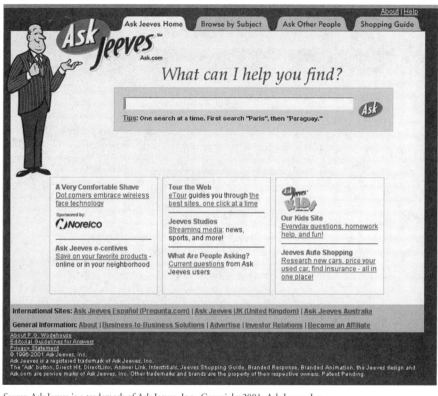

Source: Ask Jeeves is a trademark of Ask Jeeves, Inc., Copyright 2001, Ask Jeeves, Inc.

search engines frequently provide a lot of information that is irrelevant. Robots are in the developing stages, and most can be purchased as software with names such as Webtamer, Netferret, Surfbot, and Webwhacker (Mainelli, 1996). If you are interested in finding out more about robots, you might want to visit this Web site: **http://www.agentware.com.**

E-mail Once you are connected to the Internet, you will most likely want to take advantage of electronic mail, or e-mail. With e-mail you can communicate with anyone else in the world who is connected to the Internet as long as you know his or her e-mail address. E-mail addresses are always configured in the same manner (**screenname@place.domain**). The domain is the type of place: .edu is used for an educational institution, .gov is used for a government agency, .com is used for a commercial agency (company), .org is used for a nonprofit organization, .mil is used for a military site, and .net is used for a network. The place is where the e-mail is sent from, usually a service provider or ISP such as aol.com, compuserv.com, or juno.com. For example, if you received e-mail from Ishdoc@aol.com, Ishdoc is the screen name of the person sending the mail, aol is the service provider, and .com

Figure 7-5 Health Care Consumers Will Need Your Assistance

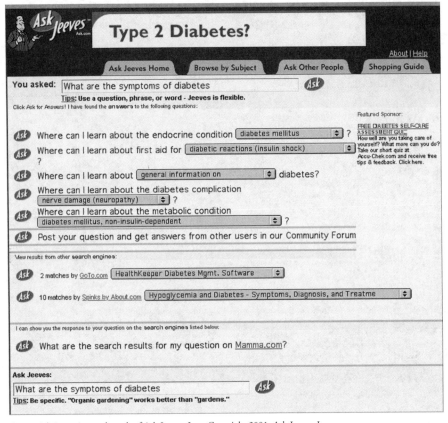

Source: Ask Jeeves is a trademark of Ask Jeeves, Inc., Copyright 2001, Ask Jeeves, Inc.

means that it is a commercial agency. Another example would be P.Jones@twu.edu, in this case, P.Jones is the person sending the mail, twu is Texas Women's University, and .edu means that it is a college or university. Most individuals with personal computers at home will have an e-mail address that ends in either a .com or a .net.

When you connect with a service provider, they will assist you in setting up an e-mail address. Once connected, you can send and receive e-mail as well as forward files, documents, and photographs! Once you are comfortable with the Web, and if you decide that you want to be adventuresome, some providers will also allow you to set up a Web page of your own. If you are connected to the Internet, you may also set up e-mail addresses free of charge through Yahoo! or through Hotmail. With a universal provider such as these, you can pick up your e-mail no matter where you are. Some specific providers will charge a long-distance fee if you try to pick up your e-mail from a location outside of your service area.

Having an e-mail address is also beneficial as a student. Many schools now require that students have e-mail addresses. That allows you and your instructors to communicate more easily. If instructors want to get a message out to all students, they can do so quite easily with e-mail. If a student is studying for an exam and suddenly comes upon a point that needs clarifying, he or she can e-mail the instructor for that clarification. Students may use the e-mail route to request specific days off on the next clinical schedule, or an instructor may notify students of an assignment modification. There are a wide variety of uses for this service while you are on your educational path.

Listservs   Another way to communicate with others is to join a mailing list or "listserv." There are thousands of mailing lists available for nearly any interest you might have. Once you become a list member, you can send messages to others on the list who share your interests. For example, if you are interested in communicating with other nursing students, there is a listserv for student nurses at listserv@list serv.acsu.buffalo.edu. In order to subscribe to it, you have to request a subscription from the listserv. You would indicate "Subscribe SNURSE-L Firstname Lastname." You will receive a return e-mail acknowledging your request. Be sure that you print and keep a copy of the original welcome message, as it will tell you how to stop your subscription from the list. You will begin receiving e-mail messages from other list members immediately. Be prepared—some lists generate almost 100 messages per day. You may want to limit the number of lists that you join or your e-mail box may be inundated!

If you are interested in learning more about what listservs are available, the following addresses will help:

- List select at http://www.liszt.com
- Several addresses can be found at http://www.tile.net/listserv/index.html
- Another option is to send e-mail to listserv@listserv.earn.net

Newsgroups   One way to communicate with others who share your interests is by Usenet newsgroups. Usenet groups are online discussion groups in which people with common interests read and post messages. Newsgroups are similar to listservs except that messages are posted to a message board that is open for all to read in a public location, while listserv messages are sent to you as an individual. Some newcomers choose to lurk for awhile before posting any messages. Lurking is reading messages that are posted without adding a message of your own. Deja News at http://www.dejanews.com allows you to search for newsgroup names. Most online services also maintain a smaller listing of available groups. Health on the Net Foundation (HON) is a nonprofit group in Geneva, Switzerland. This Web site, located at http://www.hon.ch/home.html includes a list of hospitals on the World Wide Web as well as medical support groups, newsgroups, and mailing lists.

CORE CONCEPTS   HEALTH INFORMATION

It is important to remember that there are all kinds of information available on the WWW, and, at this time, there is no quality control mechanism in place.

Some information is accurate; other information is false. It is often difficult to separate the two, because the false information may look quite plausible. This is the primary area where health care professionals must be well versed. Consumers may not have the ability to sort through all kinds of medical information to determine which information is accurate. However, the health care professional must be able to provide guidance in making decisions based on the information obtained.

Health professionals must use their professional judgment to weed out misinformation. It is important that you check out sources and confirm any information presented. Do not just "swallow it whole"; be cautious in your use of information. It is important for you to consider your professional responsibility in sharing information with consumers. You need to refer to your nurse practice act in the state in which you live. In some states it is illegal to present false information to consumers, so it is vital for you to double-check all of the information that you share with your patients.

Be alert as you surf from page to page or site to site. Even Web sites with "official"-looking names aren't necessarily what they appear to be. For example, a Web site entitled American College for Advancement in Medicine is actually a site that focuses on chelation therapy, a therapy with very limited support by conventional medicine. Avoid sites that offer cures for money, and those that claim they can treat numerous diseases with one substance.

It is important to remember that access to the Internet is not just fun and games. You need to be aware of security and privacy issues and become a responsible Internet consumer.

CORE CONCEPTS | **INTERNET PRIVACY ISSUES**

1. Never give your password to anyone! All reputable sites will not request it!
2. While surfing the Internet you may be subjected to "cookies."
    - Cookies are used by various sites to track your surfing, so that commercial sites can develop a profile of your interests.
    - Cookies embed themselves on your hard drive and have positives and negatives. For example, if you like to browse the Amazon.com bookstore (they use cookies), when you return to the site, they will suggest books that might be of interest to you based on your previous selections.
    - You need to decide whether you want to accept cookies or not.
    - Most browsers allow you to accept or reject cookies, or limit the amount of time they are stored on your hard drive.
    - Once you decide what you want to do, examine the security settings on your browser and set it to meet your privacy needs (Hinton, 1997).
3. Be careful of sending personal information over the Internet!
    - Do not give out credit card numbers unless using encryption software, or unless your browser uses encryption. Internet sites will state whether or not they have protection for your credit card number.

- Decide whether you want to share your address, telephone number, and other information when asked to register at various Web sites. If you tend to guard this personal information, you need to remember that once you share it, the potential is for millions of people to have access to it.
- If you hesitate to discuss personal or business information on a cellular or portable telephone, then you should think twice before discussing it on the Internet.
- Remember that if you send or receive e-mail at work, it is considered company property and may be accessed by others. People have been fired for sending and receiving e-mail that was derogatory to a boss or a business.
- Remember that your Internet surfing is recorded on the hard drive in the "history" file. You can change your "history" settings so that sites are deleted after a certain number of days. Your employer can look at the sites that you visit and decide whether or not they are appropriate. There have been cases of people losing their jobs because they surfed pornography sites at work.

4. Spam mail:
   - Spam mail is mail that is sent to you from various sources.
   - It is mail that you did not request and do not want.
   - The majority of spam is sent in an attempt to get you to purchase something.
   - Do not answer spam! Delete it! If you respond to spam, more information will be sent to you!
   - Your ISP may have rules about spam mail. Check them out. We need to work together to eliminate unwanted e-mail. Follow the ISP's wishes regarding reporting spammers.
   - Some spam is pornographic in nature.
   - If you have children, be sure that you set privacy settings so that they do not have access to certain Web sites and spam mail.

5. Downloading files:
   - Be certain that you have virus protection before downloading any files.
   - Do not download files from someone that you do not know.
   - Occasionally you will receive e-mail with a file attached.
   - Some files have been known to carry viruses that can destroy your computer.
   - Be sure that you are downloading information from a reputable site.

ESSENTIAL SKILLS   **WEB-USER SKILLS**

Let's do some surfing of our own so that you can acquire basic Web-user skills. You have just learned that a friend of yours has Lyme disease, and she wants to know more about it. How would you find information for her?

- Decide which search engine you want to use.
- Go to the search engine, and type in the words *Lyme disease.*
- See how many matching sites or "hits" you receive.
- Scroll down the page to see if any of the hits are worth pursuing.
- If, for example, you used Lycos as a search engine for Lyme disease, you would have received 10 hits. Only three of the hits look like they might come from a professional site (if you notice, all three originate from the same URL). Go to the site and you will discover that it is a brochure from Pfizer pharmaceuticals. It has good information, but not as detailed as you wanted.
- Try the Health A to Z search engine. Type in *Lyme disease* and you will receive 10 out of 9,060 matching documents. Which of these sites look like they are worth pursuing? Four or five of them appear to have originated from a professional site, one of which is the Centers for Disease Control and Prevention (CDC).
- Note that your search results are only as good as the search engine you choose. You may need to try more than one to get the information you desire.

Search Scenarios

1. You want to know if a new obesity drug that you read about has received Food and Drug Administration (FDA) approval.
   - Which search engine would you use (if any)?
   - What Web site would you go to?
   - Hint—don't forget the U.S. government has a number of Web sites.
   - Hint—the FDA is a government agency.

2. You have a patient who has a disease that you have never heard of before.
   - You can't find the disease in any of your textbooks.
   - Which search engine would you use (if any)?
   - What Web site would you go to?
   - Hint—if it isn't in any textbooks that you have, or in a textbook at the library, chances are it is a rare disease.
   - Hint—there is an organization that specializes in rare disorders (listed at the end of this chapter).

3. You want to learn more about multiple sclerosis.
   - Which search engine would you use (if any)?
   - What Web site would you look for?
   - Hint—you will probably find a number of sites from various search engines.
   - Hint—look for an agency that specializes in this disease such as the National MS Society.

Below are some guidelines to help you determine the accuracy of information presented on the Internet; unfortunately, they are not foolproof!

ESSENTIAL SKILLS | **INFORMATION RETRIEVAL GUIDELINES**

1. Check out the author of the material that you are reading.
   - Does the author have credentials?
   - Is the author an expert in this area?
   - There is some feeling that group-maintained Web sites might be more accurate than individually maintained sites. For example, the American Heart Association versus John Doe's heart page. However, there are a number of excellent sites that are individually maintained and have much more information than group-maintained sites.
2. Check the author's affiliation.
   - Is the author associated with a government agency, professional organization, or major national disease-specific nonprofit organization?
   - Is the author located at an educational facility?
3. If the author refers to a study or research article, check to see if the article exists.
   - See where the research is published and if it is in a reputable source.
   - Find out if the study is funded and by whom.
   - Can the information presented be validated?
4. It is important that you watch your "domain" and see if in surfing you have left the original domain.
   - For example, if you access a university site with a domain of .edu, and you link to other sites, when you find the information that interests you, has the domain changed to .com (commercial)?
   - If such a change has occurred, you will know that you are no longer at an educational site; you are now at a site that is business owned. This may or may not be reflected in the information provided. For example, Harvard University might have conducted a study on the use of antihypertensive medication in postmenopausal women. As you surf, you may access the site of a pharmaceutical company that is touting their latest antihypertensive medication.
5. Avoid sites that offer to treat a long list of diseases, or have a cure to offer for money.
   - Do you believe everything you see on infomercials?
   - There are a number of Web sites that are just like infomercials!
   - Remember that there is no quality control on the Web.
6. One Web page is available that provides information on other pages that may provide questionable advice.
   - Check it out at http://www.quackwatch.com.

A CASE IN POINT

A colleague called and explained that her nephew had been diagnosed with Berger's disease. She had diligently searched the textbooks and could only discover that it was some form of chronic kidney disease. She called knowing that we have access to the Internet. To find out more about Berger's disease, the health search engine Health A to Z at http://www.health atoz.com was used (Fig. 7-6). We discovered that another term for Berger's disease is IgA nephropathy, so in the search blank, we typed in the term *IgA Nephropathy*. Health A to Z came up with 29 related sites (Fig. 7-7) that had some information about IgA nephropathy. We clicked on the first site entitled IgA Nephropathy and were rewarded with a great deal of information about the disease, treatment, and research protocols (Fig. 7-8). The pertinent material was printed and a hard copy mailed to our colleague. We then called her to give her some basic information. Upon receipt of the information, she contacted her nephew. He was able to take the information about current treatment to his physician for his next appointment. The physician was familiar with some of the treatment but not all, and was willing to try some of the newer treatments suggested by the Web site. Not only has my colleague's nephew improved considerably, but he and his physician have also been able to keep his condition under control with some of the treatment protocols suggested by the Web site. My colleague was not only grateful for the information; she also decided that she needed Internet access as well!

Figure 7-6 Health A to Z

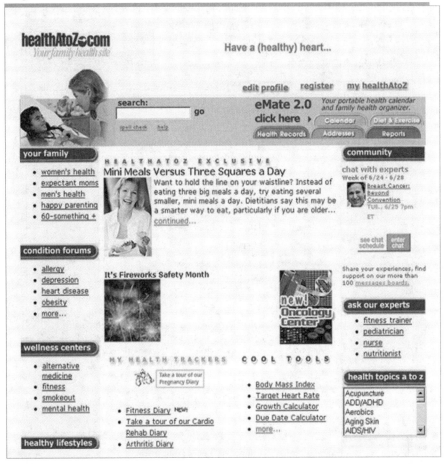

Source: Used with permission from Medical Network, Inc., www.healthatoz.com.

STOP ASK YOURSELF

1. After reading this chapter, do you have a better understanding of how to use the computer as a valuable resource? Why or why not?

   _____

   _____

2. In what ways have you resolved to use the computer to access information that will make such tasks as writing papers, learning concepts, and perhaps practicing skills easier?

   _____

   _____

Figure 7-7 Health A to Z IgA Nephropathy

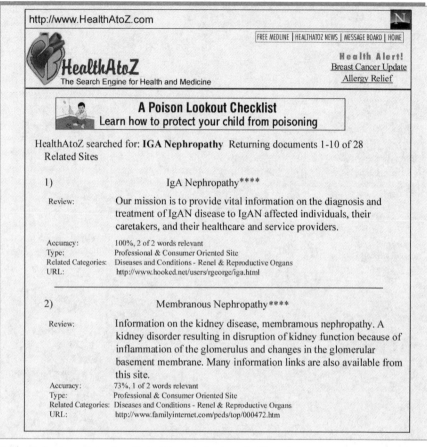

Source: Used with permission from Medical Network, Inc., www.healthatoz.com.

 CYBERLINKS: FLASH CARDS

Check to see what you now remember by making your own flash cards. Use the CD-ROM that accompanies your textbook to discover how to make flash cards for reviewing and retaining what you have learned.

 CONCEPT MAP WORD BANK

INTERNET USE
Purpose for consumers
Search engines

Figure 7-8 IgA Nephropathy Home Page

IgA Nephropathy Home Page

Home of the IgAN Foundation and IgAN E-Mail List

Site Contents

What's New

What is IgA Nephropathy?

IgAN E-Mail List subscriber information

Illustrated Kidney Function and IgAN

Kidney Disease in Perspective

Hypertension / High Blood Pressure

IgAN and Pregnancy

Current treatments for IgAN

Alternative Healthcare

Help us find a cure by understanding ourselves. Add your personal medical data

Click here for the On-line IgAN Internet Research Project Questionnaire

Make a contribution to the IgA Nephropathy Foundation

IgA **Nephropathy** or Berger's Disease is the most common non-diabetic kidney disease. Included in the diagnosis of IgAN is Henoch Schonlin Purpurea (where it involves the kidney) and sometimes other forms of glomerulenephritis. Available evidence suggests that IgA nephropathy occurs from either increased production or reduced clearance of the immune protein IgA and associated antigen complexes that are ultimately deposited within the kidney.

Many sources categorize IgAN as a rare disease afflicting 1:100,000 - 1:200,000. It seems that this esitmated level of incidence for IgAN is not accurate as a large proportion of patients who present with IgAN symptoms have mild disease which is not diagnosed via the accepted biopsy diagnosis. Some published research of random diagnostic kidney biopsies suggests IgAN may be vastly more common and may affect up to 2-4% of the human population at large. Certainly there is a dramatic variance in the prevalence of diagnosed IgAN. In Japan and France where testing for the condition is part of regular preventative medical care the disease incidence is twice that found in the USA where testing for IgAN is rarely performed as preventative medicine. Most people probably never realize they have the disease or at least do not realize it until a late stage. Amongst those diagnosed as having IgAN as many as 20%- 30% will suffer eventual kidney failure within 10-20 years. They will require life saving dialysis and/or a kidney transplant.

There are no "widely accepted" western medical treatments for IgAN save in the latest stages of the disease. There is however growing evidence that a number of therapies can be effective in delaying the deterioration of kidney function for many years. Most nephrologists with an active awareness of IgAN prescribe ACE inhibitors and fish oil at a minimum. In some cases powerful steroid treatment is utilized. For about half of those with IgAN tonsillectomy, which treats part of the underlying immune disorder, is effective. There are additional new treatments that show the promise of being a start on finding a cure for the disease.

Source: Used with permission from Russ George of the IgAN Foundation, Palo Alto, California, www.igan.org.

Search problems
INTERNET PRIVACY ISSUES
CREDIBILITY OF INFORMATION

Refer to Concept Maps and Flash Cards on pages viii–ix for an explanation of how to create and use concept maps. In addition, the CD-ROM guides you through the construction of concept maps by providing a more detailed introduction, more illustrations of examples, and key steps to follow in designing your own maps.

Legal Considerations

8

ASK YOURSELF

1. What do I already know about the meaning of standards of care?

_____

_____

2. What does the word *accountability* mean to me?

_____

_____

CYBERLINKS

Interactive Can you talk legalese? Are you savvy about how to stay out of legal trouble? Visit www.nursing.about.com. Scroll down to Legal/Political and find out about current legal issues in nursing! Other interesting and interactive links are available at this site.

Supplemental www.LPNresources.com can help enhance your learning by leading you to discover other links with more information about the topic you are studying. Becoming a masterful learner is just a few clicks away!

CORE CONCEPTS STANDARDS OF CARE

One of the most important legal concepts for you to grasp is standard of care, because many of the other legal concepts are related to standard of care. All professions have standards of care, or minimal levels of expertise, that must be delivered to the patient. Nurses are responsible for both external standards (those set on the national level) and internal standards (those set by the role of nursing). You are responsible for all standards of care as they pertain to practical or vocational nursing. You are required to maintain competence and skills after graduation by reading

65

professional journals and attending continuing education and in-service programs (programs for updating concepts and skills related to your profession).

If you are ever summoned to appear in a court of law, you will be judged by the standards of care in your community. You are responsible for delivering care that at the very least meets the standards in your community or exceeds them. By adhering to care standards, your patients will receive competent, high-quality nursing care.

According to Guido (1997), you should familiarize yourself with standards of care through the following:

- Your state nurse practice act
- Standards published by the American Nurses Association (ANA)
- Standards published by any applicable specialty organization, if you are working in that specialty area
- Federal agency guidelines and regulations such as those designated by Occupational Safety and Health Administration (OSHA)
- Employment policy and procedure manual
- Your job description

Practical/vocational nursing students are required to demonstrate the identical standard of care as licensed practical/vocational nurses. Nursing students have the ultimate responsibility for their own actions and may be liable for their own negligence. Students who are underage and not considered by state law to be adults may still be held liable for their actions.

CORE CONCEPTS   LEGAL TERMS

Whether you are a student or a licensed practical/vocational nurse, you need to be aware of the most common legal concepts or terms that are associated with the nursing role. Some of those with which you need to familiarize yourself inlude:

- *Negligence:* An act or failure to commit an act which resulted in harm to a patient. The term *reasonably prudent* is often used in the nursing profession to indicate a person who carefully uses common sense to guide his or her actions. Thus, a negligent person is one who didn't act as a reasonably prudent person would have acted under the same circumstances.
- *Malpractice:* Negligence by a professional person, whether it be a nurse, physician, or dentist. In this case, the standard of action is confined to the reasonably prudent nurse or other professional. As a nursing student, you are held to the standards of a reasonably prudent practicing LPN/LVN.
- *Assault:* Threatening to harm someone or doing something to make the person fear that you will harm him or her. Threatening a patient with the use of restraints or with a "shot" because of his or her behavior could constitute assault.

- *Battery:* Touching someone without his or her consent, whether you caused harm or not. Performing certain treatments on patients without their consent could be grounds for a battery charge.
- *False imprisonment:* Confining a person in some way without his or her consent. For the nurse, restraining a patient without following the appropriate procedure (i.e., obtaining a physician's order) could be grounds for false imprisonment. The same could be true for confining a patient in a secured Alzheimer's unit without the proper order and documentation.
- *Libel:* A written statement about someone else that is damaging to his or her character, even if the statement is true. You must make sure that all of your documentation is objective without your opinion.
- *Slander:* An oral statement about someone else that is damaging to his or her character, even if the statement is true. This could be a statement you make about a patient, another nurse, or other staff member, especially if done in a public place.
- *Abandonment:* Deserting your patient care responsibilities before another nurse can replace you to maintain the continuity of patient care. Leaving your patients before additional staff arrives to assume their care could be grounds for charges of abandonment.

ESSENTIAL SKILLS	PERFORMANCE REQUIREMENTS RELATED TO ACCOUNTABILITY

The role of the practical nursing student is one that requires the same competent care as that provided by an LPN/LVN. This requirement places a great deal of accountability on you, the student. Students are legally responsible to inform their instructor if they are unprepared or require any special assistance. Students are accountable for their skills and their knowledge. Nursing faculty members or staff nurses may be accountable for a student's lack of preparedness or competence. To help yourself provide competent care without legal consequence:

- Be certain that you know the policies and procedures of the clinical facility, and follow them at all times.
- Be adequately prepared for the clinical experience. Know your patient's treatments, interventions, and any medications.
- Be sure to inform the instructor if you are unprepared for the clinical experience. (If you don't know your patient, the treatments, surgery, medication, etc., you are unprepared!) Be aware that it might be up to the discretion of the clinical instructor to send you home from a clinical if you come unprepared and patient safety is in question.
- If you are asked to perform a procedure or give a medication that you are not familiar with, say no!
- If you have practiced a skill, procedure, or medication administration but

are unsure of yourself, ask for help from your instructor. If your instructor is unavailable, ask the nursing staff to complete the task for you.

- Know what treatments, procedures, and skills students are allowed to perform in each institution. (They are not all the same.) If asked to perform something that is not allowed, refuse! Offer to assist the staff nurse in some other way.

- If you are working in an institution as an employee, clarify what skills, if any, are allowed for employees that you are not allowed to complete as a student. Conversely, you may not practice skills as an employee that you might be trained to do as a nursing student. For instance, we have had reports of students being asked to do catheterizations when they were functioning as certified nursing assistants (CNAs) even though sterile procedures were not part of the CNA job description and were out of their scope of practice.

- Most schools require that all of their students have liability insurance (malpractice insurance) before clinical experience. Some schools will provide insurance for the student, and some schools will expect you to purchase it on your own. Nursing schools that are part of a state system might have coverage for you through the state. Be sure and clarify how liability coverage is handled for your nursing program. If your school doesn't require liability insurance, you might still consider purchasing it. Liability insurance is available through a number of insurance companies. Many companies will continue to offer coverage to you following graduation as well (Guido, 1997).

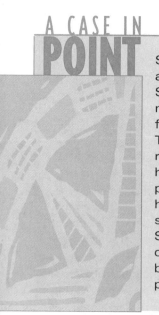

A CASE IN POINT

Susie is a student practical nurse and has been assigned a rotation in the medical–surgical unit. She perceives the charge nurse to be stern and not particularly helpful. Susie answers a call bell from a patient with whom she is not familiar. The patient wants to get up to go to the bathroom. The patient seems weak, and Susie asks him if he is allowed to get out of bed. The patient impatiently answers yes. Susie helps him to his feet and holds onto his arm, but he suddenly falls to the ground and is injured. Susie soon learns that, according to the physician's orders, the patient is not permitted out of bed because of his condition (very low blood pressure). The family threatens to sue.

GENERAL PERFORMANCE REQUIREMENTS RELATED TO AVOIDING LEGAL PROBLEMS

ESSENTIAL SKILLS

- Treat patients and family members honestly, respectfully, and openly.
- Be compassionate and professional.
- Make your patients aware of all facets of treatment and of their prognosis when appropriate.
- Know the law and incorporate it into your practice.
- Know your competence level and work to improve it through continuing education.
- Be active in your professional organizations.
- Be aware of patients who are prone to sue (refer to list in this section).
- Be aware of nurses' personality traits that trigger lawsuits (refer to list in this section) (Guido, 1997).

THE PROFILE OF PATIENTS PRONE TO SUE

CORE CONCEPTS

Vincent, Young, and Phillips (1994) found four main themes when examining why patients and their families take legal action. These four themes are:

1. *Accountability:* Wishing to see staff disciplined and called to account.
2. *Explanation:* A combination of wanting an explanation and feeling ignored or neglected after the incident.
3. *Standards of care:* Wishing to ensure that a similar incident does not happen again.
4. *Compensation:* Wanting compensation and an admission of negligence. There seems to be a profile of patients who tend to sue health care providers. The following are traits to be aware of:
   - Overly dependent
   - Hostile
   - Uncooperative
   - Noncompliant
   - Blame others
   - Insecure (Guido, 1997)

If your patient reacts in this manner, it is important that you know how to deal with him or her. Rather than react negatively, which will increase resentment and the possibility of a lawsuit, choose to be empathetic and responsive. These patients tend to experience a lot of anxiety so it helps to provide as much information as possible, and to do so repeatedly. If the patient shows any efforts at cooperation, praise these efforts. Although there is no guarantee that you will avoid a lawsuit, it helps to recognize the type of patient who might sue.

CORE CONCEPTS | TRAITS OF NURSES WHO TRIGGER LAWSUITS

The following is a profile of nurses' traits that trigger lawsuits:

- Have difficulty developing close relationships
- Insecure
- Tend to shift blame to others
- Insensitive to patient complaints
- Fail to take patient complaints seriously
- Aloof (standoffish)
- More concerned with technology and machines than the patient (Figure 8-1).
- Delegates to others to avoid patient contact (Guido, 1997)

Of the traits listed above, research has shown that the patients were most likely to sue those nurses who were insensitive to complaints and acted as if they didn't care when patients expressed their concerns. All nurses need to be aware of legal issues both at school and at work. It is important for you to learn how to protect yourself and your employer from litigation. You can tell patients that you are sorry that they feel the way that they do without admitting any liability or wrongdoing on your part or the part of the facility or other staff. All complaints should be handled professionally and referred to the proper staff for further investigation. Many larger hospitals actually have patient advocates who do just that; in other cases, it might be a social worker or chaplain. Know the policy and procedure of the facility where you are doing your clinical. You will never go wrong if you always see the importance of treating others as you or a member of your family would want to be treated.

STOP ASK YOURSELF ─────────────────────────

1. What do I especially want to remember (one to three sentences) about legal considerations for the LPN/LVN?

   _____

   _____

2. What, if any, impact or strong impression has the reading and understanding of legal considerations had on me?

   _____

   _____

CYBERLINKS: FLASH CARDS ─────────────────────

Check to see what you now remember by making your own *flash cards*. Use the CD-ROM that accompanies your textbook to discover how to make flash cards for reviewing and retaining what you have learned.

Figure 8-1 Some Nurses Are More Concerned with Technology Than with the Patient

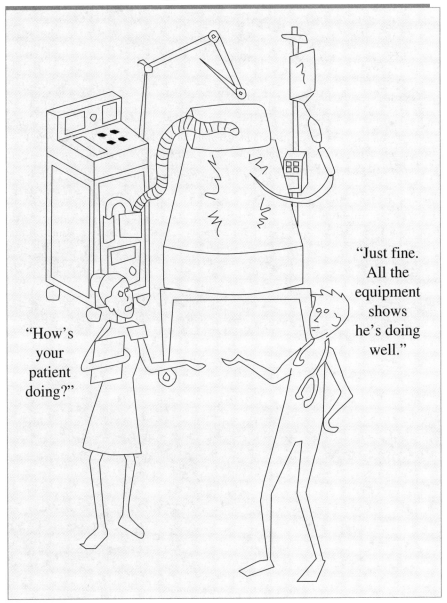

CONCEPT MAP WORD BANK ───────────────────

Accountability

Standard of care

LPN/LVN performance requirements

Patients prone to sue

Nurses' traits that trigger lawsuits

Refer to Concept Maps and Flash Cards on pages viii–ix for an explanation of how to create and use concept maps. In addition, the CD-ROM guides you through the construction of concept maps by providing a more detailed introduction, an illustration of examples, and key steps to follow in designing your own maps.

Risk Management

9

 ASK YOURSELF

1. What does the term *risk management* mean to you?

   _____

   _____

2. In what type of health care settings are you most likely to find risk managers?

   _____

   _____

 CYBERLINKS

If you are interested in more information about risk management, visit the Web site at **www.riskweb.com.**

<u>Supplemental</u> **www.LPNresources.com** can help enhance your learning by leading you to discover other links with more information about the topic you are studying.

Risk management is a specialized field within the general realm of management. Risk management in health care is similar to risk management in business as it focuses on minimizing the financial effects of accidental loss. Some of the financial losses that risk management is concerned with include property loss by fire or flood; income loss due to decrease in census; personnel loss through injury, illness, or death; machinery breakdown; and being named as a defendant in a lawsuit.

CORE CONCEPTS **ROLE RESPONSIBILITIES**

Risk managers perform frequent analyses of losses that occur within a facility. Risk managers also deal with identifying and decreasing the potential liability of the facility. Managers keep databases that reflect all losses over time. Their primary job is to stop losses from occurring or to provide means (financial) for losses that are going to occur regardless of attempts to stop them from happening. For example, in our litigious society, chances are that a health care facility may be faced with a number of lawsuits on a yearly basis. The risk manager is responsible for seeing that a certain amount of financial cushioning is provided to handle these suits.

The risk manager also serves as an insurance connection for the facility and is sometimes responsible for the automobile, property, general, professional, and workers' compensation insurance policies. The risk manager is also a legal contact for the hospital and provides information about advance directives, adoptions, questions regarding consent forms, contract reviews, and any correspondence or contact with attorneys. Risk managers may also be involved with the infection control policies of the health care facility and how they might relate to losses, especially lost time for the employee. The risk manager is not just concerned about one aspect of the health care facility, but rather with the broad picture. The risk manager has a responsibility to employees, visitors, patients, physicians, and to hospital property.

According to Cindy McClelland, risk manager, some of the things that a risk manager might be responsible for monitoring include:

- Safety
- Fire protection
- Employee health
- Incident reports
- Bomb threat procedures
- Americans with Disabilities Act (ADA) compliance
- Patient complaints
- Security
- Physician credentialing
- Damaged or lost equipment

Often, nurses are not clear about what exactly a risk manager does. As you can see, the risk manager is responsible for the day-to-day activities in the health care facility. Because of such a unique position, the risk manager can serve as a source of information about a number of things that nurses are interested in.

CORE CONCEPTS ▌ **THE RISK MANAGEMENT PLAN**

The risk manager is also responsible for developing a facility-wide plan of risk management. According to Sullivan and Decker (1992), the risk management plan might consist of some or all of the following:

- Identify potential risks by working with all departments and inspecting the facility.
- Review and monitor systems such as incident reports, audits, committee minutes, and patient complaints.

- Monitor laws and standards that relate to patient safety, consent, and care.
- Review and appraise new programs such as managed care, home health, rehabilitation, and infusion therapy.
- Eliminate or reduce a specific risk through education, policy, or insurance financing.
- Analyze trends and causes of incidents by their frequency and severity.
- Identify educational needs—staff education needs about new equipment, policies and procedures, and patient needs on admission and discharge.
- Evaluate the effectiveness of the risk management program.
- Provide reports and documentation of trends to the chief executive officer and respective committees.

Risk management is important to you for a number of reasons:

- If the facility continually loses money, you may not be able to seek employment there following graduation.
- Theft can cause the employer to stop providing necessary supplies.
- Injury and illness on the job are important to your well-being.
- The risk management program can support and provide you with information on ways to make your nursing care better and your job safer.

CORE CONCEPTS   THE CONNECTION BETWEEN RISK MANAGEMENT AND NURSING FUNCTION

Nurses tend to be involved in the areas of risk management given in the following list. It would be to your advantage to pay special attention to these areas, as well as finding out for yourself which problems occur most frequently in the area in which you work.

- Medication errors
- Complications from diagnostic or treatment procedures
- Falls
- Patient or family dissatisfaction with care
- Refusal of treatment or to sign a consent form

The risk manager can be a particularly valuable resource relating to nursing function:

- The risk manager can provide you with data about these high-risk areas for nurses.
- The risk manager can also give you specific information about the area in which you work.
- Does your area have more falls than others do? If so, why?
- What are other areas doing that your area is not?
- How can you fix the problem?

The risk manager can help you to answer questions such as those stated above and, consequently, make your area safer for you, patients, and visitors.

ESSENTIAL SKILLS   **RISK MANAGEMENT SKILLS**

1. Communicate! Let those individuals who need to know, know what is going on.
2. Document! Remember, "If you didn't chart it, you didn't do it."
3. Follow! The chain of command is there for a reason!
   - If you need help, ask your immediate supervisor.
   - If you are not satisfied with the results, ask your supervisor's immediate supervisor.
   - Do not skip steps and go directly to the chief executive officer.
4. Maintain confidentiality!
   - Keep hospital and patient information confidential.
   - Do not gossip.
5. Incident reports!
   - Always ask, and if you are still in doubt, fill one out.
   - The incident report form is a means of protecting you and the facility.
6. Communication!
   - Be honest but careful.
   - Remember, what you say can be used against you.
7. Education!
   - Stay up to date in your field.
   - You can never know too much.

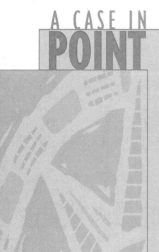

A CASE IN POINT

Barbara, a newly hired LPN/LVN, notices that during the 3 months that she has been employed by the Medical Center, five people have fallen (at different times) by tripping over a carpet mat located at the lobby entrance. She wonders if the risk manager should be consulted or if she should just "mind her own business" and assume that the risk manager already knows about this potentially dangerous situation. After all, Barbara reasons, it may not be a good idea for a brand new employee to embarrass herself.

ASK YOURSELF

1. What types of job responsibilities do you have as an LPN/LVN that might impact the medical facility in terms of financial loss if performed negligently or in an unsafe manner?

_____

_____

2. What plans or goals do you have to further your education once you become an LPN/LVN? Would you consider the field of risk management as a career choice?

_____

_____

 CYBERLINKS: FLASH CARDS

Check to see what you now remember by making your own flash cards. Use the CD-ROM that accompanies your textbook to discover how to make flash cards for reviewing and retaining what you have learned.

 CONCEPT MAP WORD BANK

RISK MANAGEMENT
Responsibilities
RISK MANAGEMENT PLAN
NURSING CONNECTION
Skills

Refer to Concept Maps and Flash Cards on pages viii–ix for an explanation of how to create and use concept maps. In addition, the CD-ROM guides you through the construction of concept maps by providing a more detailed introduction, more illustrations of examples, and key steps to follow in designing your own maps.

Section II

BEHAVIORAL COMPETENCIES

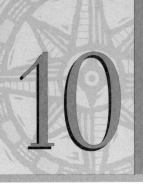

Communication

10

ASK YOURSELF

1. When you are having a conversation with someone, what do you find to be most important to you (words or feelings) in the other person's communication with you?

   _____

   _____

2. How do think the way in which you communicate with patients differs from the way you communicate with your parents or your friends?

   _____

   _____

CYBERLINKS

Interactive How would you rate your own communication skills? Check your accuracy of perception regarding these skills by taking the communication skills test at **www.queendom.com/tests/index.html** and click on the specific test.

Supplemental **www.LPNresources.com** can help enhance your learning by leading you to discover other links with more information about the topic your are studying.

Communication is an essential part of our lives. We communicate with each other constantly. As an adult, you have already witnessed ways other people communicate, and you will have developed methods of communication that feel comfortable to you. We tend to develop communication patterns that we use over and over again with the various people in our lives. We communicate one way with our parents, another way with our significant others and our children, and another way with the grocery store clerk. Although communication is a natural part of our lives, it is also a skill that must be developed and fine-tuned. In nursing, we refer to communication with patients as therapeutic communication, which is characterized by a particular set of purposeful communication skills. Some of the communication patterns that you use in nursing will be unfamiliar; others will be familiar. To develop skills in communication, you must have an interest in people and what they have to say.

| CORE CONCEPTS | **THE NATURE OF COMMUNICATION** |

Communication is basically sharing information with another person. It is letting the other person know what you think and finding out what he or she thinks. As a student nurse, you will be learning to communicate *therapeutically* with patients and *professionally* with your peers, instructors, and facility staff members. This chapter focuses on therapeutic oral communication, and the next chapter presents written communication, or documentation. Both are equally important skills in nursing. Basic communication requires that there be a sender, a receiver, and a message to be sent and received. The important thing to remember is that the message must be understood for communication to have occurred. An old saying of unknown origin states, "I know that you believe that you understand what you think I said, but I'm not sure you realize that what you heard is not what I meant." Huh? How many times have you thought you expressed yourself very well and then found that the receiver of your message totally misunderstand your point? One of the authors remembers that, as a student nurse, she was trying to communicate to a patient that he must drink more. She meant water, but she did not realize at the time that he had a problem with alcohol. When she told him he had to drink more, he looked up, very surprised, and said, "Oh? The doc said I had to cut back to a pint a day." Obviously, she had not made the point clear! In nursing, we must really work toward getting our message across to a patient and making sure we listen and understand what the patient is saying to us. It is equally important that we communicate clearly with staff, instructors and peers.

Most of our daily conversations with our peers are forms of socialization. We are spontaneous. We talk and laugh, express our views, and share our thoughts. In therapeutic communication, there is a deeper purpose to our conversation. When we are interacting therapeutically with patients, we are assessing their needs, guiding them in meeting those needs, working toward goals, and giving care and support, among other things. Therapeutic communication is a skill you will use daily as a nurse. Often, you must first think about what you want to say and how you want to say it before communicating with patients and others in the health care setting.

It is important to know what to say and how you want to say something, because underlying all communication is the expression of attitudes. As you are developing your own communication style with patients, remember what you like and dislike about the way you personally are and have been treated. You will find that some nurses treat patients as objects or things. These nurses tend to be arrogant, belittling, uncaring and lacking in warmth. You will also find other nurses who are compassionate, respectful, understanding, and caring. What kind of nurse will you be? You do have a choice!

It is essential that you treat patients and others with respect. If you adopt this respectful attitude, it will come through in your communication with each patient. Remember that patients are people too. They are not just the disease that they represent. A patient is "Mrs. Williams," who happens to be in room 107 and happens to have abdominal pain. She is not "room 107" or "abdominal pain." Treat people as you want to be treated yourself or as you would want your loved one to be treated (your mother, father, sister, brother, spouse, or child). Many times, nurses are so busy doing various tasks that they forget that there is a person behind or under the tubes, dressings, and machinery. They forget that the purpose of all of those tasks is to provide high-quality care to the patients.

The following two scenarios regarding the purchase of a pair of athletic shoes paint you a colorful picture of poor and good communication skills.

- **Scenario 1:** You go to a local sporting goods store, and as you enter the shoe department, you see three salespeople in store uniforms standing around. You walk past them and head toward the shoe department. Not one of the three employees gives you a second glance. As you approach the athletic shoes, you find that there are at least 100 different kinds—running, cross-training, walking, basketball, and tennis—as well as several different brands. Feeling totally overwhelmed, you start searching for some assistance. You finally locate an employee and request help with the selection process. The salesperson says, "Yeah, I'll be there in a minute." You wander back to the shoes and sit down to wait. After 5 minutes, you start hunting another salesperson. You locate another employee who is busy sharing details of the latest movie with other salespeople. By now, you are getting annoyed, because no one will help you. You once again ask an employee for help. The salesperson reluctantly follows you to the athletic shoes. You explain that you need help choosing a shoe for aerobic dancing in a 9 narrow. The salesperson proceeds to pull out five pairs of 9 narrow shoes from the stacks. When you ask what the differences are in the shoes the employee says, "I don't know. What difference does it make? Just find one that fits," and walks away. You feel as though no one is making an effort to help you and that the salesperson could not care less whether you are satisfied with the service or not. The employee obviously has more important things to do than to pay attention to you!

- **Scenario 2:** You decide to try a different store. You find the shoe department, and when you walk in, a salesperson comes over to you and asks, "How may I help you?" You tell her that you are trying to find a shoe for aerobic dancing in 9 narrow. As she walks you toward the end of the aisle, she explains that you are bypassing tennis, walking, and other shoes that will not provide enough support for aerobics. At the end of the aisle she points out the aerobic shoes and explains the cushioning and asks whether you have any problems with your feet. You explain that you tend to wear down the outside of your shoes very quickly. She chooses a pair of shoes for you to try and tells you that they provide a lot of lateral support. As she guides you to your selection, she smiles frequently and is extremely attentive to your facial expressions. You feel as though she is really focused on you and will stay with you and help you find the correct pair of shoes that are the best suited for you.

Now, look at the difference in the communication in each scenario. In the first one, you found employees who were uncaring, unprofessional, unhelpful, and who didn't listen. In the second, you found an employee who was caring, knowledgeable, helpful, and listened to what the customer needed. The next time you go shopping for a pair of shoes, where will you go?

ESSENTIAL SKILLS   COMMUNICATION SKILLS APPLIED TO NURSING

Although we don't often think of patients this way, they are our customers, too. They want to be treated well. If they are mistreated, they will take their business elsewhere. Many health care facilities now require that their employees take a course in customer service. They may also give patients report cards, so they can grade their hospital stay.

Mark Twain said, "Kindness is a language which the deaf ear can hear and the blind can see." Hospitals and nursing homes are businesses, and businesses have a slogan—"The customer is always right." In other words, you should do everything in your power to keep the customer happy. This means treating your patients with dignity and respect, as well as demonstrating kindness and competence in your nursing care. As a side note, research has shown that patients treated in this manner rarely sue even if something goes wrong during their hospital stay.

Verbal Messages   Effective therapeutic communication requires that you:

- Care about your patients and what they have to say. Put yourself in their shoes. This is called *empathy*.
- Listen attentively. Focus on what patients are telling you. Make eye contact with them. Give them time to express their thoughts. We had a student in a clinical once who cared for a patient the floor nurses had characterized as "confused." When the student took care of the lady, she found the patient was slow in speech but certainly not confused. The patient even told the student that the student was the first person who actually let her complete a thought!
- Value what patients tell you. You may not agree with what is said, but patients have a right to their feelings, beliefs, and thoughts. Allow them those thoughts. A good way to cut off communication is by telling a patient that what they feel is not valid. A comment such as "Oh, you shouldn't feel that way" will put an end to an interaction very quickly.
- Speak in a clear manner, using words appropriate for the individual. Do not assume you have to speak louder to older people or those with hearing aids. Be aware of the age of the patient (a 2-year-old child and a 10-year-old child

require different word choice and manner of communication). Your word choice or vocabulary should also reflect the patient's educational background and/or facility with the English language.

- What you say to patients should be goal directed. How do you want what you are saying to be interpreted by the patient? What do you want the patient to do with the information? How do you want the patient to feel after you said what you said?

Nonverbal Messages   Up until this point we have been discussing verbal communication—what we say. But we also communicate nonverbally. This includes our posture, expressions, gestures, and mannerisms. Psychologists feel that most communication is done in this manner. Remember another old saying, "It is not always what you say, but how you say it"? This type of communication comes through loud and clear, and sometimes we wish it did not!

In discussing nonverbal communication, remember that both you and your patient will be communicating in this manner. You should always be aware of your own body language as well as that of your patient.

The same qualities mentioned above for effective verbal communication are also important for nonverbal communication.

- *Communicate that you care.* How do you know when someone cares about you? They get down on your level (sit down if your patient is sitting, or pull up a chair if they are lying in bed). They nod their heads to let you know they are listening.
- *Communicate your empathy.* Use eye contact to indicate that you are listening and that you understand. Nod your head and smile as you listen to what the patient is saying.
- *Communicate that you want what is best for your patient.* If you have demonstrated that you care and are empathetic, your patient will know that you can be trusted and that you want to help. Your patients will be grateful, and your employer will be pleased.
- *Touch is important to the majority of people for communicating caring and empathy.* However, it is sometimes appropriate to ask patients if it is all right before you touch them or reach for their hands. Patients who have been subjected to physical abuse or who have certain mental disorders are often not comfortable with touch. This requires that you know your patients and their history. Consider their culture and what touch means to them before touching. Then use a light, gentle touch.

We mentioned earlier that *professional* communication with peers, instructors, and facility staff members will also be important for you. We have found that some nurses have a tendency to have more difficulty communicating with other members of the health care team than with their patients. As technology improves, more specialties develop, leaving nurses responsible for communicating with more people on a daily basis. To streamline communication for the benefit of patients, it is important for us to know which member of the health care team needs what information.

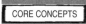 **GUIDELINES FOR COMMUNICATING WITH TEAM MEMBERS**

Patient

- Perhaps the most important team member is the patient.
- Unfortunately, many specialists want to "do for" or "do to" the patient without allowing the patient's active participation.
- As changes occur in the health care system, patients are becoming more and more knowledgeable and are demanding to be included in all aspects of their health care.
- Patients have a right and a responsibility to participate in their own health care.
- It is necessary that all members of the health care team keep patients informed so that they will be sufficiently informed to make decisions about their own health care.

Physician

- The physician is responsible for diagnosing, treating, and preventing disease.
- Typically, the doctor will use medications and/or surgery to treat patients.
- The physician used to be considered the "captain" of the health care team and was responsible for directing all aspects of care.
- Today, the doctor is considered a *member* of the health care team and needs to collaborate with other team members to provide patients with the best possible care.
- The physician needs to be informed about all aspects of the patient's care.
- It is important that you discuss with the physician any changes in health status or any changes in therapy provided by any other health team member.

Physical Therapist (PT)

- The PT focuses on problems of a musculoskeletal nature.
- The PT uses exercises and therapies to increase muscle strength and decrease loss of function.
- The PT needs to know about problems with musculoskeletal function, mobility aids, and anything else that has an impact on the patient's ability to participate in physical therapy.

Occupational Therapist (OT)

- The OT focuses on the patient's ability to maintain his or her independence in activities of daily living.

- The OT assists patients in adapting their home and/or using special equipment to continue to take care of their home or personal activities.
- The OT needs to be aware of any physical, mental, or emotional limitations the patient might have, or any problems the patient is having with activities of daily living or home maintenance.

Social Worker

- The social worker attempts to better the patient's life outside of the hospital through referrals to community agencies, counseling, or finding alternative placement.
- The social worker helps organize care for the patient at home or in short-term or long-term living facilities.
- Social workers need to be informed about the patient's physical, emotional, and mental limitations.

Dietitian

- The dietitian is responsible for providing nutrition counseling and therapy.
- The dietitian helps develop an individual nutrition plan that takes into account things such as the patient's culture, ethnicity, financial status, and health status.
- The dietitian needs to know the patient's typical diet, what type of diet the physician has ordered, and any other information that pertains to the patient's nutrition status.

Respiratory Therapist (RT)

- The RT focuses on the patient's respiratory function and treats any problems of a respiratory nature.
- In some facilities, the RT and the nurse work together to provide treatment.
- The RT needs to know about changes in respiratory function or any problems the patient is experiencing related to their respiratory treatment.

As a nurse, you will be responsible for communicating with all of these different specialists and may be responsible for coordinating information between and among them. To assist you with coordination of care, it is important that you recall two aspects of professional behavior that may impact your teamwork: advocacy and accountability.

| ESSENTIAL SKILLS | ASPECTS OF PROFESSIONAL BEHAVIOR |

Advocacy   To protect your patient's interests, you may need to be a patient advocate. Occasionally, you will find that a particular patient's needs are not being met, or the patient may actually be in jeopardy of having rights violated. It is your responsibility in either of these situations to speak on behalf of your patient. Technically, all health care team members share in this responsibility, but nurses tend to be in a better position to act as a patient advocate. This is one of the reasons that it is so important that you spend time getting to know your patient and your patient's wishes.

Accountability   As a member of the health care team, you are accountable for your own actions. You are responsible for informing your team members about any changes in the patient's status or about any information that the patient shares with you that is pertinent to the team. You are not only accountable to the patient; you are also accountable to other team members and the team as a whole.

As stated earlier, it is important that you respect your patients and treat them the way that you would want your loved ones to be treated. It is just as important that you treat other members of the health care team with respect. By encouraging mutual respect among team members, you promote the development of a professional partnership.

Since there are a number of members on each patient's health care team, roles sometimes become confused. You may run into a situation in your clinicals in which you might be given conflicting orders. It is up to you to seek clarification of each team member's role. Your clinical instructor will help you do this. Participating in patient care conferences in long-term care and extended care will also help you see the interaction between staff members and differences in their roles in planning what is best for the patient.

Confidentiality   A discussion focusing on communication would not be complete without emphasizing confidentiality once again. Whatever information you learn as part of your care for patients is confidential and should not be shared with outsiders. If patients tell you something in confidence, you must ask them if it is all right to share the information before doing so. It is a good policy to never promise a patient you will keep a secret before you know what it is. We have had diabetics who have asked students not to tell anyone they had candy bars stashed in their bedside tables! Always use the rule that information should be shared on a "need to know" basis. If others are involved in the care of your patient, they "need to know" what you have learned to ensure continuity and competent care for the patient involved. Confidentiality is also concerned with not sharing information about other staff with the patients.

It may seem that communication can be an overwhelming task, and it certainly can be. However, communication patterns are continuously evolving. With awareness of your own style of communication and how you might want to further develop your skills, communication patterns can be changed and improved. As a caretaker, your commitment should be to remember to think before you speak, respect yourself and others, treat everyone with kindness, and be genuine.

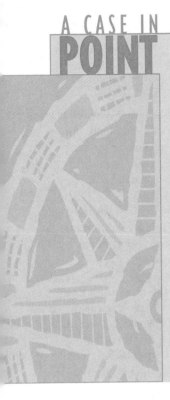

A CASE IN POINT

Mr. Smythe, a 78-year-old patient, is irritated because he has not gotten his dinner yet. The nurse acknowledges that the medical center's food service is late delivering the trays today. He says to the nurse: "Well, don't just stand there, do something about it!" Mr. Smythe's words and his tone of voice surprise the nurse. She pauses for a moment and quickly thinks about her options. She would like to just walk out but knows that would not be appropriate. Maybe she should tell him not to take his frustrations out on her. Maybe she should tell her supervisor. Maybe she should tell him that he needs to be patient. Maybe she should tell him that late trays aren't her fault or responsibility. Instead, she responds: "You must be really hungry! Let me see if I can find out what's happening with these trays. I will be right back." The nurse hears a calm "thank you" as she leaves the patient's room.

🛑 ASK YOURSELF

1. With which category of team members (patient, physician, physical therapist, etc.) do you think you will have the most difficulty communicating? Why? Which communication skills would you target for improving communication with this group?

_____

_____

2. Do you think you need to be more conscious of how you communicate nonverbally? Why or why not?

_____

_____

CYBERLINKS: FLASH CARDS

Check to see what you now remember by making your own flash cards. Use the CD-ROM that accompanies your textbook to discover how to make flash cards for reviewing and retaining what you have learned.

CONCEPT MAP WORD BANK

COMMUNICATION
Verbal messages
Nonverbal messages

COMMUNICATION WITH TEAM MEMBERS

PROFESSIONAL BEHAVIOR
Advocacy
Accountability

Refer to Concept Maps and Flash Cards on pages viii–ix for an explanation of how to create and use concept maps. In addition, the CD-ROM guides you through the construction of concept maps by providing a more detailed introduction, more illustrations of examples, and key steps to follow in designing your own maps.

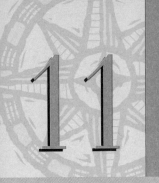

Documentation

11

 ASK YOURSELF

1. If you have some experience in documenting, either in other classes or in your clinical assignments, what have you found to be the most difficult aspect of charting or writing nurses notes?

   _____

   _____

2. What do you like most and least about inputting patient information on the medical record using the computer?

   _____

   _____

 CYBERLINKS

<u>Interactive</u> Documenting patient care is something you will spend much of your workday doing. If you are interested in current trends in charting practices or the impact of the computer on charting and in decreasing your liability related to charting, then visit **www.mednets.com.** There are articles to read on these and other subjects and opportunities for examination.

<u>Supplemental</u> **www.LPNresources.com** can help enhance your learning by leading you to discover other links with more information about the topic you are studying.

Documentation of medical records (patient record) is key to all areas of nursing practice. It is vital that nurses address individual patients' needs, problems, limitations, and progress. Unfortunately, documentation is often viewed as a chore more often than a challenge. It is important to know that documenting is a challenge because it is most likely the one issue that ends up winning or losing most lawsuits. The patient's medical record is the only comprehensive, permanent document or e-file containing all facts about a patient's care while he or she is in a medical facility.

CORE CONCEPTS	THE MEDICAL RECORD

Although nurses are not responsible for the total medical record of the patient or resident, they are considered to be the staff most responsible for having it in order. This is especially true with the "paper" chart as opposed to the computer documentation. The nurses' notes are considered to be an essential part of the medical record.

The medical record contents may differ from one facility to another. Items that may be found in a medical record are as follows:

- Face sheet with patient data such as name, address, next of kin, and insurance information
- Patient's permission to be treated
- Physician's orders
- Physician's notes of patient progress and plan of care
- Consultation reports from other physicians
- Graphic sheets or flow sheets
- Nursing Admission Assessment
- Nursing care plan
- Nurses' notes (may be called interdisciplinary notes in long-term care, as all disciplines responsible for the patient may chart in them)
- Activity flow sheets (may be certified nursing documentation of activities of daily living or might be for nursing to document routine dressing changes or other routine aspects of a patient's care)
- Medication administration records that have been completely filled in (current medication administration records are usually kept in a separate area for nursing use)
- History and physical records
- Special monitoring sheets, such as frequent vital signs
- Reports from all departments
  - Lab
  - X-ray
  - Surgery
  - Therapy departments
- Forms that are specific to long-term care
  - Permission for use of restraints
  - Mini-mental status exam
  - Record of activity attendance
  - Minimum data set, a special assessment form created by the government to help assess patient's current status and determine any problem areas the patient might be experiencing.

There are several ways that nurses communicate patient conditions and needs. Presented here are two ways: taped reports (verbal communication) and charting (written communication). Usually, the taped report relating to particular patients is a representation of what is also written (charted) in their medical records.

Taped Reports   Some facilities have the nurse who is leaving tape the end-of-shift report, which provides oncoming shift personnel with current information on all patients assigned to a particular nurse or group of nurses.

A taped report can be a good way of transferring information from one group of nurses to another. It should take no more than 3 minutes per patient. (Of course, if the oncoming nurse has not worked in a week, she or he might require a little more detail.) Each facility will require different patient information in the report depending on the focus of patient care. For example, a home health agency nurse will require much different information about his or her patients than a nurse on a hospital obstetrical unit. Our local hospitals require that the patient's DNR (Do Not Resuscitate) status and any safety precautions, like "high risk for falls," be included each shift along with current patient status. Wherever you may be working, give your report in a concise, organized manner. Think about what you would like to know as the nurse coming on. Remember the "treat others as you want to be treated" rule of nursing.

Be careful about what you say during taping. We have heard many a value judgment about patients (e.g., "That one is just a crock"). We have also heard nurses laughing and joking about recent events on the floor. Remember, the report tape can be confiscated and used against you. We often wish that patients could be present at taped reports to hear what is said about them. After all, the focus of report is to enhance exchange of information to provide better care to our patients. Follow your facility guidelines, and leave out irrelevant information.

Charting   Charting may include a handwritten record, a flow sheet, and/or a computer record. Whether a record is handwritten or entered into a computer, the same principles apply. It is important that you remember that patient records are admissible in court; therefore, you must be extremely careful in what you document.

One of the authors was called to appear in court to testify in a case in which an infant had died in a neonatal intensive care unit (NICU). Although some of the events surrounding the infant's death were able to be recalled, it had been 5 long years since she had actually worked with the infant. The only way to refresh one's memory about certain events that occurred in the past is to read nurses' notes. Luckily, this particular charting was descriptive enough to fill in any gaps in memory. However, being summoned to appear in court can be a very scary experience.

If you ever find yourself in a courtroom situation, you will probably find that your mouth is dry and your knees are knocking! If you can imagine being scared, stressed out, or a bit on the defensive with someone standing there pointing out to you any errors that you have made in charting, this picture might encourage you to chart more accurately and legibly.

[CORE CONCEPTS] **GENERAL RULES FOR DOCUMENTING** ────────

You need to be certain that in documenting you follow the policy and procedure manual of the institutions where you are assigned and that you also follow the guidelines of your state's nurse practice act. The following guidelines should also help with documentation:

- Documentation should focus on continuity of care, interventions used, and patient responses.
- If there is no change in the patient, that should also be noted at least once per shift or per visit.
- Documentation should also be concise, clear, timely, and complete.
- A complete nursing assessment should be included in the patient's record as well. In many states, LPNs/LVNs cannot complete a nursing assessment of the patient but may contribute to it.

[ESSENTIAL SKILLS] **SPECIFIC CHARTING GUIDELINES** ────────

- *Make an entry for every observation.* ***Remember the slogan, if you didn't chart it, you didn't do it.*** Some of the newer forms of charting, most notably charting-by-exception, encourage gaps in charting information. Even with charting-by-exception, you are expected to document any abnormal or significant changes that differ from the expected progress of the condition or disease process.
- *Follow up as needed.* Even if your charting is accurate and timely, you must also make and document efforts to notify others about changes in a patient's condition.
- *Read nurses' notes before giving care or charting.* As students, you are encouraged to read the chart, including the nurses' notes. As nurses, we often complain about lack of time, or we consider report as a sufficient exchange of information. However, reading the nurses' notes can provide an overall picture of how the patient is progressing or not progressing, and can also help identify any discrepancies in documentation.
- *Record entries must be timely.* As stated earlier, memories tend to fade over time, and if you are going in a hundred different directions at one time, as most nurses do, you may not recall all of the pertinent details of what happened 3 hours ago. However, charting late is better than not charting at all. Be aware that if your late charting ends up in a courtroom, questions will be raised about documenting solely to prevent liability (Figure 11-1). In other words, the attorney will make it appear that you were only trying to

Figure 11-1 The Opposing Attorney Will Make You Look Like You Did Not Know What You Were Doing

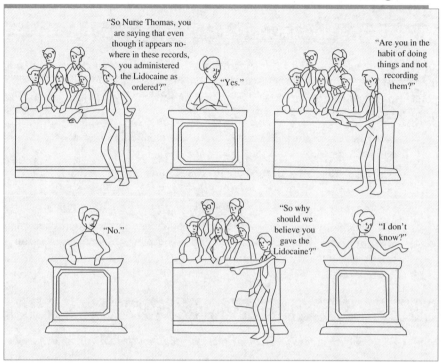

cover up an error, because something terrible happened to your patient (whether or not you did anything wrong, chances are you will appear to be guilty).

- *Chart only after the event.* Never chart prior to doing a treatment, giving medication, or anything else. More than one nurse has charted a medication prior to giving it, only to find the patient dead. Think about another of your patients going into respiratory arrest, a fire, or any number of other critical events occurring. If you chart that you gave your patient heart medication before you actually gave it, another nurse will think that it has been done, which can put your patient in jeopardy.

- *Use clear language.* Avoid using the words *seems* and *appears*. If the patient is obviously bleeding, do not chart that the patient "appears" to be bleeding. Rather, chart how much blood you observe. Do not chart that the patient "ate well," chart how much the patient actually ate. Vague references will be attacked in court, and your observation abilities will be called into question. Can you imagine charting that a patient appeared to be bleeding, and going to court because the patient hemorrhaged to death? How could you defend "appears" to be? The plaintiff's attorney will be asking you questions about your ability to identify whether a patient is bleeding or not. This is neither a pretty picture nor one that you would want to experience.

- *Be realistic and factual.* It is important that you chart a true picture of your patient without personal comments. If a patient is noncompliant, chart, "Mr. Williams refused his 9:00 A.M. medication." Do not chart, "Mr. Williams does not seem to want to improve. He is very rude and doesn't want to get better." Patients who are noncompliant or those who are abusive or threatening may perceive that they have been treated unsuccessfully or unfairly. Patients who are not pleased with their hospital stay or treatment are more likely to sue you, the doctor, or the hospital.

- *Chart only what you observe.* Do not categorize your patient's behavior; describe what you saw. For example, do not describe your patient as being "agitated." That is a conclusion. Describe the behavior: "Patient pacing halls continuously, picking at clothing, and refusing to sit down." Do not accept information from others and document it without confirming the information for yourself. Do not chart for others. You are legally responsible for what you document in a chart. As a student practical/vocational nurse, you might be documenting an action of your RN primary nurse because you observed it. Be sure you designate that. For instance if the RN administers an IV pain medication, do not chart "IV morphine given for pain," as that looks like you gave it. Instead, document, "IV morphine for pain administered by RN." Then, of course, you will also be responsible for charting the patient's response to that nursing action.

- *Chart errors.* Follow your institution policy and procedure manual regarding errors. Most facilities will ask that you draw a single line through the misspelled or wrong word and write the correct word above or to the right of it. You should also write your initials and the date and time above or to the right of the new entry. Some facilities request that you write the word "error" or "mistaken entry"; others believe that using these reflects on the entire entry, not just a single word. To protect yourself, be certain that you follow your institution guidelines. Never white out or scribble through an entry, so that what you originally wrote is illegible.

- *Identify yourself after every entry.* At the end of each entry you should write your full name and title, whether or not this information is given earlier in the chart. Some facilities have a space at the bottom or top of the page where you sign your name, title, and initials; your initials are used after each entry on the page.

- *All charting should be done in ink.* Most facilities require black ink, but there are also differences in opinion about that. It is often difficult to tell the difference between black ink originals and copies. Find out your facility policy. All entries should be legible. If you have a problem with legible handwriting, then print. We have worked with nurses who could not even read their own handwriting when asked to go back and clarify what they had written! Use only standard institution-approved abbreviations. If you are unsure about whether or not an abbreviation is approved by the facility, then write the word out. Charting should be neat and organized, using correctly spelled words and proper grammar. If your charting is sloppy and disorganized, a jury may conclude that you are sloppy and disorganized in your nursing care as well. Misspelled words and improper grammar give the impression of carelessness, which could also reflect on your nursing care. Bring a pocket dictionary to clinical if you have to. Do not leave blank spaces, or go back and try to chart between lines. Never leave a space for someone else to chart.

CORE CONCEPTS | **TYPES OF RECORD KEEPING**

There are seven types of record-keeping methods that are used for the documentation of various types of patient care. Those of greatest relevance to you will be discussed more fully. They are as follows:

- Narrative
- SOAP
- SOAPIER
- PIE
- Focus charting
- Charting-by-exception
- Computer-assisted charting

Regardless of what type of charting is used in your facility, certain basic principles apply. As part of your clinical orientation as a student, you should be instructed regarding the specifics of the charting used in each of the facilities in which you are assigned. Remember that, in most nursing programs, you will be required to have your instructor and/or the primary nurse with whom you're working review your charting before you place it into the patient's permanent record.

Flow Sheets or Checklists Most institutions rely on some flow sheets or checklists to document routine care. Vital signs have been charted on flow sheets for many years (Figure 11-2). Today, flow sheets and checklists have been developed for most areas of nursing. Rather than having to write data over and over again, the flow sheet allows the nurse to enter only pertinent data (Figure 11-3). Although these sheets can be time saving, it is important to remember that they are also legal documents and admissible in court.

We have seen many charts in which the flow sheet says one thing and the nurses' notes say another. Be certain that you check the patient yourself and that the flow sheet is accurate! We cannot begin to count the number of times we have wit-

Figure 11-2 Vital Signs

F	C	04/08/98 Day: 1					04/09/98 Day: 2									
		03	07	11	15	19	03	07	11	15	19	03	07	11	15	19
104	40.0															
103	39.4															
102	38.9															
101	38.3															
100	37.7															
99	37.2															
98	36.6															
97	36.1															
Temp			96 Orl		98 Orl		98 Orl		97 Orl							
Pulse			61		67		82		72							
Resp			20		18		20		20							
B/P			161/73		164/77		131/73		123/72							
*								*								
Wt Ht		170lb														

		NOCS	DAYS	EVES	TOTAL	NOCS	DAYS	EVES	TOTAL	NOCS	DAYS	EVES	TOTAL
I N T A K E	Oral												
	IV/Med Drips												
	TPN/Lipid												
	Tube Feed												
	Blood Product												
	Irrigants												
	TOTAL												
O U T P U T	Urine												
	Stool												
	Emesis												
	Drains												
	Blood/Drainage												
	EBL												
	TOTAL												
	NET												

nessed nurses continuing to check off the same columns as the previous shift. One time, the nurses were checking that the patient had ambulated four times a day for days, only to discover that the patient had a massive stroke and was bedridden. Of course, the nurses were aware that the patient was bedridden, but checklists are often completed while the nurse's mind is wandering or other events are occurring. Pay attention to what you are checking! Checklists and flow sheets are not mindless, time-consuming tasks. Be sure that all of your data are reliable!

Narrative Charting   Narrative charting is the traditional form of charting in which patient information and care is presented in a straightforward manner. In a hospital setting, narrative charting would usually begin and end with an assessment of the patient's status and present other data about the patient in a chronological format.

Figure 11-3 Flowsheet Charting Report

Act	active	Frg	full ROM	Obc	obeys command	Sm	small
Alt	alert	Ics	incision	Orl	oral	Spn	spontaneous
Bld	bloody	Ita	intact	Per	person	Sta	stained
Brs	brisk	Liq	liquids	Plc	place	Tme	time
Clr	clear	Nds	nondistended	Plp	palpable	Unl	unlabored
Con	continent	Nor	normal	Pnk	pink	Wrm	warm
Dry	dry	Ntn	non-tender	Reg	regular	Yel	yellow
Evn	even	O3	orient(3)	Sft	soft		

Temp	04/08							
Graph	14:35	15:07	16:00	17:19	18:04	18:55	21:08	22:22
Vital Signs								
TEMP #1		94.3F Orl		98.2F Orl				
PULSE #1		67		74				
RESPIRATIONS		18		18				
BP #1		164/77		145/73				
Neurological								
Orientation/LOC			AltO3				AltO3	
Both pupils								
Pupil Reaction								
Motor Strength								
All extremities			Nor				Nor	
Open Eyes			Spn				Spn	
Best Motor Rsp			Obc				Obc	
Best Verbal Rsp			Clr				Clr	
Respiratory								
Resp Pattern			RegEvnUnl				RegEvnUnl	
Sound/Breathing			Nor				Nor	
Cardiovascular								
Heart Rate								
Pulses								
Radial			NorPlp				NorPlp	
Gastrointestinal								
Bowel Sounds								
all quads								
Swallows			Liq				Liq	
Abdomen			SftNtnNds				SftNtnNds	
Bowel Control			Con				Con	

Narrative charting is most often used in long-term care and may be supplemented with flow sheets. In long-term care, you might not be charting chronologically but writing out a summary paragraph of the patient's condition. Long-term care charting is not done for every patient every day unless there is an acute condition that needs to be addressed. Medicare patients in long-term care are charted on every shift with specific guidelines to direct you in the items needed to be covered in your charting.

This is the easiest form of charting to do, but it is difficult to go back and pick out certain pieces of patient data without reading the entire entry. For instance, if you wanted to know how nurses on previous shifts had described the patient's respiratory status, you would not be able to pinpoint that information without reading all that the nurse had written.

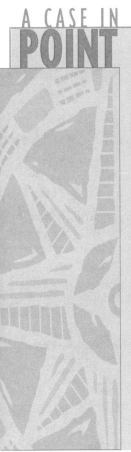

A CASE IN POINT

7:30 A.M. Forty-six-year-old white female admitted to 4SA for evaluation. Pt transferred from ER after commenting that she "Is tired of it all and would be better off dead." Dr. Creed visited pt and completed pt history. Pt oriented to unit and introduced to staff. Pt is coherent, communicates her needs, and is cooperative. Pt is dressed appropriately and is wearing appropriate makeup.

8:00 A.M. Pt served breakfast on the unit. She ate 75%. Pt has not made any suicidal statements.

9:00 A.M. Pt attended music therapy and interacted with other patients. She smiled during group and participated by choosing a song to sing.

10:00 A.M. Pt attended education group. She openly discussed her medications and how she adheres to a dosing schedule. Pt helped others see the need for continuing therapy even when feeling well.

11:00 A.M. Pt discussed current depressive episode with RN. Stated that she felt "overwhelmed by a teenage son and daughter and an unfaithful husband." Pt also stated that "My mother died a month ago and I don't think I'm handling it very well."

Charting-by-Exception Charting-by-exception is a fairly new way of charting that encourages the nurse to chart only significant or abnormal findings rather than documenting normal findings over and over again.

- Document only significant or abnormal findings.
- Progress or lack of progress reflected in clinical pathways, nursing diagnosis–based standardized care plans and protocols, flow sheets, and checklists.
- Very streamlined and efficient.
- May leave major gaps when problems occur and the nurse is unable to thoroughly document all that was done for a patient.

Focus Charting This may also be referred to as DAR charting, as you are documenting patient **d**ata, nursing **a**ctions, and patient **r**esponse. This type of charting uses key words, or focuses, so you can organize your charting. The nurses' notes sheet allows you to identify the focus of each entry separately. A focus may be any of the following:

- The patient's current condition
- Any significant change in the patient's condition or behavior
- Nursing diagnosis
- Body system
- Sign or symptom noted on your shift
- Summary of comments by patient regarding their concerns
- An event, such as physician visit, therapy report, lab work or x-rays done
- A medical condition might be used, but it is preferred that you use patient needs and conditions that might be associated with the medical condition.

The data part of the documentation may be subjective or objective information that is related to your focus. The action piece refers to your nursing actions or plans for nursing actions based on the data you received. The response portion of the entry refers to the patient's response to your actions. (See Figure 11-4.)

Focus charting is very flexible and allows you to chart on a variety of issues. It is helpful in organizing your data and easy for future health care providers to track specific problems or conditions.

SOAP Charting   Documenting in the SOAP format emphasizes a problem-solving approach to planning patient care. The initials stand for the following:

Subjective information, received from the patient or his or her family

Objective information, based on your own observations

Assessment, or analysis, of the patient's problems

Plan of care developed to meet the needs of the patient

To use this type of documentation, there has to be an initial database of patient information, problem list developed on admission, and an initial nursing care plan.

Figure 11-4 Focus Charting Example

Date	Time	Focus	Progress Notes
7/13/01	1000	Pain	D. Pt c/o pain at incisional site. On a scale of 1 to 10, pt describes pain as an "8."
			A. Administered 50 mg Demerol IM as per physician order. Assisted patient with repositioning.
			R. Pt reports pain level decreased to a "3" within 30 mins after injection.
			Nurse's signature

A number of flow sheets are used to supplement patient data. Changes to the care plan may be needed as the patient's condition changes.

This is a frequently used type of charting, because it meets JCAHO (Joint Commission on Accreditation of Healthcare Organizations) standards for incorporating a nursing care plan into daily documentation. JCAHO is the organization that accredits hospitals by conducting annual on-site reviews of the hospital and its staff and determining if they meet JCAHO standards. There is no chronological order associated with this type of charting.

PIE Charting   PIE charting is similar to SOAP charting, because it is problem based. It also tries to include the nursing care plan in the daily documentation. The initials stand for the following:

>   **P**roblem (Admission data is used to identify patient problem areas. These problems are written as nursing diagnoses.)
>
>   **I**nterventions (These may be ones you are currently doing or ones you plan to do.)
>
>   **E**valuation (Each problem must be evaluated every 8 hours.)

This type of charting also ensures that a facility will meet JCAHO standards. It provides organization for nursing documentation but also leads to repetition in nursing entries with the frequent evaluation of each problem.

SOAPIER Charting   This format may be incorporated into the charting-by-exception method of documentation described earlier. It is an extension of the SOAP charting. The initials "IER" refer to the following:

>   **I**nterventions, or nursing actions, you are currently doing
>
>   **E**valuation of your actions in regards to patient's response
>
>   **R**evisions that might be made in the original plan of care

Computer-Assisted Charting   Computers have developed into a lifeline for most facilities. Computers can be used for everything, including admission histories (see Figures 11-5 and 11-6) and many other types of data. Physicians can access patient records from their offices and transmit orders directly to the lab, pharmacy, and nurses.

- Nurses usually have access to a microcomputer through a video display terminal or a handheld portable terminal.
- Nurses are provided with computer training during orientation or other education program.
- Once a nurse is trained in the use of the computer, an access code is given.
- This access code is secured and is only to be used by the individual nurse who receives it.
- Allowing anyone else to use your access code number may result in termination of your employment.

Figure 11-5 Admission History

```
                                                      04/09/99 10:13
                                                          Page: 1
                            Admission History
        From 04/07/99 07:00            To 04/09/99 07:00
    -------------------------------------------

    4068-A Name: _____ MD: _____
    Sex: ____ Age: _____ Adm: 04/08/99 01:15  Patient Id:_____ Med Rec No: _____
```

Admission History

Religious Denominations
04/08 09:30   Religious Denomination: Episcopal. (CAL)
Admitted
04/08 09:30   Admitted ambulatory from admitting. Accompanied by: spouse/SO. Informant: patient/self. (CAL)
     09:30   ID bracelet on. (CAL)
Medications
04/08 09:30   Current med: Atenolol 50 mg q am Procardia XL 30 mg q HS. Last dose of this medication was taken: yesterday. Current med: Premarin po and 1.25 ng. Last dose of this medication was taken: yesterday. Current med: Synthroid 0.1 mg Tylenol Child. (CAL)
     09:30   Current med: Synthroid 0.1 mg q day. Last dose of this medication was taken: yesterday. (CAL)
Allergies/Adverse Reactions
04/08 09:30   Allergies/Adverse Reactions: PCN, Codeine—reaction—rash Dilaudid—reaction—spaced out. (CAL)
Reason for Admission
04/08 09:30   Reason for admission: (patient's understanding) patient to have surgery/procedure—bronchoscopy and cholecystectomy. (CAL)
Advanced Directives Information
04/08 09:30   Patient has not executed an Advance Directive. Information on Advance Directives: refused by patient. (CAL)
Prevous Hospitalizations
04/08 09:30   Previous hospitalizations/out-patient treatments: year—1977. Reason: surgery—bladder suspension. Previous hospitalizations/outpatient treatments: year—1975. Reason: surgery—hernia repair—hiatal. (CAL)
Assistive Devices
04/08 09:30   Assistive devices: patient has none. (CAL)
Discharge Planning
04/08 09:30   Plans have been made for discharge. (CAL)
Care Provider: CAL

• Staff are usually limited to the screens that are appropriate for their position.

Some computers have a keyboard with which information is typed in; others use a penlight or other scanning device. Some of the newer computers have a bar-code reader that can scan a patient's ID bracelet prior to giving care or medications. If a medication is given in error or at the wrong time, the nurse is notified immediately on a video screen.

Figure 11-6 Cumulative Care Plans

```
                                              04/09/99 10:14
                                                   Page: 2
                        Cumulative Care Plan
          From 04/08/99 07:00          To 04/09/99 10:13
          -------------------------------------

  Name:_____ MD:_____
  Sex: _____ Age: _____ Adm: _____ 01:15 Patient Id: _____ Med Rec No: _____

  Cumulative Care Plan
  Active        Inactive     Freq  NURSING DIAGNOSIS
  04/08 (NH )                       1. Pain: Acute
                                        Defining Characteristics:
  04/08 (NH )                             — c/o pain
                                        Related to
  04/08 (NH )                             — surgical wound
                                        Secondary to
  04/08 (NH )                             — cholecystitis
                                        Goals:
  04/08 (NH )              PRN            — Verbalizes a reasonable level of comfort
                                        Interventions:
  04/08 (NH )              PRN            — Administer pain medication per following plan,
                                            document response:
                                              instruct patient to request pain medication
                                              before pain becomes severe and administer
                                              medication before pain becomes severe.
                                        Assessments:
  04/08                    PRN            — Assess effectiveness of pain control measures
  Care Providers:
  Nancy Hay, R.N.
```

CORE CONCEPTS

THE POSITIVES AND NEGATIVES OF COMPUTER CHARTING

There are several truisms regarding the use of computers in health care.

Positives

- Computer charting will definitely be health care's documentation choice in the future. It not only streamlines our entries, it also generates typed, up-to-the-minute information.
- Information tends to be more accurate and error free, as the computer may prompt the nurse to fill in gaps or challenge conflicting information.

Negatives

- Computer charting has the potential of causing problems with confidentiality. Having access codes and limited computer screens are methods of dealing with this problem.

- There could be a possible delay between the time a medication is administered and the time the computer permanently records the administration.

Some of these problems (the negatives) are being addressed, and new software is being developed to handle them.

Documentation is one of the most important things you will do as a nurse. The way you document can save you or hang you in a courtroom. Documentation can also be perceived as tiresome, boring, and time consuming. It is a bit like any other repetitive task; it becomes what you make it. If you find charting boring, you will have a tendency to be sloppy and not pay much attention to it. If you look at it as a challenge, you will pay attention and do a good job. Think about having your instructors organize a mock trial. Use some of your own charting or that of a fellow student. Look at it as a lawyer would. Are there any gaps? Are there any unapproved abbreviations? Make it an adventure!

 ASK YOURSELF

1. What concerns you most about charting nurses' notes?

   _____

   _____

2. After reviewing the charting guidelines listed in this chapter, which, if any, of these guidelines do you think (or have you observed) are most often ignored? What resolve will you make to ensure you adhere to these guidelines?

   _____

   _____

 CYBERLINKS: FLASH CARDS

Check to see what you now remember by making your own flash cards. Use the CD-ROM that accompanies your textbook to discover how to make flash cards for reviewing and retaining what you have learned.

 CONCEPT MAP WORD BANK

DOCUMENTATION
Taped reports
Charting
TYPES OF CHARTING
TYPES OF RECORD KEEPING
COMPUTER DOCUMENTATION

Refer to Concept Maps and Flash Cards on pages viii–ix for an explanation of how to create and use concept maps. In addition, the CD-ROM guides you through the construction of concept maps by providing a more detailed introduction, more illustrations of examples, and key steps to follow in designing your own maps.

12

Patient Teaching

 ASK YOURSELF

1. What experience have you had as a teacher in any capacity—tutoring or other formal or informal teaching situations?

   _____

   _____

2. Referring to your response to question 1, what did you like best and least about your experience?

   _____

   _____

 CYBERLINKS

<u>Interactive</u> Information is available to you that will help you help your patients. One of the most valuable interactive sites for obtaining information about health matters is **www.thriveonline.com**, which contains many tools and quizzes that would be appropriate for patient teaching.

<u>Supplemental</u> **www.LPNresources.com** can help enhance your learning by leading you to discover other links with more information about the topic you are studying.

When a friend of ours applied for a teaching position in a nursing school, she was asked what teaching experience she had. Her reply was, "Every nurse is a teacher." This is true of the student nurse as well. As you are learning yourself, you will be teaching others. It is a proven fact that, in teaching others, you enhance your own learning. In other words, you learn, you teach, you learn. Learning from our patients is integral to teaching them.

Patient teaching requires that you have good observation skills to assess the need for learning; good communication skills to help meet learning needs; and creativity to ensure that the teaching will be effective for that particular patient.

As a student, you will be doing two types of teaching. One will be on an informal level, and one will be on a formal level. Both of these will be discussed. First, however, some general background information is required.

CORE CONCEPTS   PATIENT'S LEARNING NEEDS

Recognizing a patient's learning needs requires that you be very observant of your patients and their behavior. When you are gathering data on your patients, you need to look for signs that they are in need of further learning. There are several clues to help you reach that conclusion:

- The patient is a new admission.
- The patient has a new diagnosis.
- The patient has a new medication.
- The patient is scheduled for a new diagnostic test, treatment, or therapy.
- The patient is scheduled for surgery.
- The patient is scheduled for discharge.
- The patient asks questions.

Any time a patient is in a new situation, there is an opportunity to teach. Any time patients ask you questions about their condition or care, there is an opportunity to teach.

CORE CONCEPTS   TIME TO TEACH

Not every moment is a teachable moment. As nursing students, you need to determine a good time to teach. The following situations would not be good times to teach:

- The patient has a room full of company.
- The patient has just been given some upsetting news.
- The patient is sedated.
- The patient is having pain or other types of discomfort, such as breathing problems.
- The patient just received a meal tray.
- The patient is exhausted from therapy.

You get the idea. If the patient is visiting, sedated, uncomfortable, eating, or tired, whatever teaching you try to do will be lost.

Choose a time when the patient is comfortable (perhaps 30 minutes after pain medication), relaxed, and alone, or perhaps has one family member present. Sometimes, as a nursing student, it is appropriate to teach family members as well, especially if the patient is being discharged soon.

When you are teaching in response to a patient question, you do not need to wait for the "perfect moment" to answer the question. Answer the question and, if the time is right, spend more time elaborating on associated information. If the question arises during one of the situations listed above, give the patient the information he or she is seeking and offer to come back later to discuss it further.

ESSENTIAL SKILLS **PREPARING TO TEACH**

Most students cannot just begin teaching as soon as they walk into a patient's room. There are some steps of preparation.

- *Be knowledgeable yourself.* That is why your nursing instructors will require that you research your patients, their medications, and conditions before beginning your care. We require our students to come in the day before care to gather a lot of preliminary information. In preconference, students have the opportunity to ask any unanswered questions before the shift begins. We require that students make their own drug cards on each medication the patient will be taking. Students need to be prepared to answer their instructors' questions as well as their patients'!

- *Find your patient's level of knowledge.* You will find most patients who have had a disease or condition for a long time have a lot of knowledge about their conditions. Listen to them and learn. It will help you in your care of them as well as your care for future patients with similar conditions. One of the authors once asked a patient with an ileostomy how she liked to take care of it. She looked at her with a bright smile and said, "I've had this for 20 years. You're the first nurse who has asked me how I like to take care of it." That gave both patient and nurse a boost! Find your patient's baseline knowledge, and build on it.

- *Find out what your patients think they need to know.* Sometimes nursing students proceed with what they think patients need to know instead of what patients themselves feel that they need to know. Establish priorities. Start with the patient's ideas of learning needs; then, build on that base to include things you feel are also important.

- *Set goals of learning.* Before you begin, set the goals you want to accomplish in learning. If you do not do that, you will not be able to evaluate whether you have achieved your goals. If you are teaching a newly diagnosed diabetic patient how to do a blood sugar, the goal will be that the patient will be able to perform that test accurately and safely and be able to interpret the results. Base your teaching on *how* the patient can achieve that goal.

- *Set a time frame for achieving your goal.* Remember that not all teaching can be done in one sitting. You may have to break your teaching down into stages. Or you may have to pass your teaching along to someone else to complete. Many health care facilities now have patient teaching flow sheets. Nurses or nursing students initial what they have been able to teach, so that the next nurse coming on can look at the sheet and know where to begin. This provides continuity for the patient. However, you need to keep track of when the patient will be discharged. We remember assisting a nursing student to teach a newly diagnosed diabetic patient on giving his own insulin injections. It had to be done very quickly, because the physician discharged the patient unexpectedly, and no teaching had been done. This was an uncomfortable situation for all involved. We had to communicate with the home health nurse to let her know she would have to supervise the administration of insulin in the home that evening and continue with the teaching.

- *Know what teaching resources are available within the health care setting.* Do not try to reinvent the wheel. If the facility has pamphlets, videotapes, or teaching tools available, use them. Many hospitals have access to written teaching information via the Internet for specific diseases or conditions; pharmacists have teaching sheets available on new medications; dietitians have teaching sheets on diet.

- *Try to determine your patients' learning style.* You may need to ask them some questions about how they learn best. Also, try to get a "feel" for their level of education. If you are thinking of using written teaching materials, consider that most studies show that many people in the United States read at only a 4th or 5th grade reading level. Consider patients who have another language as their primary language as well. Sometimes pictures or illustrations work better for all.

- *Try to put all teaching into "layman's" terms.* My mother told me of a roommate she had in the hospital many years ago. The nurse kept asking her all day if she had "voided." The patient said "yes." Many hours later, she turned to my mother and told her how uncomfortable she was, because she had not been able to "pee" all day. Watch your language, and plan your teaching in words your patient can understand. Shy patients may not tell you they do not understand what you are talking about.

ESSENTIAL SKILLS   **FORMAL VERSUS INFORMAL TEACHING**

Informal Teaching   Informal teaching occurs as the situation arises. This is the teaching you will be doing on a daily basis every time your patients ask you questions. It is not planned but just happens. That is why you should be prepared for clinical. We have had patients quiz the nursing student on each one of their medications only to find out the patient knew exactly what the medications were. The patient just wanted to know if the student knew! However, in teaching, the student learned the medications a lot better. Informal teaching is the most common form of patient teaching that the practical/vocational nursing student will be doing.

Formal Teaching   Formal teaching requires more extensive preparation than informal. In this type of teaching, you know ahead of time what you need to teach the patient. As mentioned previously, it might be that you need to teach the newly diagnosed diabetic how to do his or her own blood glucose monitoring. In this situation, you would need to:

1. Discuss with the patient what the *objectives* would be. Examples would be to learn: names of the pieces of equipment to be used; how to set the machine; the functions of the machine; how to insert the lancet into the penlet; how to insert the chemstrip into the machine; how to obtain a blood sample and apply it to the chemstrip; how to read the blood sugar; what to do with the information.

2. Decide on your *approach*. Will you give the patient information to read about the procedure first? Will you obtain a video to show? Will you demonstrate the technique on yourself or on your patient? Will you write up the procedure yourself with pictures to illustrate?

3. *Prepare* the patient for the learning situation. Tell the patient what you will be doing and when. The patient may want to have family members there to learn as well. Find out what they already know, and start from there.

4. Do the teaching in whatever manner you have decided will work best for your patient based on the information given in the Preparing to Teach section.

5. After you have concluded the teaching, *give the patient the opportunity to ask questions* and then return the demonstrations to you if they are ready to do so. Some patients may need more time to think it over before showing you what they know. They will need encouragement and reassurance that it is okay to make a mistake. It is better to make a mistake while you are watching and can give them more teaching than to make it while they are home alone. Always look back at the objectives you set up to make sure you have met them all.

6. *Reassess what happened in the teaching process.* If the patient is having difficulty learning the procedure, try to find out why. Is there some other method you can try? This is where your creativity comes in. Do not get stuck in a "box," but try new ways that might work for this particular patient.

Formal teaching may also be needed when you are preparing presentations for your classroom. Keep the above steps in mind for your classmates as well.

Teaching others may be uncomfortable for you at times, especially as a new nursing student, or perhaps even as a graduate. If you view patient teaching as an incredible challenge, however, the experience will stretch your mind and talents far beyond what you ever imagined!

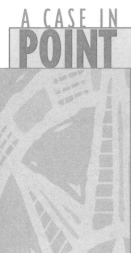

A CASE IN POINT

Pauline, an LPN, is assigned the care of a newly diagnosed diabetic. Pauline's supervisor has asked her to teach the patient how to self-administer insulin. Pauline assembles the equipment, the printed material with instructions for self-administration, and an orange. She approaches the patient's bedside. Pauline begins to tell the patient that she is going to be helping him learn to give his own medication. The patient says he hates "shots" and asks how long he will have to have them. Pauline thinks that the patient seems confused. She decides to begin by asking the patient what he already knows about diabetes.

 ASK YOURSELF

1. Do you think that it is usually helpful to patients to have visual aids when learning procedures or other information? Why or why not?

    _____

    _____

2. After reading this chapter, do you think you will be involved in more informal or more formal patient teaching? What is the reason for your response?

    _____

    _____

 CYBERLINKS: FLASH CARDS

Check to see what you now remember by making your own flash cards. Use the CD-ROM that accompanies your textbook to discover how to make flash cards for reviewing and retaining what you have learned.

 CONCEPT MAP WORD BANK

PATIENT LEARNING NEEDS
TEACHING PREPARATION
TEACHING OPPORTUNITES

TYPES
Informal
Formal

Refer to Concept Maps and Flash Cards on pages viii–ix for an explanation of how to create and use concept maps. In addition, the CD-ROM guides you through the construction of concept maps by providing a more detailed introduction, more illustrations of examples, and key steps to follow in designing your own maps.

Critical Thinking

13

ASK YOURSELF

1. Have you heard the term *critical thinking* before? In what circumstance was it used?

   _____

   _____

2. Do you enjoy analyzing and dissecting information or being deep in thought? Why or why not?

   _____

   _____

CYBERLINKS

Interactive Visit **www.before-after.com/quizz/taketest** to learn your creativity strengths and weaknesses and how to generally improve your thinking performance. Although this particular site is sponsored by a mind tools company, the test is offered free of charge.

Supplemental **www.LPNresources.com** can help enhance your learning by leading you to discover other links with more information about the topic you are studying.

Critical thinking is a term that you will hear frequently. At present, there are numerous definitions of critical thinking. A saying by Confucius reads in part, "He who learns but does not think is lost; he who thinks but does not learn is in danger." Perhaps that statement best characterizes critical thinking. Critical thinking is an interaction between thinking, knowledge, and experience. It is thinking based on the knowledge that you already have. It is thinking that allows you to look at all sides of the picture, evaluate what you see and feel, and make a decision based on your past experience and current knowledge. It is a thinking that allows you to look at a problem creatively, think "outside of the box," and generate new solutions. It is included in the unit on getting your point across, because critical thinking is the basis for a lot of your communication in nursing. As a matter of fact, it should be

113

the basis for all of your nursing decisions and actions as well. This method of thinking will be further expanded in Chapter 14 when we discuss the nursing process and clinical pathways.

Critical thinking is a central theme throughout nursing programs. Find out how your faculty defines critical thinking, and have them explain their expectations of your abilities to do and use critical thinking.

Even though we do not know exactly how your faculty defines critical thinking, let's explore highlights of the topic and see what you may expect. To start, you may want to know why this is such an important issue.

CORE CONCEPTS | THE DEVELOPMENT OF CRITICAL THINKING

There are three main reasons why the development of critical thinking is so important:

1. *It is required.* All programs that are accredited by the National League for Nursing Accrediting Commission (NLNAC) have to demonstrate that their graduates possess critical thinking skills. Not all practical/vocational schools have obtained this accreditation. However, the requirements of the NLNAC provide basic guidelines for nonaccredited nursing programs as well. In the near future, as more state Boards of Nursing remove themselves from the accreditation process, it is possible that all practical/vocational nursing programs will be required to attain the accreditation of a national agency.

2. *Critical thinking is essential for successfully answering questions on the National Council Licensure Examination (NCLEX).* Passing this state exam results in obtaining your license.

3. *Your success and survival as a practitioner will depend on your critical thinking abilities.* Among other things, you will be required to keep your knowledge base current, make decisions in complex situations, evaluate nursing interventions and patient outcomes, and quickly identify priorities. The foundation for these activities is critical thinking.

The development of critical thinking, regardless of how it is specifically defined in your program, is an important part of your curriculum. The reason we said earlier that you must have your faculty define critical thinking is that the NLNAC leaves the specific definition up to faculty in each nursing program. That definition should indicate how the faculty measures or evaluates your ability to reason, analyze, and make decisions.

Because any kind of thinking (daydreaming, reasoning, problem solving, etc.) cannot be observed directly, faculty will use various observable ways to evaluate your critical thinking skills. One of the most frequently used evaluation tools is the nursing process, the basis for the nursing care plan. How you complete nursing process assignments tells faculty a great deal about your critical thinking skills. For example, your written care plans give insight into your critical thinking capacity in such areas as ability to identify and collect valid data: objective (what you identify with your five senses) and subjective (what the patient tells you). The manner in which your care plans are written also gives insight into how you make logical conclusions based on your data collection, and then how you decide on nursing interventions based on those conclusions. In other words, the nursing process is one form of critical thinking that utilizes problem-solving abilities.

Agreement among faculty is that critical thinking involves more than problem solving. Let's look at a small sample of other expanded views of critical thinking. Paul (1993) states that critical thinking involves the "intellectually disciplined process of actively and skillfully conceptualizing, applying, analyzing, synthesizing, or evaluating information gathered from, or generated by, observation, experience, reflection, reasoning, or communication, as a guide to belief and action" (p. 110). This definition probably requires that you reread and devote some thought to grasp its full meaning. Table 13-1 contains additional information on characteristics of

| TABLE 13-1 | Four Perspectives on Critical Thinking |

Characteristics of a Critical Thinker[a]
- Being open to views that are new and to different viewpoints.
- Being able to express and present ideas in an organized manner.
- Having evidence and logical reasoning to support ideas and views.
- Listening to others but thinking for oneself.

View of a Critical Thinker[b]
- Separates relevant from irrelevant information.
- Spots inconsistencies in a line of reasoning.
- Identifies and challenges assumptions.
- Separates verifiable facts from value claims.
- Identifies doubtful or unclear claims and arguments.

Characteristics of a Critical Thinker[c]
- Recognizes and challenges statements or ideas accepted as true without supporting data (these unchallenged ideas are assumptions).
- Identifies and explores as many alternatives as possible when analyzing a situation.
- Utilizes logical reasoning skills.

Questions a Critical Thinker Asks[d]
- What is the purpose of my thinking?
- How well am I articulating the question I am trying to answer?
- What is my frame of reference?
- What am I taking for granted (what assumption am I making)?
- Once I have come to a conclusion, what are the implications?

[a]*Source:* Chaffee, J. *Thinking critically, first edition.* Copyright © 1985 by Houghton Mifflin Company. Used with permission.
[b]*Source:* Beyer, B. K. (1987). *Practical strategies for the teaching of thinking.* Boston: Allyn & Bacon.
[c]*Source:* Brookfield, S. D. (1987). *Developing critical thinkers: Challenging adults to explore alternative ways of thinking and acting.* Jossey-Bass. This material is used by permission of John Wiley and Sons, Inc.
[d]*Source:* Paul, R. W. (1993). *Critical thinking: How to prepare your students for a rapidly changing role.* Dillon Beach, CA: Foundation for Critical Thinking. www.criticalthinking.org

critical thinking and critical thinkers by four individuals who are considered experts in the field. Although this table presents four separate views, do you see anything that the four views have in common? Notice that although critical thinking requires a knowledge base, the crucial part is how you use that knowledge. Knowing facts is not enough; it is how you put those facts together that is important.

CORE CONCEPTS	**THE EVALUATION OF CRITICAL THINKING SKILLS**

You can see from this very brief overview that critical thinking is a complex concept. You, no doubt, already have some critical thinking skills on which to build. How one expands this skill is not well established. One essential element in its development, however, is a sound knowledge base. Without this base, critical thinking about a specific problem or situation is not possible. So, your critical thinking skills will start with learning specific information. In early nursing courses, faculty will have exercises and exams that require only that you recall the knowledge. However, faculty will expect you to demonstrate your knowledge base in clinical situations, written assignments, class discussions, and exams in more complex ways. For example, faculty in maternity nursing could have a multiple-choice question on the age at which the anterior fontanel (soft spot) normally closes. Such a question, however, indicates only your ability to recall the information. A question aimed at evaluating your critical thinking skills would be far different. For example, faculty could provide you with the following data: You are caring for a 25-month-old child. On examination, you find a smiling child with a soft spot in the area of the anterior fontanel. Based on this information, faculty might:

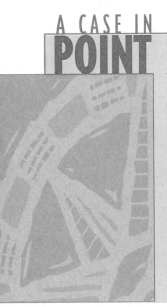

A CASE IN POINT

Mary Ann is a school nurse. It is January and the weather has been cold. On Thursday, one of the 11th grade girls comes to her office. She is wearing jeans and a long baggy shirt. She states that she has been feeling sick to her stomach in the mornings, with dizziness and headaches. She tells Mary Ann that by the time her second class is over she feels better. She asks Mary Ann what could be causing this and how she can avoid getting sick in the morning since it is interfering with her early classes. Mary Ann begins to examine the student, beginning with the respiratory system. However, in her head, Mary Ann is already considering potential causes for the illness.

- Ask you to describe (written or oral) your actions in order of priority with your reason for each action. Your responses provide faculty not only with information on your knowledge regarding the anterior fontanel, but also with information such as your ability to prioritize and your written or oral communication skills.
- Provide you with multiple-choice options in which you must pick the best action. This means that all of the answers are correct but one response is better than the others for various reasons. This type of question requires that you know the significance of an open anterior fontanel and the normal age for closure of the anterior fontanel, and can distinguish between the options and identify the one action that is the most important.

This type of question is the type that you as a student may not like. You may feel that it is unfair, since all the responses are essentially correct. However, the focus of this type of question is an indication of critical thinking skills. Be prepared for this type of question in school and on the NCLEX-PN.

The depth of your response to cases or questions posed in which there is one most correct answer will help faculty evaluate how well you are able to use your knowledge base. Early in your studies you may be expected only to ask the student described in the above Case in Point about her menstrual cycles. If this situation were presented in a later, advanced nursing class, however, faculty would expect much more such as:

1. In addition to the student's complaints, are you concerned with any other data in the situation? If so, what and why?
2. Are you curious why the symptoms seem to clear during her second class?
3. Do you display in any of your responses consideration of ethical and legal issues associated with the role of a school nurse?

In place of a written or verbal response to this situation, faculty might instead have written the case in this form on a test: It is January and the weather is cold. A student comes to the school nurse with complaints of feeling sick to her stomach, dizziness, and headaches that last about halfway through her second class. She has had these symptoms for several days now. In addition to assessments regarding this student's menstrual cycle, what information is essential for the nurse to obtain at this time?

   a. overall nutrition status
  * b. health of family members
   c. vital signs
   d. date of last menstrual cycle

The answer is (b), for the following reason. Although the student's complaints are often signs of early pregnancy, they are also manifestations of carbon monoxide poisoning. (Note the major piece of information about the weather.) If this family has gas heat and if other family members have similar complaints, there may be a leak in the heating system. Responses (a) and (c) may be part of the assessment but there are no data to indicate that they are essential at this time. Response (d) is included in the stem of the question. Note that in both of the above situations (the oral questions or the test question), you are pulling together information from more than one source or data bank. This is typical of critical thinking. Remember that *if you can go to a page in a text and find the answer, it is not critical thinking;* it is basic recall of information.

Thus, critical thinking is gaining prominence in all levels of schools of nursing as an essential skill for today's graduate. The amount of formal class time and content devoted to the topic is limited, but a demonstration of your effective usage of critical thinking should be visible throughout all of your courses, especially as you reach the conclusion of your program. To learn more about this topic, you might want to read some of the sources listed at the end of this chapter.

 ASK YOURSELF

1. Are you satisfied with your own critical thinking skills? If not, which skills would you like to improve?

_____

_____

2. In reference to question number one, what will you do to improve your skills?

_____

_____

 CYBERLINKS: FLASH CARDS

Check to see what you now remember by making your own flash cards. Use the CD-ROM that accompanies your textbook to discover how to make flash cards for reviewing and retaining what you have learned.

 CONCEPT MAP WORD BANK

CRITICAL THINKING
Definition
Characteristics
Evaluation

Refer to Concept Maps and Flash Cards on pages viii–ix for an explanation of how to create and use concept maps. In addition, the CD-ROM guides you through the construction of concept maps by providing a more detailed introduction, more illustrations of examples, and key steps to follow in designing your own maps.

Nursing Process and Clinical Pathways

14

 ASK YOURSELF

1. How would you define the terms *nursing process* and *clinical pathway*?

   _____

   _____

2. What relevance do you think these topics have to you in your role as an LPN?

   _____

   _____

   _____

 CYBERLINKS

A wealth of information about nursing process and standards is available at www.nursingworld.com. It is most definitely worth a visit.

In addition, www.LPNresources.com can help enhance your learning by leading you to discover other links with even more information about the topics you are studying.

The nursing process and clinical pathways (also called critical pathways) are two ways that your critical thinking skills might be put into action. They are both organized ways of determining what needs a patient has and how the nurse can best meet those needs. It is the nursing approach to using the scientific method you may have studied earlier in your education. The term *nursing process* has been used in nursing schools since 1967. *Clinical pathways* is a newer term and is now used in many medical–surgical textbooks and in many hospitals to direct the care of patients with specific conditions. This chapter will illustrate both types of critical thinking processes.

The majority of complaints received from nursing students relate to the value of the nursing process. Students frequently want to know why nurses have to do all the paperwork or busy work. Often, the nursing process is seen as a waste of time until it is used in patient care. Unfortunately, some facilities reinforce this idea by requiring that care plans be up-to-date just prior to visits by the Joint Commission on Accreditation of Healthcare Organizations (JCAHO). In some situations, nurses are sitting at a desk filling in 3 weeks worth of nursing care plans on patients who have already been discharged because of a planned JCAHO site visit. It is unfortunate that the nursing process is not seen in a more positive light. Long-term care facilities are probably more up-to-date with resident care plans, as these must be updated every three months in an interdisciplinary patient care plan conference attended by representatives from nursing, dietary, social work, activities, and the therapies. Often family members and/or residents themselves are present for the conference.

To illustrate the nursing process, let us look at your situation in making decisions about your nursing education. When you decided to go to nursing school, you were probably directed to an advisor. The advisor spoke to you about your needs, plans, and goals. You discussed your high school courses or general equivalency diploma (GED) and possibly previous college education. You took placement tests. You told the advisor whether or not you wanted to become a practical/vocational nurse or whether your final goal was that of an RN with an associate degree. Having gathered all of this information about you, the advisor then gave you an educational plan based on your goals and previous education. The plan provided you with information about what courses you had to take and when you needed to take them in order to graduate. If you had prerequisites to take prior to admission into the practical/vocational nursing program, you received that information as well. You may have also been given an option for completing your associate degree in nursing following your practical/vocational nurses' education. This whole process involved assessing data about yourself, deciding on your needs based on this data, establishing goals, and then developing a plan to help you meet your educational goals. At the conclusion of your nursing education, you will be able to evaluate whether or not your goals were met and how well they were met. This process is similar to the nursing process for your patients.

CORE CONCEPTS　　**THE NATURE OF THE NURSING PROCESS** ——————

The nursing process is a way of organizing data about patients. It also provides a blueprint, or map, for caring for the patient. Imagine what would happen if nursing schools did not have educational plans. Trying to get your certificate or associate degree would be extremely confusing. Think about registration and choosing courses that you thought might lead you to your goal without being sure. Attempting to reach your goal of graduation without an educational plan would be similar to trying to care for a patient without the nursing process or a care plan. Many educational and clinical facilities still use the nursing process in the form of nursing care plans, although some have chosen to use clinical pathways instead.

The nursing process generally begins with a patient history and assessment in order to develop a nursing care plan. The history and assessment varies depending on many factors.

**FACTORS THAT INFLUENCE
THE HISTORY AND ASSESSMENT**

In most states, practical/vocational nurses are not allowed to do initial history and assessments on patients who are new admissions. They are allowed to contribute information to the assessment initially and on an ongoing basis. However, as a practical/vocational nursing student, your clinical instructor will most likely expect you to conduct your own history and physical of each patient for whom you provide care. This does not become part of the clinical facility records but serves several purposes:

1. It allows you to systematically *prepare for your patient's care.* It guides your thinking to help you develop the knowledge base you will need to efficiently and effectively provide care.
2. It allows you to *develop your knowledge base for the future.* After you have done a history and assessment on three or four patients with congestive heart failure, you will begin to see patterns emerge that will help you in caring for other patients with congestive heart failure in the future.
3. It gives your instructor a *basis for evaluating your critical thinking skills.* It also provides her/him with a base on which to build suggestions that will help to improve your care.

No matter how varied history and assessments are, they are used to gather information about a patient and the patient's apparent need for health care. Your attitude and approach to the history and assessment can make a big difference in the ease with which you obtain important information. If you believe that the assessment is a big waste of time and its only purpose is to create paperwork for an assignment, then it is doubtful that you will have an easy time of gathering information. If, however, you view the assessment process as a way of getting to know your patient better and as a means of obtaining vital information, then you will probably see its value. Keep the following things in mind while taking a patient history or making an assessment:

- Determine the objectives of the assessment. This is the first step of the nursing process and serves as the basis for the rest of the nursing care plan. Although the assessment includes medical data, it should not duplicate a medical examination. Nursing should be looking for patients' responses to their problems.
- The history and assessment should be conducted in a holistic manner. This means that you evaluate all observable data related to the patient. What do you observe about the patient's appearance, posture, manner of speech, and orientation? What are the patient's verbal *and* nonverbal responses to your questions? How can they be interpreted?
- Listen and look for clues about other concerns the patient might have, for

example, psychosocial concerns such as payment for the hospitalization, possible loss of job, child care, and home care worries after discharge.

• Do not use the patient only as a means to gathering the information. There might be support people such as family and friends who can provide valuable information and insight. In addition, the client record containing comments by the physician and auxiliary personnel, and texts and journals about the patient condition are all informative sources.

Generally, the nursing history and assessment are like a detective novel: You have to read the patient, fill in between the lines, and solve the puzzle. It is challenging and can be a lot of fun!

The nursing care plan usually consists of four to seven columns that help you organize assessment information and project some type of plan of care for your patient.

CORE CONCEPTS | **NURSING CARE PLAN COLUMNS** —————

Examples of the information used in the nursing care plan are as follows.

Assessment

• *Subjective* (what the patient tells you) data. This may be referred to as "symptoms."

• *Objective* (what you observe or read in the chart, lab values, vital signs, etc.) data. Objective data is information that can be observed the same way by anyone caring for the patient. This may be referred to as "signs."

• Data may then be clustered to indicate problem areas. For instance, a school may choose to use Maslow's Hierarchy of Needs on which to structure problems. This makes it easy to prioritize problems. In other words, Maslow helps you to see which problems are probably the most important and the ones that should be dealt with first. A patient who is having difficulties with respiration and problems with eating and drinking because of them would find all of these problems categorized in the physiological needs level of Maslow's hierarchy. If that same patient were also anxious and demanding, those needs would fall under the safety and security level. Based on Maslow, the physiological needs require the most immediate interventions.

Analysis

• This may also be called *problem identification* or *nursing diagnosis*. Some schools allow students to use only nursing diagnoses from an approved list such as North American Nursing Diagnosis Association (NANDA); others may encourage students to creatively develop their own diagnoses in an accepted format.

- This may be a two-part statement using human response (response to a health care problem) and related factors (cause of the problem) or a three-part statement using human response, related factors, and evidence of the problem. Examples would be: "Pain related to (R/T) inflammatory process" (two-part statement) or "Pain R/T inflammatory process as evidenced by (AEB) patient reports of pain and facial grimacing when ambulating" (three-part statement).

Planning

- *Goal or outcome.* Stated as "The patient will . . ." The patient is always the focus of the goal. It is not your goal.
- *Short-term.* This goal can usually be accomplished in less than 48 hours.
- *Long-term.* This goal is sometimes not completed until discharge.
- The goal needs to be specific and describe what is to be done, when it is to be done, how, where, and how well. A goal of "Patient will ambulate on my shift" is not specific enough. "Patient will ambulate 25 feet with a walker and assistance of one two times on my shift" is better. Avoid using vague words such as *decrease, increase, improve,* and so on, since they are terms that cannot be measured.

Strategies, or Nursing Interventions

- How the nurse is going to help the patient accomplish the goals.
- Some schools break down strategies into those that the nurse (student) can accomplish on his or her own and others where the nurse is dependent on other caregivers (such as physical therapy).

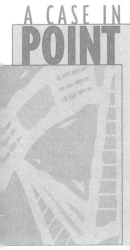

A CASE IN POINT

Leslie is a 24-year-old female who was admitted to the acute psychiatric unit following a suicide attempt. Leslie is divorced and has one child. She appears to be sullen and sad. Both wrists are bandaged, and the ER reports major lacerations with possible tendon damage. Leslie was admitted 5 years ago with a diagnosis of major depression, and her current medical diagnosis is major depression. You have been assigned to care for Leslie during your next clinical day and have been asked to develop a care plan for her (Figure 14-1).

Figure 14-1 Care Plan for Leslie

Assessment Subj. Data	Planning Short-Term Goal	Strategies	Rationale	Implementation	Evaluation
"I don't have anything to live for. If only they hadn't found me when they did."	By the end of my shift the pt will state one thing worth living for.	1. Establish a therapeutic relationship.	1. Establishing trust allows the pt to share information in a confidential manner (Burgess, 1997, p. 175).	1. Had three 30 min one-on-one sessions with pt.	Goal Met: Pt stated that her child was worth living for.
Obj. Data Sad affect Crying Bandaged wrists (each wrist required 20 stitches) Disheveled Poor Hygiene	By the end of my shift the pt will comply with all suicide precautions. During my shift the patient will make no attempts to harm herself.	2. Provide close observation. 3. Encourage pt to sign a no-suicide contract.	2. Protecting patients from suicidal impulses is critical (p. 574). 3. A no-suicide contract is a time-limited verbal or written promise (p 275).	2. Checked on pt every 15 min when not with her. 3. Pt signed a no-suicide contract.	Goal met. Pt was compliant with suicide precautions and signed a no-suicide contract. Goal met: pt did not try to harm herself.
Nurs. Diag. Self-Directed Violence related to feelings of hopelessness as evidenced by recent suicide attempt.	**Long-Term Goal** By discharge the pt will verbalize a desire to live and willingly attend outpatient therapy.	4. Use active listening techniques. 5. Provide an activity to release tension.	4. Nurses need to express concern and establish an alliance with the pt (p. 573. 5. Use positive interest and build mutual trust (p. 578.)	4. Used active listening. 5. Pt used the punching bag for 10 min and created a clay figure in OT.	

- If you are unsure as to whether or not an intervention is appropriate, ask yourself if that intervention will help your patient achieve the desired goal. We have nursing students write down great interventions, but they are inappropriate for the goal the patient is trying to reach. To turn, cough, and deep breathe a patient is a good nursing intervention, but if the goal is for the patient to be able to eat 75% of lunch, this is not an appropriate intervention for that problem and goal!

Rationales

- The nurse justifies why, or provides a rationale for, the actions he or she chooses to use.
- The rationale is the scientific evidence to support a specific nursing action.
- Ask yourself, "Why will this intervention help my patient to achieve the goal?" If you cannot answer that question, then the intervention is probably not appropriate.
- Your instructors may ask you to document from a specific page in a text or nursing journal to support your rationale.
- Some programs allow use of faculty lectures and/or common sense.

Figure 14-2 Home "Patient" Care Plan

Nursing Student's House

Assessment	Diagnosis	Planning Short-Term Goal	Strategies	Implementation	Evaluation
Subjective: "I can't even see my floors. "There are books everywhere!" *Objective:* 20 piles of unwashed clothes and 2 sinks full of unwashed dishes	Alteration in home maintenance related to nursing school attendance as evidenced by unwashed dishes and clothes, unmade beds.	1. The house will have no dishes in the sinks by 2 pm Wednesday. 2. The house will have clean floors by 9 am Thursday. *Long-Term Goal:* The house will remain clean and free of clutter.	1. The student will wash one load of clothes daily for 3 weeks. 2. The student will purchase necessary cleaning supplies. 3. The student will wash dishes daily. 4. The student will wash one floor area daily. 5. The student will develop a plan to limit clutter.	1. I washed one load of clothes yesterday and today. 2. I went to the store and bought cleaning supplies. 3. I washed all of the dishes today. 4. I washed the kitchen floor. 5. I wrote down the places in the house that tend to collect clutter.	Goal 1 met 100%: All dishes are clean. Goal 2 partially met: only one floor is clean.

Implementation

- What the nurse actually did for the patient.

Evaluation

- Evaluation and reevaluation of movement towards the original goals.
- Look at your goal, and decide whether or not it was met. If it was not, you might make suggestions as to why it wasn't met and possibly suggest a change in your interventions that might work better. For example, if your patient's goal of ambulating 25 feet twice on your shift was not met, you might explain that the patient was having some difficulty breathing and could not tolerate the distance. Or, sometimes, you might state that in reevaluating the goal, you believe it was unrealistic. In the above example, a goal of 10 feet might have been a more appropriate starting point for your patient.

A humorous "nursing" care plan that most students can relate to can be found in Figure 14-2. The "patient" is the home of a nursing student.

| CORE CONCEPTS | **CARE PLAN PITFALLS**

There can be several pitfalls in any nursing care plan. Examples include:

- Getting bogged down in the paperwork part of the nursing process rather than following a logical step-by-step process.

- Difficulty focusing on one diagnosis and tending to want to include all they have learned about a patient in one care plan. It is better for students to simplify the process by focusing on just one diagnosis at a time.
- Losing focus and wandering off to other problems during the process. For example, a nursing diagnosis might be anxiety, but halfway through the care plan, the student will develop strategies that deal with alterations in diet or incontinence, which would be better served by a separate nursing care plan.
- Making a problem out of just one piece of supportive data. We require a minimum of three pieces of assessment data to support the fact that there is a problem.
- Using published nursing care plan textbooks without individualizing them to your patient. Remember that these textbooks serve a very useful purpose, but they are to be used solely as a guide for you. The writers of the textbook do not know your patient or your patient circumstances. We have had students write that they would monitor the results of arterial blood gases (ABGs) as a nursing intervention when no such test had ever been ordered for their patient. It was only a textbook suggestion. The same holds true for generic nursing care plans that the clinical sites might have on hand to save time. These still have to be tailored to fit the needs of specific patients.

CORE CONCEPTS | CLINICAL PATHWAYS

The guiding tool in delivering nursing care in some health care facilities is the clinical pathway (i.e., critical pathway, care maps, interdisciplinary (action) plans, anticipated recovery plans) rather than a nursing care plan. Regardless of the terminology, these pathways outline an anticipated progression for a patient with a specific condition. The pathways are used most successfully for patient conditions that have relatively predictable outcomes (Figures 14-3 and 14-4). Each pathway will "establish the sequence and timing of interdisciplinary interventions, and incorporate education, discharge planning, assessment, consultations, nutrition, medications, activities, diagnostics, therapeutics, and treatments" (Beyea, 1996, p. 3).

In addition to acute care settings, pathways are being used in a variety of settings such as home health, outpatient, rehabilitation, and long-term care.

Although publications are now available with pathways for many patient conditions, several institutions develop pathways that reflect their specific patient populations. Both sources of pathways tend to have the following four features (Burrell, Gerlach, & Pless, 1997):

1. They identify patient outcomes expected at various points along the pathway and at time of discharge.
2. The pathways have timelines, and sequencing of interventions is indicated.
3. Pathways reflect interdisciplinary teamwork and interventions.

Figure 14-3 Vaginal Delivery Critical Pathway: Infant

Date of Birth:_____   Time of Birth:_____

		0-6 Hours	7-12 Hours	13-18 Hours
Laboratory/ Diagnostic Tests		Coombs, Maternal Hep B status		
Treatments/ Procedures		Stabilization, Baby ID, Vital signs as per patient standard, Weight = _____ gm, Bath	Circumcision permit, Hep B permit	
Medications/IVs		Triple dye to cord, Vitamin K, Erythromycin ointment to eyes	HBIG if mother Hep B positive or status unknown, Hep B vaccine	
Consultations				
Activity		Radiant warmer until stable temp	Open crib	Open crib
Nutrition		Breastfeeding/or Glucose H2O	Breastfeeding per policy / care plan or formula at least q 4hrs	
Assessments		Apgar at 1 and 5 minutes, Gestational age, Nursing assessment for VS, feeding, voiding, bonding	I + O, Nursing assessment for VS, feeding, voiding, bonding	I + O, Assess circumcision site
Education/ Discharge Planning		See mother pathway		
Home Care				
Variances Order Reason Order Reason				

RN Signature: _____   _____   _____

Target discharge status =   Feeding well
Maintaining temperature
Voiding & stooling adequately
Bonding

(Continues)

4. They track holistic aspects of care such as diagnostic tests, nutrition, mobility, and patient education.

However, regardless of which pathways are used (individual institution or a generic publication), some patients will not progress as anticipated. When this occurs, it is called a variance. Three reasons that a variance might occur are (Beyea, 1996):

1. *System variance:* In this case, the health care institution or community is unable to provide the needed care (for example, the patient may need to travel 50 to 60 miles to have an MRI because the institution does not have one).

2. *Provider/clinician variance:* In this case, the health care provider's actions affect the patient's outcomes (for example, a nurse's poor handwashing practices leading to a nosocomial wound infection).

Figure 14-3 Vaginal Delivery Critical Pathway: Infant (Continued)

	19-24 Hours	Within 2 Hours of Discharge	Home 24-48 Hrs. Post Discharge
			Target LOS= 24-48 Hours
Laboratory/ Diagnostic Tests	◄············· PKU and bilirubin at age 24 hours ·············► Coombs results Maternal RPR status at delivery		PKU, if initial PKU done before 24 hrs Bilirubin if > 5 at age 24 hours or if baby jaundiced by home health nurse; report results to by pediatrician
Treatments/ Procedures	Circumcision care if circumcision done		
Medications/IVs			
Consultations			
Activity	Open crib	Open crib	
Nutrition	Breast–feeding/or formula at least q 4hrs	Breast–feeding/or formula	
Assessments	Physician assessment of body systems Nursing assessment for VS, feeding, voiding, stooling, bonding		HHC nurse assessment of physical environment and baby, including VS, feeding, voiding, stooling, bonding, jaundice
Education/ Discharge Planning		Instructions to parents	
Home Care			
Variances Order Reason Order Reason			

Confirmed by pediatrician:

_____   _____
Signature   Date

Source: Thomas Jefferson University Hospital; Women and Children Care Program; Philadelphia

Source: Allen, C. V. *Nursing process in collaborative practice: A problem-solving approach* (2nd ed.). © Reprinted by permission of Pearson Education, Inc. Upper Saddle River, NJ 07458.

3. *Patient variance:* In this case, the patient factors affect outcomes (for example, a patient may not be taking a prescribed medication).

The nursing process and clinical pathways that you are exposed to in the facilities where you do your clinicals may vary from what has been presented here. It is important to remember that as students, flexibility is key to your learning. You will most likely be exposed to many different interpretations of these concepts. Be certain that you know what is expected of you in whatever facility you are in at any

Figure 14-4 Vaginal Delivery Critical Pathway: Mother

Date of Birth: _____

	Prenatal Record to L&D by 36 weeks	Labor, Delivery, Recovery	0-12 Hours
Laboratory/ Diagnostic Tests	H + H Type + Screen Rubella RPR HBSAG	CBC per order MS BOS per order RPR	H+H or CBC if ordered Determine Rhogam and Rubella status

Treatments/ Assessments		Receive medical record from MD's
		    office by 36 weeks
		Assessment, vital signs and EFM
		    per patient care standard
			Post partum assessment per
			    patient care standard
			Peri care
			Hygiene + comfort measures
			Anesthesia follow-up if indicated

Medications/IVs	Prenatal vitamins	Analgesia/Anesthesia per order Pitocin per order	IV discontinued Analgesics as needed for pain
Consultations	Social Work per guidelines		Lactation consult if breastfeeding Social Work PRN Pediatrician visit with mother ┅▶
Activity		OOB unless contraindicated	OOB with assistance Shower Voiding without difficulty Rest
Nutrition	Appropriate weight gain	Clear liquids per order Ice	Regular diet

Education/ Discharge Planning	Childbirth preparation classes
	Parentcraft classes
	Breast–feeding class if BF
	Orient to discharge program tour
	Contraceptive planning
	Select pediatrician
	*Preparing for Your Baby's Birth
	    at Jefferson*
	"Baby Talk" video
		Comfort measures and
		    relaxation techniques
		Orient to EFM
		2nd stage pushing
		Initial breast–feeding instruction
		    if breast–feeding
		Breast–feeding
			Handwashing
			Orient to baby's crib
			Infant positioning, feeding,
			    changing

Home Care	Referral to home care		
Variances *Order* *Reason* *Order* *Reason* *Order* *Reason*			

RN Signature: _____   _____   _____

Target discharge status = Minimal vaginal bleeding
Demonstrates parenting skills
Minimal physical discomfort

(Continues)

particular time. If you are in doubt, ask your clinical instructor and refer to the policy and procedure manual.

STOP   ASK YOURSELF

1. After reading this chapter, how would you now respond to Ask Yourself question 2 at the beginning of the chapter?

_____

_____

Figure 14-4 Vaginal Delivery Critical Pathway: Mother (Continued)

		Target Post Delivery LOS = 24-48 Hours	
	Time of Birth: _____		
	13-24 Hours	Within 2 hrs. of Discharge	Home
Laboratory/ Diagnostic Tests	☐ Rhogam if Rh negative and baby Rh positive ☐ RPR results ☐ Rubella if not immune		
Treatments/ Assessments	☐ Assess parenting skills ☐ Post partum assessment per patient care standard ☐ Peri care ☐ Hygiene + comfort measures ☐ Anesthesia follow-up if indicated		☐ Follow-up phone call at 3-5 days post discharge by maternity nurse to assess ☐ Assessment by HHC nurse
Medications/IVs	☐ Stool softener as ordered ☐ Analgesics as needed for pain		
Consultations	problem (per BF Care Plan and Supplementation Policy/Procedure) ⋯⋯⋯⋯⋯⋯⋯⋯▸		☐ Lactation consult if breast-feeding problem ☐ Social work consult if needed
Activity	☐ OOB with assistance ☐ Voiding without difficulty ☐ Rest	☐ Escort mother and baby to car	
Nutrition	☐ Regular diet	☐ Regular diet	
Education/ Discharge Planning	☐ Sitz bath ☐ Infant care class ☐ Discharge planning ☐ Infant safety ☐ S&S of dehydration and infection ☐ Circumcision care if baby circumcized ☐ Breast pump if needed	☐ Discharge instructions ☐ Gift pack ☐ Infant car seat requirement ☐ Smoke detector ☐ Follow-up appointments ☐ Educational needs summary	☐ Reinforce teaching of infant and self–care by HHC nurse
Home Care	☐ Notify home care of delivery	☐ Home care contact in hospital	☐ Scheduled home care visits 24-48 hours post discharge
Variances Order Reason Order Reason Order Reason	☐	☐	☐ Earlier home care if needed ☐ 2nd home care visit if needed
RN Signature:	_____ _____ _____	_____ _____ _____	_____ _____ _____

Confirmed postdelivery by obstetrician:

_____   _____
Signature   Date

Source: Thomas Jefferson University Hospital; Women and Children Care; Philadelphia

Source: Allen, C. V. (1997). *Nursing process in collaborative practice: A problem-solving approach* (2nd ed.). © Reprinted by permission of Pearson Education, Inc. Upper Saddle River, NJ 07458.

2. Do you think that writing a nursing care plan is an absolutely necessary task for ensuring the highest quality patient care?

_____

_____

CYBERLINKS: FLASH CARDS ————————————

Check to see what you now remember by making your own flash cards. Use the CD-ROM that accompanies your textbook to discover how to make flash cards for reviewing and retaining what you have learned.

 CONCEPT MAP WORD BANK ————————————

HISTORY AND ASSESSMENT

NURSING CARE PLANS

CASE MANAGEMENT

Refer to Concept Maps and Flash Cards on pages viii–ix for an explanation of how to create and use concept maps. In addition, the CD-ROM guides you through the construction of concept maps by providing a more detailed introduction, more illustrations of examples, and key steps to follow in designing your own maps.

CORE ISSUES

15

Stress

 ASK YOURSELF

1. Has your stress level increased since you began your educational program? If so, how or why?

   _____

   _____

2. How are you coping with stress (and if you responded affirmatively to question one, how are you coping with the added stress)?

   _____

   _____

 CYBERLINKS

Interactive www.healthfinder.gov/ is the site to visit for some healthy self-assessment such as how you are doing juggling family and work. Once at the site, go to today's online checkups and then click on S for Stress.

Supplemental www.LPNresources.com can help enhance your learning by leading you to discover other links with more information about the topic you are studying.

All human beings experience stress. Without stress we wouldn't be alive! Unfortunately, most of us experience more stress than we need. The growth of technology has changed our lives forever. Many of us rely on cellular phones, pagers, faxes, and e-mail to keep in touch with our place of work. Some of us maintain 24-hour contact with our jobs. Stress has contributed to the development of many of the diseases experienced in our society. Some of the major diseases that have been linked to stress are asthma, coronary artery disease, hypertension, strokes, tension headaches, backaches, irritable bowel syndrome, colitis, arthritis, and diabetes.

| CORE CONCEPTS | **COPING WITH STRESS** |

To deal with stress, we adopt coping behaviors to help us handle life's stressors. For example, we may use ego-defense mechanisms. These help us to defend ourselves against threats to our psychological well-being. Denial (refusal to accept a problem as real) and rationalization (making up excuses for our failures) are two commonly used ones. We may also make use of other behaviors that have worked for us in the past. Table 15-1 lists various positive mental strategies to handle stress. Some of us may choose negative coping behaviors. Since the continued use of the same defense mechanisms and coping behaviors develop into habits, it is important to choose positive coping strategies that will allow you to succeed as a nursing student and as an LPN/LVN.

For example, starting nursing school is a stressful event for most students. Student A copes by trying to get as much information as possible about each class, organizing a calendar, and thinking positively. Student B copes by drinking heavily on weekends and complaining about the amount of work expected to anyone who will listen. Student A is attempting to problem-solve, which is positive. Student B is reducing tension, which is not as healthy. Both students are coping with stress, but Student A is coping more positively.

We all use certain behaviors to deal with stress. Some examples are:

- Overuse of alcohol and drugs
- Overeating
- Humor
- Swearing
- Crying
- Self-pity
- Exercising
- Sharing with others

Some of us tend to deal with stress better than others. It is possible for an individual to develop stress resistance (an increased ability to tolerate stress) (Figure 15-1). Some of the things that help to increase our resistance to stress are under our control and others are not. For example, we can change our lifestyle, but we cannot change our genetic structure. Genetics may make us more susceptible to stress. For example, if we are born with a heart valve defect, the defect cannot be altered to increase our stress resistance. If, on the other hand, we smoke, we can increase stress resistance by stopping smoking.

| CORE CONCEPTS | **STRESS MANAGEMENT** |

Obviously, we can learn to increase our stress resistance by focusing on those areas that we *can* control such as lifestyle, sense of humor, safety and security, self-confidence, and adequate social and material resources. We can do this for ourselves and for patients. Listed below are a number of factors that can increase our resistance to stress:

TABLE 15-1	Various Thought Strategies to Handle Stress and Their Rationale

Mental Response	Definition and Rationale
Use of knowledge	Learn causes of stress and ways to prevent or manage situations. Know personal limits. If the problem is beyond your control and cannot be changed now, accept the situation until it can be changed.
Objectivity	Sort out, compare, and validate events, ideas, and emotions to gain a (reality orientation) total perspective and better understanding on the basis of facts, not just feelings; maintain realistic perception.
Analysis	Study logically and systematically the components of a situation to arrive at realistic explanations and answers; manage part if not all of situation.
Concentration	Deliberately set aside thoughts and feelings unrelated to the situation (mental self-control) to master tension, save energy, find answers, and make necessary decisions for the task at hand.
Planning	Think through situation before acting to release tension, promote problem solving, and avoid unnecessary use of energy, error, and consequent frustration. Avoid too many deadlines. Decide what drudgery chore you want to complete and do it as quickly as possible, so it does not become a focus. Make a list of tasks and check off as they are accomplished.
Reconstruction	Review a recent stressful event, writing ways it could have been better and ways it could have been worse. Write what could have been done to make it better, thus improving sense of challenge and control.
Fantasize (daydream)	Visualize release of tension and successful achievement rather than dwelling on fear of failure to plan strategy, ensure goal-directed action, cope with stressors, and relieve tension.
Rehearsal	Fantasize or anticipate event or another's response before stressful event to practice what you will think and how you will act. This allows you to gain confidence in your ability to manage.
Substitution of thoughts and emotions	State ideas and feelings that are different from your real ones to avoid adding to stressful situation or to meet demands of the situation. Focus on one good thing that happened during the day.

TABLE 15-1	**Various Thought Strategies to Handle Stress and Their Rationale (Continued)**
Suppression	Hold thoughts and emotions in abeyance (put them "on hold") or momentarily forget to wait until it is more timely to change behavior, attack a problem, or implement a solution. Deliberately push all stress-producing thoughts aside for 60 seconds.
Valuing	Establish or reaffirm religious or sociocultural values to foster a sense of balance and relaxation in face of stressors. Value and believe in yourself. Take an hour each day for yourself.
Empathy	Imagine how others in the situation are feeling so that behavior can take these feelings into account.
Humor	Point out inconsistencies in situation, laugh at self, and use past feelings, ideas, and behavior to be playful, keep objective distance from a problem, reduce anxiety, maintain self-identity, enrich solution, and add enjoyment to life.
Tolerance of ambiguity (Vagueness)	Function in a way that lays the basis for eventual effective solutions when the situation is so complex that it cannot be fully understood or clear choices cannot be made now.

Source: Murray, R. B., Zentner, J. P. (1997). *Health assessment and promotion strategies through the life span* (6th ed.) Reprinted by permission of Pearson Education, Inc. Upper Saddle River, NJ.

1. Healthy lifestyle
   - Balanced diet
   - Regular exercise
   - Regular sleep
   - Avoidance of alcohol
   - Avoidance of tobacco and drugs
   - Keeping a routine of balanced activities
2. Sense of humor
   - Laughing at ourselves and others
   - Not taking life too seriously
3. Self-confidence
   - Feeling good about ourselves
   - Feeling good about our abilities
   - Feeling good about our relationships with others
4. Safety and security
   - Feeling safe at home and in our communities

Figure 15-1 It Is Possible to Develop Stress Resistance

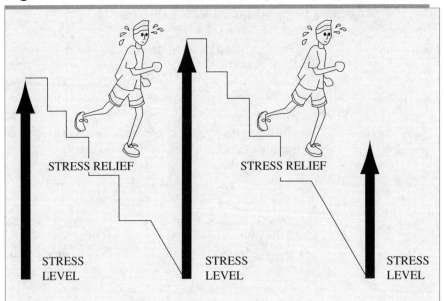

5. Adequate social and material resources
   • Having enough money, food, shelter, clothing
   • Having help from others (Berger & Williams, 1999)

ESSENTIAL SKILLS

HELPING THE PATIENT WITH STRESS MANAGEMENT

Unfortunately, we do not always have control over the stressful events in our lives, but we do have control over how we respond to them. Focusing on the benefits of an experience is not always easy, but it can be done; it just takes practice! Likewise, helping patients cope with stress requires careful attention:

1. *Assess major life stressors* (those things that cause you stress), and identify the ones that affect you the most. There are a number of assessment tools available to measure stress. One of the most common of these tools lists life events that may cause you stress, such as death of a spouse, and assigns a number to the event. Add up the numbers of the events you have experienced this past year. The higher the number, the more stress you have had. Starting school and any changes in your life circumstances are among the stressors! Do you think being a new nursing student qualifies you? Most facilities have at least one instrument to measure stress, or you can find one in most psychiatric or fundamentals nursing textbooks. Help your patients to do the same.

2. *Review the physical and psychological signs and symptoms of stress* both for yourself and for your patients to help you understand them more clearly:
   - Increased heart rate
   - Increased blood pressure
   - Increased glucose
   - Hyperventilation
   - Delayed healing
   - Increased hostility
   - Increased sadness
   - Increased reliance on alcohol or drugs

3. Identify your own support system and your usual manner of coping with stressful situations.

4. Determine if the patient has adequate support systems and how the patient usually copes with stressful situations.
   - Help patients to focus on a balance in daily activities including diet, exercise, and rest (Figure 15-2).
   - Help patients to change negative thoughts about stress to positive ones. Was there one positive point the patient could take out of a negative, stressful experience?

CORE CONCEPTS | **NURSING AND STRESS**

Nurses are often much better at giving patients information to follow than following it themselves. Have you ever seen an obese health care provider telling an obese patient that the patient needs to lose weight? Have you ever seen a health care provider stress the need for a good diet to a patient and then head for the vending machine on his or her next break?

Nursing tends to be a very stressful profession, and nurses need to follow their own advice. Often, nurses are working under conditions that produce stress including shift work, long hours, inadequate staffing, and dealing with people who are needy and suffering. The fact that we confront death and disease on a daily basis tends to threaten our sense of safety and security. Some patients will die; so, we must face the fact that we will die too. Nurses are held responsible for their patients' lives and for vast amounts of technical information. After paperwork and other responsibilities, many nurses are dissatisfied with the amount of quality time that is left to spend with patients. New graduates also experience reality shock as they make the transition from school to work.

Nurses who do work long hours and/or work in highly stressed areas such as critical care often experience burnout. *Burnout* is a term meaning mental, physical, and emotional exhaustion. There are a number of facts regarding burnout:

- It is easier to recognize burnout in others than it is to recognize it in oneself.

Figure 15-2 Helps Your Patient Learn How to Balance Daily Activities

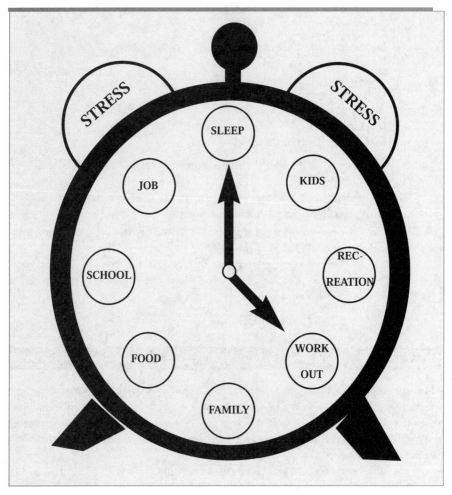

- Burned-out nurses are apathetic and uncaring and may also experience a number of stress-related symptoms.
- Burnout, once recognized, can be reversed with time and stress-reduction techniques.

Some nurses find that a change in job is beneficial. Perhaps a move from an acute medical–surgical floor in the hospital to long-term care or a physician's office might help. Nurses are lucky that there is such variety of opportunities in the profession. There are any number of job possibilities, and most of us can find a place where we can be happy and where burnout is less likely. If you find yourself in a job in which you are not happy, keep looking! Sooner or later, you will find a job that is right for you.

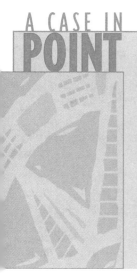

A CASE IN POINT

There is a severe nursing shortage in the medical center where Mary works. She has been asked to come in on her days off and very frequently works overtime. It is difficult for Mary to say no, especially since the supervisor views her as exceptionally dependable. Her family, however, tells her that she needs to stop working so much. They are worried about her and repeatedly remark that she looks tired, seems tense, and has lost her sense of humor. Mary feels that they just don't understand. She has been unhappy in her work but prides herself on "grinning and bearing it."

ESSENTIAL SKILLS

GUIDELINES FOR NURSES FOR OVERCOMING STRESS

1. Live in the moment!
   - Most of us try to do five things at once and feel stressed as a result.
   - Concentrating on one thing can help decrease anxious feelings.
   - Appreciate the now!
2. Balance your life!
   - Give some of you to work, some of you to your personal life, and some of you to your spiritual life.
   - This does not mean 80% work, 10% family, and 10% spiritual; it means balanced.
3. Don't sweat the small stuff!
   - Does it really matter if there are no tickets available to the movie that you want to see? Could you see a different one? Could you go see it next week? Does it really matter if the copier ran out of paper? Does it really matter that your co-worker has to leave 10 minutes early? Does it really matter that you have to wait in line 5 minutes at the grocery store?
   - Think about the long-term scheme of things.
   - These minor hassles can cause major stress if you let them.
   - Learn which things are of value to you—focus on those and forget the rest.
4. Decide what things are important to you, and focus on those things.
   - The things that are important to most people are health, family, friends, work, home, and religious beliefs.
   - Avoid the things that are not important.

5. Try meditation!
   - Meditation can help you relax and feel ready to face the world again.
   - It does not have to last 30 minutes or an hour to be helpful.
   - Ten minutes of controlled breathing are enough to slow your pulse rate, your breathing, and even lower your blood pressure.
   - Meditation can also help clear your mind of thoughts and worries.

6. Keep a journal!
   - Write down the things that bother you—get it all out—even if you have to burn it when you're finished.

7. Laugh!
   - Laughter can reduce stress, so take time to see that new comedy.
   - Find a funny friend, call the joke hotline, or do whatever you need to do to have a chuckle.
   - Keep a humor file, and fill it with cartoons, funny cards, jokes, or anything else that "tickles your fancy." Look at it from time to time when you need a lift.

8. Organize and manage your time.
   - Prioritize important tasks.
   - Do unpleasant things first and get them out of the way.
   - Carry your day planner with you.

9. Use positive self-talk.
   - Start your day with positive affirmations, a "pep talk" about your abilities. Post them on your bathroom mirror if you have to.
   - End your day the same way.

CORE CONCEPTS | **NURSING STUDENTS AND STRESS**

Nursing students have stressors unique to their life situations. Sources of stress may be outside stressors (family, friends, finances, etc.) or school stressors (grades, coursework, clinical, faculty, etc.).

Family Family stressors can be the result of poor planning, or they can be unexpected. Nursing school is extremely demanding, and families need to be prepared for what is ahead. Spouses need to realize that the student will be gone (at odd hours) for long periods of time. They need to know that studying is a priority and that household chores need to become a joint responsibility. You will need to keep channels of communication open and be flexible. So will your spouse! Talk things out, and take time for each other. The divorce rate among student nurses and graduates is high. If your marriage was good prior to school, it will most likely survive. If you and your spouse were having problems, they will most likely intensify. Seek help early! We have seen some students lose a marriage and flunk out in the same semester.

Children also need to know that school is demanding. Young children often feel abandoned when a parent is in nursing school. When not at school, the parent is usually busy studying or trying to fit too much into too little time. Remember that your children will be there long after you finish nursing school. They are more important than school, and they need you to keep that in perspective. Sure, you are trying to provide them with a better life, but if they do not feel loved, they will resent the time that school requires. Do fun things with your children. Do your homework together. You will serve as a great role model. Be there when they need you. Help them to understand when you have important work to do for school. Sometimes, you might even be able to ask and receive their help. Children love to be patients on whom Mom or Dad can practice.

Friends   Your friends will either lend their support or complain that you no longer have time for them. You will need the supportive ones. Set aside time for your friends. You are not entering a monastery or being confined to jail. There is a life outside of nursing school. Make time for it, or you will find your stress building.

Finances   All schools of practical/vocational nursing offer financial assistance through grants, scholarships, and loans. If you need financial assistance, find the financial aid office and go there. You are not seeking a handout. These schools are required to give a certain amount of financial aid each year. If you don't ask for it, someone else will get it anyway. Talk to your department head or faculty. Ask questions! For your own good, go check it out. Apply for any scholarships that are available. You may have to write an essay as part of the requirements, but you have nothing to lose and much to gain.

Grades   Another stressor that seems to stand out above all others is grades. Not everyone in class will get all A's. Some students are not satisfied unless they get an A; not making an A will become a significant source of stress for these students. We have had students fall apart because they got a 95% grade on an exam. We have had students who wanted to rewrite a paper because they only received a 97%. You are not your grade. Whether you make a C or an A, you will still graduate and receive the same certificate. If settling for a lower grade means that your marriage might survive nursing school, and that your kids will remember who you are, it is worth it to give up the A. Would you rather be a nurse with straight-A grades or one who has a life? Some students can have both, but most have to give up one or the other. Which one is worth more to you? On the other hand, we do realize that, for some students, excelling in all subjects is their priority. If they do not excel, stress results. We respect that difference, and our thoughts are not to put down the student who has high grades as a focus. We just encourage students to prioritize their values and their goals. A good goal for all is to learn the material presented in class, and be fully prepared to provide the best nursing care that you possibly can.

Stress is something that we all have to deal with. It is important to control and decrease our stress levels whenever possible. Nursing and nursing school are both very stressful. Learning how to control your stress is essential to both your health and that of your family.

ASK YOURSELF

1. What new ways of dealing with stress have you learned from reading this chapter?

   _____

   _____

2. Have you identified any ways in which you deal with stress that you now perceive to be unhealthy? What will you do to acquire more healthy strategies?

   _____

   _____

 CYBERLINKS: FLASH CARDS

Check to see what you now remember by making your own flash cards.

Use the CD-ROM that accompanies your textbook to discover how to make flash cards for reviewing and retaining what you have learned.

CONCEPT MAP WORD BANK

STRESS

COPING MECHANISMS

PATIENT STRESS MANAGEMENT

NURSE STRESS MANAGEMENT

STUDENT STRESS MANAGEMENT

Refer to the Concept Maps and Flash Cards on pages viii–ix for an explanation of how to create and use concept maps. In addition, the CD-ROM guides you through the construction of concept maps providing a more detailed introduction, more illustrations of examples, and key steps to follow in designing your own maps.

Pain

16

 ASK YOURSELF

Think of a time when you have experienced physical pain.

1. How did you deal with it emotionally?

   _____

   _____

2. What methods, traditional (medication, etc.) or alternative (meditation, etc.), did you use to relieve your pain?

   _____

   _____

 CYBERLINKS

Interactive Pain is a symptom that accompanies most illnesses. However, because pain is subjective, it is one of the most difficult symptoms to assess. www.ipl.org offers a number of pain assessment tools that are helpful in interpreting the patient's pain. Once at the site, go to Reference Center, then Health and Medical Science. Scroll down to Nursing, and finally click on "City of Hope Pain Resource Center."

Supplemental www.LPNresources.com can help enhance your learning by leading you to discover other links with more information about the topic you are studying.

Pain is a fact of life that you will encounter in almost all clinical environments and is one of the most studied human experiences. Even if, as a graduate, you manage to work in a setting with healthy individuals who have no periods of pain, you will be exposed to pain away from work: pain felt by yourself, by relatives, and by friends. Perhaps it is because pain is so common and yet complex that providing effective interventions is often a great nursing challenge. It is a difficult concept for both the patient and the caregiver. Patients often have trouble understanding why they are having pain or severe pain and why it can't be better controlled. The caregiver often has difficulty assessing pain—just how bad is the patient's pain? Pain is, after all, a subjective symptom.

CORE CONCEPTS   **THE NATURE OF PAIN**

People respond to unrelieved pain in many different ways. Think of those responses to pain laying out on a continuous path, with minor responses on one end progressing to major responses on the other. This path is referred to as a continuum. Some of the minor, common reactions are irritability, restlessness, and anorexia, or loss of appetite. At the opposite end of the continuum is suicide. And the fear of uncontrollable pain is one of the major factors in the current national debate on physician-assisted suicide and euthanasia.

As of January 1, 2001, the Joint Commission on Accreditation of Healthcare Organizations (JCAHO) released pain standards that require all hospitals to identify patients with pain and effectively manage that pain. The JCAHO standards cover issues such as assessment of pain in all patients, education of staff and patients on pain control, and the appropriate treatment of the pain. Pain is now considered to be a "fifth vital sign."

Pain can be analyzed from many viewpoints including duration (acute or chronic), location, etiology (cause), and severity. Pain is often the single most common symptom that causes a patient to seek help. In one respect, nature is kind to us in relation to pain. At the time the pain is experienced, we are miserable. However, after the pain is gone, we remember only how miserable we were; we do not reexperience the pain. Pain is also the one human sensation for which there is such a wide variety of vastly different intervention techniques for relief.

There are three **basic components** of pain:

1. *Reception at the site of origin to the brain.* Nociceptors are the nerve fibers that carry the pain impulse to the spinal column.

2. *Perception of the pain.* This occurs at two levels.
   - Physiologic perception: Brain reception and interpretation of the pain impulse (dull, sharp, aching, etc.).
   - Psychological perception: The individual's mental interpretation of the pain based on such factors as past experiences with pain, current situation, anxiety, culture, gender, and age.

3. *Response to the pain perception.* This also has two basic levels.
   - Physiologic response: Changes in body physiology such as pulse rate, respiratory rate, and blood pressure.
   - Behavioral response: The objective indicators of the pain including pacing, gritting the teeth, crying, irritability, groaning, inability to keep still, and facial grimacing.

A list of objective indicators could be very lengthy, because behavioral responses will be individual and influenced by the psychological factors at the perception level.

The list can also be very short, because there are individuals who present very few objective indicators of pain.

| ESSENTIAL SKILLS | ASSESSING PAIN: THREE METHODS |

When dealing with patients who are experiencing pain, the first nursing action is to assess the pain.

Determine the Pain's Etiology

- Where is the pain?
- When did you first notice the pain?
- What does it feel like?
- What causes the pain?
- Does anything make it better? Worse?
- Are there any other changes you notice when you have the pain?

On the surface, this last question may sound rather silly. After all, if a patient just had surgery, we expect him or her to have pain. Many a nurse, however, making such an assumption, has medicated a patient only to discover later that the pain was not related to the surgery. The patient, in fact, was developing a pulmonary embolus (blood clot in the lung) or having cardiac pain and, therefore, proper medical intervention was delayed. On the other hand, the pain could be related to a condition as simple as constipation, requiring a totally different intervention than for postoperative pain.

Determine the Severity of the Pain Experienced

- There are a number of pain assessment tools useful with adults and a few for young children.
- One of the more common tools used with adults is a numerical rating scale based on 0 (no pain) to 10 (maximum or severe pain).
- Another tool used with adults is a Simple Descriptive Pain Intensity Scale with pain being verbally described as none, mild, moderate, severe, very severe, and worst possible.
- A common scale for children is the Wong–Baker Faces Rating Scale (Figure 16-1). This scale is sometimes used with hearing-impaired patients or non–English-speaking patients. However, more research needs to be conducted on its validity in other groups.
- Some staff on Alzheimer's units have developed individual pain scales for each resident based on their knowledge of the residents and their knowledge of common pain responses in elderly people.
- There is no valid assessment tool for evaluating pain in newborns.

The key to using any pain assessment tool is consistency. All individuals working with the patient should use the same pain-rating system. This helps to cre-

Figure 16-1 The Wong–Baker FACES Rating Scale

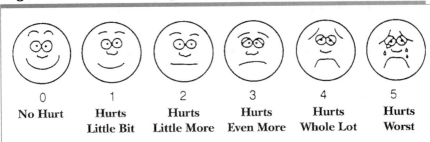

0	1	2	3	4	5
No Hurt	Hurts Little Bit	Hurts Little More	Hurts Even More	Hurts Whole Lot	Hurts Worst

Explain to the patient that each face is for a person who feels happy because he has no pain (hurt) or sad because he has some or a lot of pain. Face 0 is very happy because he doesn't hurt at all. Face 1 hurts just a little bit. Face 2 hurts a little more. Face 3 hurts even more. Face 4 hurts a whole lot. Face 5 hurts as much as you can imagine, although you do not have to be crying to feel this bad. Ask the person to choose the face that best describes how he is feeling. Rating scale is recommended for persons age 3 years and older.

Source: Wong, D. L., Hockenberry-Eaton, M., Wilson, D., Winkelstein, M. L., and Schwartz, P. *Wong's essentials of pediatric nursing* (6th ed.) St. Louis, 2001, p. 1301. Copyright by Mosby, Inc. Reprinted by permission.

ate uniformity in assessment and documentation of pain and the effectiveness of intervention. As your nursing skills improve with experience, you will be able to combine your assessments of pain etiology and severity into one.

Determine the Effectiveness of Your Interventions (e.g., Medications, Massage, Distraction)

- This is done approximately 30 minutes after the intervention.
- One of the most common indicators of effectiveness is again a pain-rating scale.
- The scale used in the first assessment should be used to evaluate effectiveness. Figure 16-2 presents, in descending order of importance, pain-rating guidelines, which apply at all stages of pain management.

CORE CONCEPTS   THE CONCEPT OF PAIN THRESHOLD

There are many phrases associated with pain. One of these is pain threshold. This describes the point at which the patient feels pain. According to controlled laboratory experiments, the pain threshold is fairly consistent in all people, regardless of age or sex. However, you will hear certain terms regularly in health care settings. These are two red flags that come up in relation to pain. They are, "This patient has a low pain threshold," and its opposite, "This patient has a high pain threshold."

Figure 16-2 Pain-Rating Guidelines

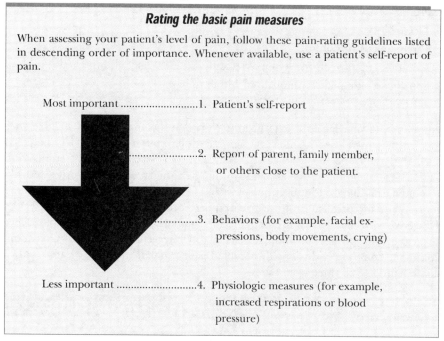

Rating the basic pain measures

When assessing your patient's level of pain, follow these pain-rating guidelines listed in descending order of importance. Whenever available, use a patient's self-report of pain.

Most important ....1. Patient's self-report

..........................2. Report of parent, family member, or others close to the patient.

..........................3. Behaviors (for example, facial expressions, body movements, crying)

Less important ....4. Physiologic measures (for example, increased respirations or blood pressure)

Source: McCattery, M. Pain management handbook. *Nursing 97, 27*(4): 42–45. Used with permission.

The first phrase is basically another way of saying, "This patient sure asks for pain medication a lot; he or she is probably addicted." This is a red flag that the health care team does not have the latest information about pain management.

When a patient has what is commonly considered a painful condition and the opposite phrase, "This patient sure has a high pain threshold," is used, the second red flag goes up. Not seeing any of the anticipated behavioral pain indicators, the physician and/or nurse may conclude that the patient experiences less pain than the "average" individual in a similar situation. In this case, personal perceptions of the physician or nurse could result in the patient's not receiving the needed pain medication. The patient may have had a poor pain assessment by the health care team, or the patient may have excellent individual coping skills for pain due to cultural beliefs that showing pain to others is not acceptable.

Health care workers should accept the patient's statement of pain. If patients state they are in pain, they are in pain. Only patients themselves can fully know the intensity of their pain.

CORE CONCEPTS   INTERVENTIONS FOR PAIN RELIEF

There are a great variety of interventions for pain relief. These interventions can be placed into three main categories: surgical (Table 16-1), pharmacological (Table 16-2), and nonpharmacological (Table 16-3). Each table contains only the most

TABLE 16-1	Surgical Interventions

- Nerve blocks
- Percutaneous cordotomy
- Commissural myelotomy hypophysectomy
- Spinal cord stimulation (implanted TENS units)

common interventions for each category. Note that the interventions in Table 16-1 are generally used after the nonsurgical methods have been tried and have not been successful. Also be aware that the trancutaneous electrical nerve stimulation (TENS) intervention can be implanted (a surgical intervention) or worn externally (a nonpharmacological intervention) (Table 16-3). The current interventions used most often for pain control are in the pharmacological category (Table 16-2). However, with the increasing acceptance and popularity of alternative approaches to health care, the use of nonpharmacological interventions are becoming more common. Some individuals with complex pain problems may be treated with a combination of all three techniques.

CORE CONCEPTS	THREE COMPLICATIONS OF PAIN CONTROL

Since the primary intervention you will be using for pain control with your patients is pharmacological, questions may arise about addiction, drug tolerance and psychological dependence. You need to have an understanding of these terms both for your own benefit and for educating your patients as well. Many patients do not want to take medications for pain relief because of their fear of becoming addicted.

Addiction

- This is a physical or psychological dependence (or a combination of the two) on a drug usually in the opioid group.

TABLE 16-2	Pharmacological Pain Interventions

1. Nonopioids
    Acetaminophen
    Salicylates
    NSAIDs (nonsteroidal anti-inflammatory drugs)
    Supportive
        Antianxiety
        Antidepressants
        Corticosteriods
2. Opioids

TABLE 16-3	Common Nonpharmacological Interventions

- External TENS units
- Distraction
- Relaxation
- Imagery
- Biofeedback
- Acupuncture
- Hypnosis
- Behavior modification
- Meditation

- For an addict, the drug is sought out at all costs only for its emotional and psychological effects and not for pain relief.
- If the drug is discontinued for any reason, physiological withdrawal symptoms will occur.
- When opioids are used for pain relief, the patient experiences a therapeutic response and doesn't become addicted when the drug is used for short periods of time; even a terminally ill cancer patient taking high doses of the opioids to control pain is not considered to be an addict. The cancer patient may require up to 8,000 mg of morphine every 24 hours to achieve pain relief that was originally obtained at 60 mg every 24 hours. (The 8,000 mg is not a misprint.) The extremely high dose is required for adequate pain relief.

Drug Tolerance

- This is the body's physiologic adjustment to a drug, so that greater amounts of the drug are required to produce the desired physiologic response.
- Tolerance occurs rather quickly with opioids; it may also occur with non-opioid drugs.
- A physician may be reluctant to increase the dosage of a medication for fear of an addiction developing; however, for individuals with chronic, severe pain, of any etiology, the indication for a medication dose change should be the patient's response—is the pain at a tolerable level and are adverse reactions acceptable—not whether or not the patient is receiving the recommended dosage.

Habituation

- This is the body's psychological dependence on the drug, which is often seen as a patient's intense desire or compulsion to continue taking the drug.
- There are no physical or withdrawal effects if the drug is stopped.

It is confusion over these physical responses and the fear of creating an addict that leads to patients being undermedicated for pain. In addition, in many states, physicians who have prescribed long-term use of opioids for individuals with chronic, unrelieved pain have found themselves before their state medical board facing disciplinary action. As research sheds more light on pain and treatment options, as medical and nursing schools include pain control in the curricula, and as practitioners who have been in the field for a number of years become aware of pain treatment advances, undermedication of those in pain will hopefully decrease.

At one time, medical literature contained little information on pain control. This, of course, is no longer true. In addition to professional publications, lay literature (books, newspapers, magazines, information on the Internet) contains a vast amount of information on the nature of pain, as well as pain control techniques. It is clear that patients are becoming very aware that pain is controllable, and they are being educated to expect adequate treatment. With the new pain standards set forth by JCAHO, health care facilities have also been mandated to recognize and effectively treat and control pain.

ESSENTIAL SKILLS | **ASSISTING THE PATIENT WITH PAIN MANAGEMENT**

There are a number of ways to help the patient in relieving pain and controlling pain.

1. It is essential that the caregiver not be judgmental.
   - Pain is what the patient says it is.
   - Placebos should never be given as a way to prove or disprove the existence of pain. Many health care workers look for certain behavioral or outward responses to pain. If these responses are absent, the nurse or physician automatically jumps to the conclusion that the patient does not have "real" pain. There was a time when such a patient was given a placebo to prove he or she really did not have any pain. The current standard is for some nurses to be the *keeper of the keys* (i.e., having access to, and control of, pain medications), which creates a sense of power. If the pain medication order states it may be administered no sooner than every 4 hours, that is what the nurse does, despite evidence that the patient is not receiving adequate pain relief. This is changing, though, as many health care facilities increase the use of the patient controlled analgesia (PCA) pumps, which allow the patient control over the administration of pain medication. These pumps are set up to deliver opioids intravenously when the patient presses a control button. Patients cannot overdose on the drugs, because the pumps have been programmed for maximum dosages and time intervals for delivering the drug (Ellis & Nowlis, 1994). These pumps put patients in charge of their pain relief.

2. The caregiver can help the patient (and often his or her family) understand the following:

- Pain does not have to be tolerated. But on the other hand, the patients with chronic pain may need help understanding that it may not be possible to be totally pain free. Perhaps the goal is to reduce the pain level to a 1 or 2 on the 10-point rating scale.
- Taking opioids for pain may lead to tolerance and dependency but not addiction.
- There are many interventions for pain.
- Patients often need encouragement to try some of the nontraditional interventions.
- Pain intervention used should be initiated before the pain becomes severe.
- Some patients may need a referral to a local pain clinic.

3. Medication can be given around the clock (ATC).

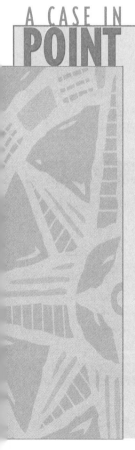

A CASE IN POINT

David, a 33-year-old patient who is one day postop for removal of a mass in his left lung, is complaining of severe pain. His pain is being managed with controlled release morphine (pump). Wendy, the LPN assisting with David's care, notices that he is grimacing, restless, colorless, and almost inaudible when he speaks. He had been repeatedly telling her that he was in a lot of pain. Wendy reported her observations and the patient's complaints to the nurse, but the nurse explained that David had recently had something for pain and that, in addition, he should just be encouraged to press the control button for morphine. In addition, the nurse tells Wendy that some pain is expected even with morphine, and that probably the patient had a low pain threshold. Soon after her conversation with the nurse, Wendy's shift ended. The next morning, during change-of-shift report, Wendy learns that David had been in so much pain because his morphine pump had been malfunctioning, and the alarm bell (which usually signals this occurrence) was malfunctioning also. David had not received morphine for 18 hours.

- Medicating the patient around the clock will keep the blood level of the pain medication consistent, providing the best pain control.
- The patient may need to be awakened to receive a night dose.
- Caregivers may need help realizing that waking the patient is more important to pain relief than uninterrupted sleep.

Before we leave the topic of pain, we will spend a few words on *phantom limb pain*. There are many theories regarding phantom limb pain, but to date, this is a phenomenon that is not well understood. Most explanations found in textbooks agree that the nerves at the amputation site continue to send impulses to the spinal cord and then on to the brain where perception occurs. This does not, however, explain why or how some paraplegics with complete breaks of the spinal cord experience leg pain. Since the spinal cord damage prevents transmission of impulses to the brain, how do impulses get to the brain? So, although much progress has been made on the physiology of pain, phantom limb pain is an area with many unanswered questions.

Continuing research by Melzack (1998) has generated additional information to the experience of phantom pain. Melzack has studied individuals who were born without a limb. Approximately 20% of the group "reported feeling—often vividly—in an arm or leg they had never had or known" (p. 20). Although current theories may explain some aspects of phantom pain, the perceptions of some individuals born without a limb indicate that a great deal is still unknown.

And like the experience of phantom pain, pain in general, remains a topic that requires further research. In addition to the work being done with neonates, other groups require research, such as the elderly, who often receive poor pain management. Mechanisms of pain, and techniques to manage it, will continue to be developed. Pain will be one of the topics that you will encounter throughout your nursing career.

 ASK YOURSELF

1. Has the reading of this chapter changed your perception of the concept of pain threshold? If so, how?

   _____

   _____

2. What key concepts related to pain have made the greatest impression on you?

   _____

   _____

 CYBERLINKS: FLASH CARDS

Check to see what you now remember by making your own flash cards. Use the CD-ROM that accompanies your textbook to discover how to make flash cards for reviewing and retaining what you have learned.

CONCEPT MAP WORD BANK

PAIN
Understanding
Components
Assessment

PAIN CONTROL
Management
Complications

Refer to Concept Maps and Flash Cards on pages viii–ix for an explanation of how to create and use concept maps. In addition, the CD-ROM guides you through the construction of concept maps by providing a more detailed introduction, more illustrations of examples, and key steps to follow in designing our own maps.

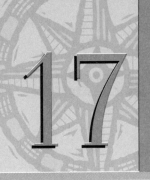

Rehabilitation

 ASK YOURSELF

Think of a time when you had a chronic illness or injury that interrupted your "normal life."

1. How did you react emotionally to this situation?
   _____
   _____

2. How did family and friends react? Did any of their reactions have a negative physical, psychological, or emotional effect on you?
   _____
   _____

 CYBERLINKS

Interactive As the aging population increases in number, so does the need increase for rehabilitative services aimed at dealing with patients' altered function. Rehabilitation information related to all ages in all situations can be found at www.ipl.org Go to Reference Center and then to Health and Medical Sciences, and then to Disabilities. Scroll down to NARIC (National Rehabilitation Info Center).

Supplemental www.LPNresources.com can enhance your learning by leading you to discover other links with even more information about the topic you are studying.

Rehabilitation is essential to many areas of nursing practice. As the aging population continues to grow, the number of individuals with chronic illnesses will increase. A number of chronic illnesses lead to altered functional ability and, as a result, altered lifestyles. Rehabilitation nursing uses a problem-solving approach to diagnose and treat the responses of individuals with actual or potential health problems that occur as a result of the changes brought on by chronic illness or injury

(Habel, 1997). As a practical/vocational nursing student, you will be involved in rehabilitation both in long-term care facilities and in the acute care hospital, especially in the specialty areas of orthopedics and neurology.

| CORE CONCEPTS | **THE ROLE OF THE REHABILITATION NURSE** |

- Focus on the patient's physical and mental status as well as his or her emotional responses to pain, disability, and alterations in self-concept.
- Assess self-care abilities and work with both the patient and the family to assess their ability to cope with changes.
- Understand the value of preventing complications and teach the individual and the family prevention techniques.
- Coordinate the efforts of the rehabilitation team and serve as the case manager. (LPN/LVNs will usually not be found in the role of a case manager.)

Frequently, nurses find that patients can be less than cooperative; therefore, they need to recognize when patients and their families are having a natural reaction to an illness or injury versus a true problem. It is important for nurses to prevent complications and deformities, start rehabilitation activities early, teach patients and family, and refer to other professionals and agencies as ordered by the physician.

The term *chronic illness* indicates that we are dealing with an illness or injury that is most likely permanent and that will last at least 3 months or more. Individuals with chronic illness or injuries are forced to deal with many lifestyle changes. The focus of the rehabilitation team is to help the patient to learn to live with the chronic, and often debilitating, injury or illness. As nurses, we want patients to be the best that they can be given the limitations imposed by their condition.

| CORE CONCEPTS | **LIFESTYLE CHANGES AND RESPONSES OF CHRONICALLY ILL PATIENTS** |

All of the following changes cause additional stress, frustration, and often, fatigue.

- Health status
- Body image
- Loss of self-esteem
- Relationships and roles
- Activities and leisure pursuits
- Sexual functioning
- Loss of income or financial stressors
- Multiple doctor or hospital visits
- Multiple laboratory tests and medication trials
- Exacerbation (worsening) of the illness

Patient responses to injury or changes associated with a chronic condition depend on the following:

- Patient's personality and attitude
- How quickly the changes occur (e.g., spinal cord injury versus arthritis)
- How significant the changes are to that individual
- Coping mechanisms in place
- Presence of additional illnesses or injuries
- Presence of other stressors
- Availability of treatment and resources

It is important for the nurse to remember that our society emphasizes wholeness, youth, and beauty. Your patient is trying to deal with changes and put the new "self" into some perspective. The new self will also need to be accepted by the patient and society, and be viewed as worthwhile. Some patients never make the adjustments necessary to adapt and accept the new person. Patients with chronic illness or injuries may experience reactions similar to patients who are grieving a loss. They may initially feel shock, but it soon becomes apparent that a change has occurred and they may feel angry, depressed, anxious, and hopeless. Often, the anger and hostility these patients feel toward themselves for becoming ill is projected onto others. Patients may also respond with anger and hostility as a result of their loss of power to make choices. In this situation, the nurse must offer choices in areas where patients can make them. For instance, asking patients when they would like to bathe, what they would like to wear, and whether or not they would like to attend an activity are choices the patient can make. They do not seem like much, but they are putting *some* control back into the hands of the patient who may feel as if he or she has lost *all* control.

Nurses need to recognize that patients will experience a variety of feelings that are not easy to deal with. Following an injury or diagnosis, the patient may cope by using denial, an unconscious defense mechanism. There are different levels of denial, and its use can be healthy or unhealthy. Initially, the use of denial is considered healthy as the individual retreats into him- or herself to reduce the threat of what has occurred to his or her self-concept. Over time, the individual is usually able to recognize that a change has occurred but may continue to use denial. You may hear a patient say, "I know that I'll never be able to snow ski again, but that isn't so bad. I can live with that." Other patients might ignore the problem by saying, "I know the doctor said I have high blood pressure, but these pills are for my kidneys." Unhealthy denial occurs when a patient continues to verbally deny that which is obvious.

When a patient is in extreme denial, it is very important to get the patient to share how he or she views the illness or injury. Some patients may need more information about the present changes or those that will occur. It is unfortunate that denial occurs at a time when most patients are experiencing a number of physical assaults. The physical condition becomes the priority of most health care professionals, leaving patients to deal with the psychological changes on their own. As the

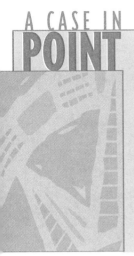

A CASE IN
POINT

A young male patient suffered a spinal cord injury as a result of a diving accident. He was only 28 years old when he became paralyzed from the level of the 5th cervical vertebra, a C5 quadriplegic. He kept telling everyone who came into his room, "I can feel my legs, watch, I'll move them for you." The nurses would leave the room without commenting whenever he said this. They felt at a loss as to what to do. They thought that his belief that he could move his legs made him happy, and that made the nurses happy.

patient's physical condition improves, health care professionals often move on to the next patient whose physical care is a priority. Patients need care at all stages of recovery, both physical and psychological!

Eventually, the individual is able to progress through the denial and acknowledges that in order to survive, certain changes will have to occur. At this time, individuals require a great deal of emotional support as they learn to focus on the reality of their situation. They must analyze who they were before, who they are now, and who they will become in the future. This entire process can be very distressing.

Finally, the individual is able to rebuild a new life, incorporating the changes brought on by the chronic illness or injury. For example, we know a young man, Sam, who became a paraplegic as a result of a horseback-riding accident. An athletic man prior to his accident, he decided to take up paraskiing (Figure 17-1) as a sport following a period of rehabilitation. Although Sam was excited and pleased to be accomplishing new things, he still regretted the fact that he could no longer ski on his own two legs. Experiencing two very opposite emotions, such as pleasure and regret, may leave individuals feeling confused, helpless, and frustrated. They need to share these feelings with people they trust. These individuals will also be highly sensitive to how others treat them. If you or someone else regards the patient with pity or disgust, the patient will know it, and you or others will be unable to help the patient through this change process. Individuals need to know that even though they are changed, they are still worthwhile people. Focus on the positive—what they can do, what they can learn. Remind them that they will develop other social relationships, create a redeveloped self-esteem, and create a new social identity based on the changed "them."

CORE CONCEPTS   **MOBILITY** ─────────────

Impaired mobility is the most common problem with patients involved in rehabilitation. One of the priorities of rehabilitation is to get the patient to become as

Figure 17-1 Participation in Sports Before and After Accidental injury

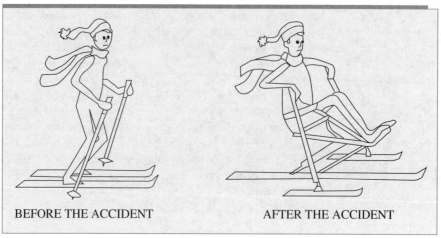

BEFORE THE ACCIDENT   AFTER THE ACCIDENT

mobile as possible. As a nurse, you should remember that there are positives and negatives associated with a patient's mobility.

1. Responsibilities of the nurse
   - Reinforcing correct techniques
   - Offering encouragement
   - Assisting with exercises
2. Mobility positives
   - Be physically active
   - Become physically fit
   - Build self-esteem
   - Contribute to developing an activity and rest schedule that will allow for continued improvement

It is important to note here that some patients with deteriorating neuromuscular diseases such as amyotrophic lateral sclerosis (ALS), multiple sclerosis (MS), and muscular dystrophy (MD) may not experience improvement despite physical activity. These patients should be encouraged to be realistic in their expectations. Mobility negatives include:

- Decreased mobility and physical activity can lead to increased stress
- Withdrawal and apathy will delay recovery
- Decreased social contact
- Decreased chance to control their interactions with others

For example, for a patient who is bedridden, the only people the patient sees are ones who come to see the patient. The patient has no control over getting out and initiating contact with others. His or her world shrinks to just a few individuals. Imagine seeing the same people over and over only when they want to see you!

Nurses need to be tuned in to changes in a patient's mobility status. It is important for you to have a mobility baseline assessment. Once the baseline is established, it will be easier for you to determine whether the patient is making progress. Remember, however, that some patients will not experience much progress. Patients with certain neuromuscular disorders may become more disabled over time regardless of intervention. It is important to remember that any progress (no matter how small) is positive. Whether your patient was formerly an Olympic athlete or relatively inactive, each individual will progress at different rates. For the former Olympic athlete who is now a quadriplegic, moving a finger may be a giant step. Adjusting your expectations to small steps is essential to your ability to become satisfied with rehabilitation nursing. You may see the occasional giant step, but they usually come slowly (Figure 17-2).

Figure 17-2   Changes May Come Slowly During
Rehabilitation

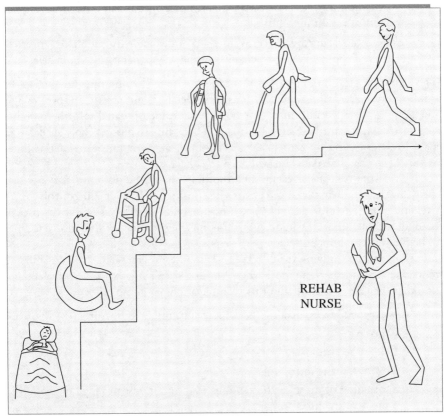

REHAB
NURSE

ESSENTIAL SKILLS	MOBILITY HISTORY ASSESSMENT

One way for you to establish a mobility baseline is through a mobility history and assessment. A number of good tools are available to help you gather this information. The basic areas of assessment include the following.

1. Vocational: Type of work, how much physical effort required

2. Home and family: Relationships, ability to perform home maintenance, such as cooking, cleaning, and other daily activities

3. Social: Leisure activities (past and present); how the illness has changed these

4. Sexual: Satisfaction with relationships; how the illness has affected sexual functioning

5. Activities of daily living:
   • Exercise: How much, what kind, how illness has affected methods of exercise choices
   • Sleep: How much, any problems
   • Nutrition: Eating habits; how has the illness affected them, intake of beverages, tobacco use
   • Medications: What is used regularly, prescription, and over-the-counter; any affect on mobility

6. Psychological: Any concerns, method of dealing with problems, effectiveness of coping strategies; changes in the way patient feels about self

The actual physical mobility assessment focuses on evaluating integumentary (the skin), pulmonary, cardiovascular, musculoskeletal, neurologic, and psychologic functioning. Detailed information is obtained and incorporated into the mobility history to construct a baseline assessment. There are established tools available to assist in determining the patient's risk for skin breakdown and functional abilities as part of the baseline data you will need to collect.

Once the baseline is established, nothing should be done for patients that they can do for themselves. Every activity, no matter how small, contributes to strengthening. The old adage of "Use it or lose it" is especially true for the patient needing rehabilitation. If you do everything for the patient, it will reinforce feelings of helplessness and hopelessness.

You will be studying the effects of immobility in great detail in your nursing fundamentals course. Remember when working with patients requiring rehabilitation that they are at risk for all of the complications of immobility:

• Weakened bones, making them more susceptible to fractures (osteoporosis)
• Constipation
• Urinary retention
• Muscle wasting (atrophy)
• Shortening of muscles and tendons resulting in loss of range of motion in joints (contractures)

- Pulmonary emboli (blood clots in the lungs)
- Pneumonia
- Skin breakdown

CORE CONCEPTS **IMPACT OF MOBILITY ON SEXUALITY**

Changes in mobility have the potential to alter sexual satisfaction. The sexual changes that occur may be a result of fatigue, loss of independence, or inability to adapt to illness or bodily changes. During the time a patient is hospitalized, sexual satisfaction is often overlooked, but potential problems and concerns should be addressed prior to discharge. If a patient requires extended rehabilitation, sexual outlets need to be provided. Caring staff members can provide for necessary privacy.

Changes in Self-Concept Patients and their partners frequently experience conflict as a result of added tensions listed below:

- Feeling that they are no longer desirable
- Fearing the reactions of their partner
- Fear may lead to a decrease in sex drive
- Possible withdrawal due to a fear of rejection

It is important for you to inform both the patient and the partner that this conflict is not abnormal. Your compassion and knowledge can help them both overcome the tension. Patients may also need information about how to make sexual activity a part of their new lives. Simple changes in positioning may be all that is needed for the patient to continue to have satisfying sexual relations. The patient may also need to know about ways of anchoring or removing catheters prior to intercourse. Sometimes, the timing of prescription medication (for spasticity, etc.) or taking a warm bath can enhance ability to perform. Your patients will have many questions about their changed sexuality, whether or not they ask. You need to provide an environment where the patient feels comfortable in expressing concerns. As a nursing student, you are not expected to be able to answer all questions and concerns, but you should be aware of the appropriate staff member to refer patients to for answers to their more intimate questions.

CORE CONCEPTS **MOTIVATING FOR CHANGE**

Rehabilitation involves significant changes in almost every area of life. Motivation is the key to successful rehabilitation. Individuals who have been extremely independent and believe that they are in control of their lives tend to participate more readily in the rehabilitation process. However, all patients will require external reinforcement and support, especially during the early stages of rehabilitation.

Enhance Motivation

1. Listening: Be sure that you listen intently to both the verbal and nonverbal cues that the patient gives you. Active listening will help you gain an understanding of exactly what might motivate the patient. Remember that we are all different. I might be motivated by an ice cream sundae; someone else might be motivated by some quiet time alone (Figure 17-3).

   • It is up to you to figure out what the patient's motivating factors are.
   • Remember you do not know what the patient is going through. Do you have the same disability? Do you think/feel/believe the same?
   • Do not assume you know what the patient is experiencing.

2. Actively participating: The patient needs to participate in goal setting. Work on establishing a goal that has meaning for the patient. For example, if the patient was an accomplished horsewoman, then perhaps a goal of getting back on horseback will have the most meaning. Do not assume that achieving any goal is impossible for the patient. There are numerous hippotherapy centers (therapeutic riding) across the country. Plastering the room with pictures of horses may help reinforce this goal for the patient. Often, if individuals have a strong enough desire to accomplish a

Figure 17-3 What Motivates the Patient May Be Very Different from What the Nurse Perceives as Motivating Factors

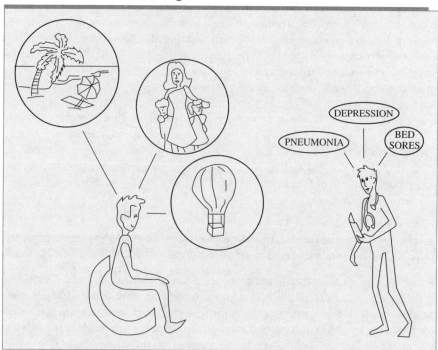

goal, nothing will stand in their way. We have seen numerous patients who were told that they would never walk again, walk, and even complete a marathon.

3. Making choices: Allow the patient to make personal choices. This will give the patient an increased sense of control. Even small choices or forced choices are still choices, for example, "Lucy, would you prefer to bathe in the morning or in the afternoon?" or "Would you prefer to wear your green shirt or the blue one?" or "Would you rather have cake or ice cream for dessert?" These choices might seem insignificant to you, but they can help your patient regain some semblance of control as well as enhance their feelings of self-worth.

4. Making a contract: A written or verbal contract can help the patient to work toward specific goals. Keeping a diary or journal can also help the patient to see progress when it is difficult to notice. For example, a patient might make a contract to walk one length of the parallel bars by the end of 1 month. Each step is significant—each pick-up, put-down of a foot. If the patient notes that "I took one step today," "four today," "six today," he or she can look back and see progress. Sometimes, the change is so small that it is difficult for the patient to see any improvement. With a diary or journal, the patient has no doubt that progress is being made.

5. Working together: Work with other team members. A group effort with everyone focusing on the same outcomes is best for the patient.

CORE CONCEPTS   **COMPLICATIONS**

Often, in chronic illness, complications cause more problems than the original disability. It is vital that you work hard to prevent, or at least recognize early, any potential complications. Not only do complications cause problems, but they also can cause more financial expenditure, increased discomfort, and potentially, death. Some examples of problems that can be prevented with good nursing care include:

- Dehydration
- Distended or full bladder
- Rectal impaction
- Incontinence of bladder or bowels
- Decubiti (bed sores)
- Deformities from disuse
- Emotional distress

You also need to keep an eye out for depression, isolation, and fatigue. You provide nursing care to the patient, but the patient decides whether to accept or refuse it. Let the patient and family know why you are doing what you are doing and why it is necessary. Explain about decreased mobility and physical changes that occur as a result such as contractures, what they are, and how they are preventable.

Rehabilitation is challenging in both chronic illness and injury. In order to succeed in rehabilitation nursing, a nurse must be patient, creative, and caring. You will need to develop an understanding of the rehabilitation experience from the patient's standpoint and be empathetic and genuine. The patient in need of rehabilitation will be extremely sensitive to rejection and will need your constant reassurance.

 ASK YOURSELF

1. Do you agree with the statement at the beginning of this chapter that says that our society emphasizes wholeness, youth, and beauty? Why or why not?

_____

_____

2. Do you think some form of rehabilitation is involved in the recovery of illness for every patient? Why or why not?

_____

_____

 CYBERLINKS: FLASH CARDS

Check to see what you now remember by making your own flash cards. Use the CD-ROM that accompanies your textbook to discover how to make flash cards for reviewing and retaining what you have learned.

 CONCEPT MAP WORD BANK

REHABILITATION
Nursing role
Patient need

TYPES
Mobility
Mobility assessment

IMPACT OF IMMOBILITY

MOTIVATING CHANGE

COMPLICATIONS

Refer to Concept Maps and Flash Cards on pages viii–ix for an explanation of how to create and use concept maps. In addition, the CD-ROM guides you through the construction of concept maps by providing a more detailed introduction, more illustrations of examples, and key steps to follow in designing your own maps.

Ageism

 ASK YOURSELF

1. Do you have any fears related to your own aging?

   _____

   _____

2. Do you think that dementia is something that happens to all old people eventually? Why or why not?

   _____

   _____

 CYBERLINKS

Interactive Did you know that in your lifetime, most of society's health care dollars will be spent on care for the elderly? However, not all elderly individuals need care or the same extent of care. At **www.healthanswers.com,** an informative and useful tool, an extended care needs assessment, is available.

Supplemental **www.LPNresources.com** can help enhance your learning by leading you to discover other links with even more information about the topic you are studying.

It is no secret that the population of older adults is increasing. According to the 2000 United States census, there are approximately 35 million adults 65 years of age and older. By 2020, it is estimated that this number will increase to 59 million, including approximately 266,000 individuals who will be 100 years old or older. You should, therefore, realize that a high percentage of your patients in the near future will be older adults. This will be true in most settings where you will be doing clinicals (except OB and pediatrics!!!).

CORE CONCEPTS	DEFINING OLD AGE

We begin our discussion of aging by exploring the meaning of *old, elderly, aged, senior citizen.* The first, most obvious observation, is that "old" is a relative term. To the 3-year-old child, anyone who is 5 years old is old; and this view tends to continue through the ages. Old applies only to those who are ahead of us in birthdays. The second observation is that many terms and phrases are used to refer to basically the same group of individuals. There are two objective ways to describe old.

1. *Chronological age:* Selects an age as "old" and compares an individual's age to this number as a standard. Since the 1965 amendment to the Social Security Act, 65 has been the standard definition of old age. In addition, 65 was established as the minimum age for Medicare health care benefits, while the Age Discrimination in Employment Act establishes 70 as mandatory retirement age. Many commercial establishments also use chronological age to offer certain customers special benefits such as discounts on purchases. For example, 50, 55, and 60 are common ages businesses have selected as the number that fits a customer into the "senior citizen discount" group. So, it is this chronological age that tells us when to have a birthday party. It is the age that makes us eligible to vote, to a number we put on a form that has a space for "age," and provides the opportunity to get a free coffee or soft drink at one of the many fast food restaurants. Although chronological age offers quick and convenient ways to determine who is "old," it does not give any indication of the individual's functioning or performance skills and abilities.

2. *Functional age:* Also referred to by some as biologic age. This approach requires individual assessment on several levels rather than a number. It is not an easy concept to measure or define in a few words.

In an attempt to create more uniformity, there is a trend in gerontology (the study of aging) to use a single set of terms as reference points for definitions of old (Table 18-1). However, these definitions are not universal yet.

Another term worth exploring is *ageism.* This is a term that was coined by Dr. Robert Butler, President and CEO of The International Longevity Center, in 1968. He equated the stereotyping of and discrimination against the elderly with racism and sexism that involve discrimination because of race or gender (Butler, 1969).

TABLE 18-1	Various Definitions of Age	
Age (years)	**Category**	**Definition**
65–74	Early old age	Young–old
75–84	Middle old age	Middle–old
85+	Late old age	Old–old, frail elderly

You have, no doubt, identified ageism in others. How about in yourself? Remember the next time you are assigned to care for an older patient and you groan ever so softly: "Oh no. Not another geriatric!", you too are expressing ageism.

Ageism is a complex subject that is easier to define than it is to understand. Stereotyping of the elderly—assuming certain things are true because of the person's age—can lead to inferior medical and nursing care. All too often, the elderly patient's problems are seen as a direct result of the aging process and thus assumed by some health care workers to be inevitable and untreatable. In one way, ageism might be seen as an "occupational hazard" for health care workers since we see so many older patients who are ill, frail, confused, and hospitalized, or in long-term care facilities. We fall into the generalization trap and do not separate facts from myths. A major myth is that all older adults are like those we see in our daily practice. Statistics tell us that only 5% of the older population are actually in long-term care facilities; the other 95% continue to live in the community. Additional myths (Farrell, 1990) are listed in Table 18-2.

Research has provided us with some disturbing information regarding the elderly and health care, including the fact that elderly patients do not receive as much attention from health professionals as younger patients do. The elderly are seldom successful in having their concerns addressed. However, this long-standing situation is changing. One reason for the evolving change is that, although mainstream advertisements of all forms (TV, paper, radio, magazines), are aimed at the young, the focus of many ads now target older adults. A second reason is the explosion of information aimed at the elderly. Books, TV programs, special segments of news broadcasts, popular magazine articles, specialty magazines, organizations, and the Internet are readily accessed by the older generation. These sources provide the elderly with vast amounts of information on such topics as pain control, dietary needs, activity, sexuality, end-of-life decisions, what to expect (and sometimes demand)

TABLE 18-2   Common Myths About Aging

- Old age is a disease.
- Old age begins at 65.
- Senility is part of aging.
- Old people are all alike.
- Older people are usually unhappy.
- Older people are set in their ways and unable to change.
- Older people have no power.
- Older people are sexless.
- Most old people are poor.
- People become more religious as they age.
- In general, older people are lonely and socially isolated.
- Most older workers cannot work as effectively as younger workers.

from health care providers. The list goes on. The point is, the elderly population is growing in number and, at the same time, becoming more active participants in many aspects of their lives. They are not willing to quietly accept less than that received by the "younger" generation.

CORE CONCEPTS | **PROMINENT THEORIES OF WHY WE AGE**

For all cultures, and through the millennia, the process of aging has been of great interest. Currently, there are at least seven prominent theories of why we age (Table 18-3). We will look at the basic premise of each. Remember that each theory is complex and has various amounts of research to support it.

1. *Immunity and autoimmunity*
   - Explains aging on basis that the immune system begins to develop antibodies to destroy older cells that have mutated and are unrecognizable
   - Decline of the immune system contributes to the development of age-related diseases
2. *Cross-linkage*
   - Based on chemical reactions creating damage to deoxyribonucleic acid (DNA)
   - If DNA strand is unable to repair itself, cell death will occur, or abnormal cells will be produced
3. *Free radicals*
   - Thought that environmental pollutants cause molecules to break off cells
   - Believed that these free-floating electrons will then damage various cell structures
4. *Wear and tear*
   - Proposes that the body has a time schedule and wears out as its time winds down
   - Stress and damage play a role in this theory

TABLE 18-3 | **Common Theories of Aging**

- Immunity and autoimmunity
- Cross-linkage
- Free radicals
- Wear and tear
- Nutritional restriction
- Error
- Biologic programming

5. *Nutritional restrictions*
   - Based on research that shows that laboratory animals maintained on restricted diets outlive their regular-diet counterparts
6. *Error*
   - Thought to be due to cells receiving wrong messages from the cell nucleus resulting in cell mutations
7. *Biologic programming*
   - Claims that life expectancy is governed by heredity
   - Humans have a preset biologic clock that determines the onset of aging and life span

The fact that there are so many theories of aging, each with its own research base, tells us that there are apparently many factors involved in aging and that eternal youth is not possible. Aging just occurs! If nothing else, there are three accepted characteristics of aging according to Matteson, McConnell, & Linton (1997):

1. Aging is common to all members of a given species.
2. Aging is aggressive.
3. Aging is deleterious, ultimately leading to death.

In addition to theories that try to explain why humans experience specific physical changes with aging, various theories exist that describe developmental changes that occur at various stages of life. A few of the more prominent developmental theories are by Erikson, Peck, Havighurst, Ebersole, and Butler.

If aging is inevitable, are there changes we can make to prolong the lives of us and our patients? Like the many theories of aging, there are many theories about how to affect longevity including diet, exercise, vitamins, antioxidants, and anti-aging therapies. Hayflick (1994) believes that no study has ever shown, without a shadow of a doubt, that aging can be stopped, slowed, or reversed or the life span changed by "any medical intervention, lifestyle change, nutritional factor, or other substance . . ." (p. 313). Hayflick notes, "We still do not know how to slow the aging process in humans, but we do know how to increase our life expansion by eliminating or reducing causes of death" (p. 341).

Many systematic, scientific studies have been conducted concerning the process of aging. After reviewing the data produced by the Baltimore Longitudinal Study of Aging (BLSA), Hayflick states that one major factor is apparent, "Older humans show a greater range of individual variation in many physiological and psychological measurements than do younger adults" (Hayflick, 1994, p. 140). The notion that all old people are essentially the same is a myth! Everyone ages differently and at an individual rate. Think of your parents or grandparents. How are they aging?

Nonetheless, from the BLSA and other research, we are learning a great deal about the aging process. Some of the findings support long-held beliefs, while a great deal of the new findings are shattering many others. (Thus, for some the study has come to be called the "myth buster.")

A small sample of current information on aging from the BLSA follows.

- Predominant characteristics of old age are: (a) a reduced capacity to adapt, (b) reduced speed of performance, and (c) an increased susceptibility to disease.
- Maximum heart rate diminishes with age—this is not a health problem.
- When disease-free, the heart of an older person pumps just about as well as a young healthy heart.
- Short-term memory declines with age.
- Vocabulary scores do not change with age.
- In the absence of disease, personality traits remain essentially the same throughout life.
- The common belief that as people age they become crankier or mellower is a myth.
- Lifestyle habits, such as low-cholesterol diets and not smoking, can influence the development or progression of some age-associated diseases, but there is no evidence of a direct effect on the fundamental aging process.
- Relative frequency of sexual activity does not change with age.
- The ability to identify odors declines earlier and more rapidly in men than in women.

The BLSA, and other research on aging, is providing data that distinguish between age-related normal changes and age-related illnesses. Table 18-4 lists some examples. Again, although there are many age-related conditions, they are not a part of the normal aging process. Hayflick (1994) points out this distinction between normal age changes and age-related illnesses. He writes that "physiological losses character-

| TABLE 18-4 | Normal Changes with Aging Versus Age-Related Illness |

Age-Related Normal Changes	Age-Related Illnesses
• Loss of strength and stamina	• Cancer
• New hair growth in ears and nose	• Heart disease
• Decline in short-term memory	• Alzheimer's disease
• Balding	• Strokes
• Loss of bone mass	• Dementia
• Decrease in height	• Arthritis
• Hearing decline	• Parkinson's disease
• Reduction in visual acuity	
• Renal blood flow and glomerular filtration rate (GFR)	
• Liver spots on skin	

istic of aging eventually occur in the cells, tissues, and organs of all older members of a species, while changes due to disease occur only in some members" (p. 48). Note that although many of the normal age-related changes increase the older adult's risk to specific diseases, normal aging and age-related disease are not the same things! This is often the basis for the confusion that exists about two terms that might be incorrectly interchanged—geriatrics and gerontology. Geriatrics is the study and practice of dealing with elderly patients who have an age-related illness or condition; gerontology is the term to indicate the study and practice of normal, age-related problems and changes. Although they are two distinct areas, it is possible to be dealing with both areas in the same patient.

At times, a common difficulty for caregivers of the older adult is deciding if the patient is becoming ill. A good rule of thumb is the appearance of a functional loss in "active, previously unimpaired elders" even though there are " no typical symptoms and signs of disease" (Besdine, 1990, p. 3). In other words, when an older adult suddenly demonstrates problems with mobility, cognition, continence, or nutrition, there is cause for further assessment and evaluation to identify the source of the problem. For many older individuals, loss of functional ability may not be seen until the individual is under stress, either physical or emotional. The most common functions to be affected are cognition (ability to know and learn), memory, and ability to remain continent or walk. Loss of one specific function (especially suddenly) is often the red flag of illness. So, for an individual who is 80 years old, well oriented, and continent, sudden incontinence may be the initial symptom of pneumonia. The older individual is more likely to demonstrate a sudden onset of confusion with an illness than the onset of fever as you might find in a younger person. We had one elderly gentleman in long-term care who used to lean to the side in his wheelchair whenever he had a urinary tract infection! Remember that in the older person, there is usually a poor correlation between the type and severity of problem (functional ability) they present and the etiology (source of the problem).

| CORE CONCEPTS | **TWO COMMON ASSESSMENTS SPECIFIC TO THE ELDERLY** |

As with many distinct patient populations, there are a number of assessments specific to the elderly. Two of the most common and initially most useful ones are ADL and IADL assessments.

1. *Activities of daily living (ADLs):* Activities necessary for self-care such as bathing, toileting, dressing, and transferring. There are a number of ADL assessment tools. One well-known ADL tool is the **Katz Index.** This tool assesses patients' actual performance on ADLs versus what they do that requires help provided in controlled settings. Another tool used to measure ADLs is the **Barthel Index.** This tool assigns numbers to various activities based on the patient's degree of independence. If you are working in long-term care or in an in-hospital rehabilitation unit, the assessment tool being

used is the Minimum Data Set (MDS), which needs to be completed on every new resident within 14 days of admission. This not only reviews a resident's functional abilities in regards to ADLs but looks at at least 18 areas of concern.

2. *Instrumental activities of daily living (IADLs):* A must for the elderly patient living in the community. This is an expansion of ADLs. Assesses items such as ability to carry out various household activities such as shopping or taking of medications.

There are multiple issues associated with the older adult. In the following sections we will explore several specific ones: urinary incontinence, polypharmacy, abuse, restraints, sexuality, and dementia.

| CORE CONCEPTS | **URINARY INCONTINENCE** |

Urinary incontinence (UI) is considered the involuntary escape of urine to such a degree that it causes a problem. Nurses usually only think of urinary incontinence as something that occurs in elderly, nonambulatory, institutionalized patients. Research has, however, revealed that in addition to the 1.5 million incontinent nursing home residents, UI occurs in 15% to 30% of noninstitutionalized individuals over age 60. For all of these individuals, UI has mental, physical, social, and economic consequences. Individuals with UI must cope with problems of skin breakdown, urinary tract infections, depression, and social isolation to the tune of about $15 billion annually. UI is the leading cause of admissions to long-term care facilities.

Like so many other situations, successful interventions for UI depend on identifying its etiology. For too long, this etiology was considered the individual's old age. However, UI is no longer considered a natural part of aging. Rather, at least 10 causes for UI have been identified (Table 18-5). UI can also be placed into a type. Each type provides a description of the circumstances when the incontinence occurs.

There are five types of urinary incontinence:

1. *Urge incontinence*
   • Involuntary incontinence that occurs as soon as a strong need to void is identified.

| TABLE 18-5 | **Etiologies of Urinary Incontinence** |

• Urinary tract infections	• Weak bladder sphincters
• Vaginal infections and irritation	• Neurologic disorders
• Constipation	• Immobility
• Medications	• Benign prostatic hypertrophy
• Weak bladder muscles	• Impaired cognition

- Frequently associated with involuntary detrusor (muscle of the bladder) contractions.
- May be accompanied by frequency and nocturia (having to void three or more times during the night) as well.
- These individuals cannot get to the bathroom fast enough.

2. *Stress incontinence*
   - Involuntary incontinence that occurs with increased intra-abdominal pressure without detrusor muscle contraction.
   - Usually associated with weakened pelvic muscles or a damaged bladder neck.
   - Multiple births, obesity, and menopause are frequent causes.
   - Examples are coughing, sneezing, laughing, assuming an upright position, and physical exertion such as exercise or lifting heavy objects.

3. *Overflow incontinence*
   - Incontinence occurs when the bladder is not completely emptied, usually due to an obstruction of some kind, and urine dribbles out to prevent bladder damage.
   - This type is more common in males, especially those with an enlarged prostate.

4. *Functional incontinence*
   - Involuntary incontinence that occurs in individuals with normal bladder functioning who have difficulty getting to the bathroom.
   - Seen in patients with cognitive disorders and those with impaired physical mobility.

5. *Transient incontinence* (may include any of the above types)
   - Incontinence that is associated with an acute treatable condition that, once corrected, eliminates the incontinence.
   - Causes could be delirium (temporary confusion), urinary tract infection or inflammation, depression, fecal impaction, and certain medications.

If you look at the table of etiologies, you will see that the types of UI are associated with specific etiologies. As mentioned, benign prostatic hyperplasia (BPH) or fecal impaction can contribute to overflow incontinence, detrusor hyperreflexia from a stroke can create urge incontinence, and a severe head injury may lead to functional incontinence. Therefore, UI can be caused by pathologic, anatomic, or physiologic factors and, at times, more than one factor may be operating.

Because the etiologies for each type of UI vary, so will interventions. One of the greater challenges for the nurse is to convince patients that they do not have to tolerate UI. Urinary incontinence is not considered normal or an accepted part of aging. Once individuals accept this fact, they need to discuss their situation with their physician and determine the etiology. The problem, however, is that there are reports that many physicians do not respond when informed of the incontinence. If this happens, it means that you need to help the patient educate his or her physi-

TABLE 18-6	Treatment Options for Urinary Incontinence

- Medications
- Surgery
- Bladder training
- Pelvic muscle (Kegel) exercises
- Biofeedback
- Catheterization
    Intermittent
    Indwelling
- External collection devices
- Absorbent products

cian or find another one (preferably a urologist or gerontologist). Once the patient has an understanding physician, the diagnostic process will start with a history and physical exam with special emphasis on the urinary system. Based on the history and physical, any number of specific urologic tests may be conducted from the simple to the complex.

Identification of the type of UI and the specific etiology is the foundation for treatment choice, which again will range from simple to complex. The most common treatment modalities of UI are listed in Table 18-6.

CORE CONCEPTS | POLYPHARMACY

Many elderly individuals take more than one medication due to multiple medical conditions. Polypharmacy is the name given to the use of numerous medications at the same time. The latest statistics show that, although Americans over the age of 65 make up only 12.4% of the population, they take 30% of all prescription medications and 40% of the over-the-counter (OTC) medications. This often involves taking four to five prescription medications concurrently.

There are a number of reasons why polypharmacy can have harmful effects for the elderly. Aging affects the way that the body absorbs, metabolizes, and excretes drugs, making the elderly more susceptible to adverse drug reactions and causing them to have unexpected responses to certain medications. Polypharmacy is the number one reason for adverse drug reactions. Combining a number of these drugs leaves the patient more prone to drug interactions as well. The more drugs individuals take, the more likely they are to experience drug interactions. Having multiple chronic illnesses compounds the problem, as disease will also alter the individual's response to drugs.

The elderly have more of a tendency to visit a number of different health practitioners, obtaining prescriptions from each one. Then, they may have the prescriptions filled at different pharmacies, making it difficult for the pharmacist to identify possible drug interactions. In addition, elderly husbands and wives may also share prescriptions if they have similar symptoms.

Keep all of these things in mind when obtaining a medication history on your patients. Be sure you ask about the use of over-the-counter medications as well. Many individuals do not think of listing such common OTCs as ibuprofen, milk of magnesia, and Benadryl, and yet these can interact with many medications. Medication self-administration is an important area of teaching for the LPN/LVN as well as the PN/VN nursing student.

| CORE CONCEPTS | ABUSE |

Elder abuse (which is also referred to as elder mistreatment) is a very serious and prevalent problem that can occur at several levels. Like child abuse, the most obvious form is physical abuse such as slapping, hitting, and pushing. Physical abuse can also include neglect such as lack of physical care, inappropriate physical care, and inadequate nutrition. Physical abuse provides objective evidence. However, other less obvious forms of abuse include verbal abuse, exploitation, financial and psychological abuse, and sexual abuse. Although more literature is appearing on elder abuse, it remains a topic with little research. We do not know much about such topics as the nature of the problem, its causes, characteristics of the abuser and the elder, and aspects of prevention. Table 18-7 identifies factors for both the elder and the abuser that increase the possibility of elder abuse.

Because nurses have such frequent contact with elderly patients, they are often the first ones to suspect some form of abuse. With few exceptions, almost every state requires that anyone who is aware of elder mistreatment, or has strong reason to suspect it, is required by law to report it to proper authorities. In most states this authority has the title of Adult Protective Services (APS), and its number appears in local papers and government listings in telephone books, and can also be located through the telephone information operator. Once notified, it is up to the authorities to investigate and take appropriate action. If, however, you have reported a sit-

TABLE 18-7	Risk Factors for Elder Abuse		
Risk Factor		**Victim**	**Abuser**
• History of mental illness		•	•
• Shared living arrangements		•	•
• Family history of violence		•	•
• Isolation		•	
• Stressful events			•
• Poor health		•	
• Cognitive impairment		•	
• Substance abuse			•
• Dependency		•	•
• Lack of financial resources		•	•

Source: Lynch, S. H. (1997). Elder abuse: What to look for, how to intervene. *AJN 97(I):*29.

uation and continue to see or suspect that the mistreatment is continuing, report it again! History has demonstrated that problems are not always corrected in a timely manner. If abuse is suspected within a long-term care facility, reporting may be done to the nursing home administrative staff and then to the state health department and to the local ombudsman for further investigation. Abuse may also occur within acute care facilities and needs to be reported to the hospital administration.

The dynamics of elder abuse are complex. One factor, however, that seems to be related to mistreatment is caregiver stress. Some research has shown a correlation between the two. If the nurse identifies caregiver stress and provides interventions to relieve that stress, abuse may be avoided. In addition, some neglect problems may be corrected with caregiver teaching. Table 18-8 illustrates other intervention strategies. If you are involved in a home health situation, you need to be able to recognize signs of caregiver stress. Signs of depression, irritability, complaints of sleeping

---

TABLE 18-8 | **Strategies for Intervention(s) with Elder Abuse**

Patient Refuses Treatment
- Allow patient to make choice of refusal.
- Remain nonjudgmental.
- Educate regarding available services and incidence and severity of abuse increasing over time.
- Provide emergency contact numbers
- Contact Adult Protective Services (APS) in accordance with state law.

Patient Lacks Mental Capacity
- Contact APS.
- Arrange for provisions to be made regarding guardianship, financial assistance, foster care, and court proceedings.

Patient Accepts Intervention
- Examine positive and negative aspects of change.
- Discuss safety options, such as hospitalization, changing living arrangements, obtaining orders of protection, changing locks, and pressing charges.
- As appropriate, refer to hospital social services, home health care, respite care, education, chaplains, and supportive counseling.
- Refer to APS for assistance contacting appropriate resources, such as case workers, counselors, and legal services.
- Allow patient to express feelings and fears.

For Abusers
- Remove victim from danger, relieving abuser of caregiving responsibility and stress.
- Provide support services, such as counseling, education, and rehabilitation for drug or alcohol abuse.

Source: Lynch, S. H. (1997). Elder abuse: What to look for, how to intervene. *AJN 97*(1):29.

difficulties, and the smell of alcohol on the caregiver are often indicators that the caregiving role is becoming too burdensome and requires intervention.

Keep in mind that it is not always someone else who carries out the mistreatment. There is a form of mistreatment classified as *self-neglect*. The individual does not seek out medical care, refuses care, is noncompliant, has poor nutrition, and lives in a dirty environment. All these actions are a result of the individual's choice. These situations often create more challenges than those situations in which another person causes the mistreatment. Until declared legally incompetent, the older person has the right to accept or reject care, including help with nutrition, medication, and living conditions. Many ethical factors need to be considered before making the decision to seek legal intervention. Nurses, as well as families, struggle with issues of self-neglect. There is no one or easy answer to the problem of elder abuse in any form.

| CORE CONCEPTS | **RESTRAINTS** |

Over the years, nursing's answer to the elderly who were cognitively impaired and had behaviors that were considered potentially or actually dangerous to the individual (falling, wandering away, pulling at various tubes, etc.) was to use restraints. Restraint devices at that time included such things as special restraint vests, sheets, belts, side rails, wrist restraints, and geri-chairs. Most of the time, the devices were utilized solely at the nurse's discretion. (If the nurse was not satisfied with the effectiveness of the restraints, she or he would often ask and receive from the physician an order for some sort of chemical restraint such as sedatives and tranquilizers.) Despite their use, however, the problems that restraints were supposed to cure have remained! Eventually, some nurses began to doubt the wisdom of restraints, and research to explore the consequences of restraints began. It soon became apparent that the use of restraints created as many, or more, problems as they were intended to prevent. As nurses began to doubt the wisdom of restraints, so did society. Many individuals and groups became involved in issues regarding the elderly. One of the most recent and influential developments was the *Omnibus Budget Reconciliation Act,* commonly known as OBRA, passed by Congress in 1987. This legislation addressed many issues regarding quality of care in long-term care facilities, including residents' rights. Chief among these rights is the right to be free of restraint (physical and chemical).

When the legislation regarding restraints became law, most nurses in long-term care facilities threw up their hands and said it could not be done, that the elderly "need restraints for their own good." It has not been an easy road, but time has proven those nurses wrong. With very few exceptions, safe, competent nursing care does not have to include the use of restraints.

One of the most striking changes with OBRA has been that the use of restraints now requires a physician's written order. The order must state the specific type of restraint to be used (e.g., vest or waist). The corresponding charting regarding use of restraints is extensive. For example, the charting must indicate not only the reason for the restraints (specific behavior) but indicate what alternative interventions were tried prior to the restraints. (Note that "lack of staff" to watch the

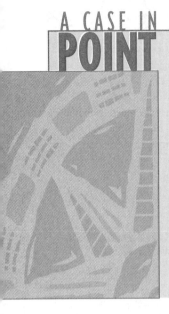

A CASE IN
POINT

Leona, a 95-year-old widow in failing health but mentally competent, lives alone in her own home. Her husband recently died of lung cancer. Leona and her husband had been married for 65 years and had no children. Soon after Leona's husband died, her niece decided that she should no longer live on her own and that she should be placed in a nursing home. Leona knows that it has become harder for her to take care of herself. However, she refuses to leave her home of 65 years. She says she wants to die in her own bed, in her own home. One evening, Leona takes a dose of barbituates and dies in her sleep. Since Leona is 95, the coroner does not do an autopsy and rules that Leona died of natural causes.

patient is not an acceptable reason for restraints.) The documentation must also include such data as the times the patient was monitored, the patient's response to the restraints, care given during the restrained period, and reasons for prolonged use. The usual guidelines are that restraints must be checked every 30 minutes and removed every 2 hours for the resident or patient to be repositioned, toileted, and offered food or water.

Guidelines for chemical restraints have become just as extensive. Physicians must review their orders for any psychoactive medications, such as tranquilizers, on a regular basis and explain why the continued use of them is required. They must specify the type of behavior that will require the use of the medication. The nursing staff must then document observations of patient behavior that required the use of the chemical restraint. Medicating a patient as well as physically restraining is considered a "double restraint" and is viewed very closely by the health department, which monitors the conditions within all long-term care facilities.

Today, there are some long-term care facilities that are almost totally restraint free. Although OBRA addressed care in long-term care facilities, its influence has spread to other areas such as acute care facilities, adult day care, and home care. These areas of care, including various levels of intensive care units, are realizing that alternative actions to restraints are desirable and possible.

| CORE CONCEPTS | SEXUALITY |

Although definitions of sexuality vary, they all convey the idea that there are more than physical activities associated with sex. It "encompasses the manner in which individuals use their own roles, relationships, values, customs, and maleness or femaleness" (O'Toole, 1997, p. 1473). Figure 18-1 indicates major factors that influence sexuality. For many individuals born in the first half of the twentieth century, sexuality was associated only with the sexual act. They were raised to believe that sex was an activity for married couples only; and after the childbearing years, sex was generally considered unnecessary and/or impossible. When it was discovered that an older man or woman wanted to or actually participated in sexual activities, he or she was labeled as a "dirty old man" or a "dirty old woman." This generation of individuals is today's patients, who are in the age range of about 55 years and older. One of the major mistakes nurses make with this group is assuming that because of the patients' backgrounds, issues of sexuality and sexual activity can be deleted from their care. This is a mistake! Although many patients in this age group may in fact "be done" with sexual intercourse, they may have many concerns regarding their sexuality (Table 18-9).

Needless to say, during the second half of this century, society's attitude toward sex has changed. Sex before, outside of, and without marriage for a large

Figure 18-1 Major Variables Influencing a Patient's Sexuality

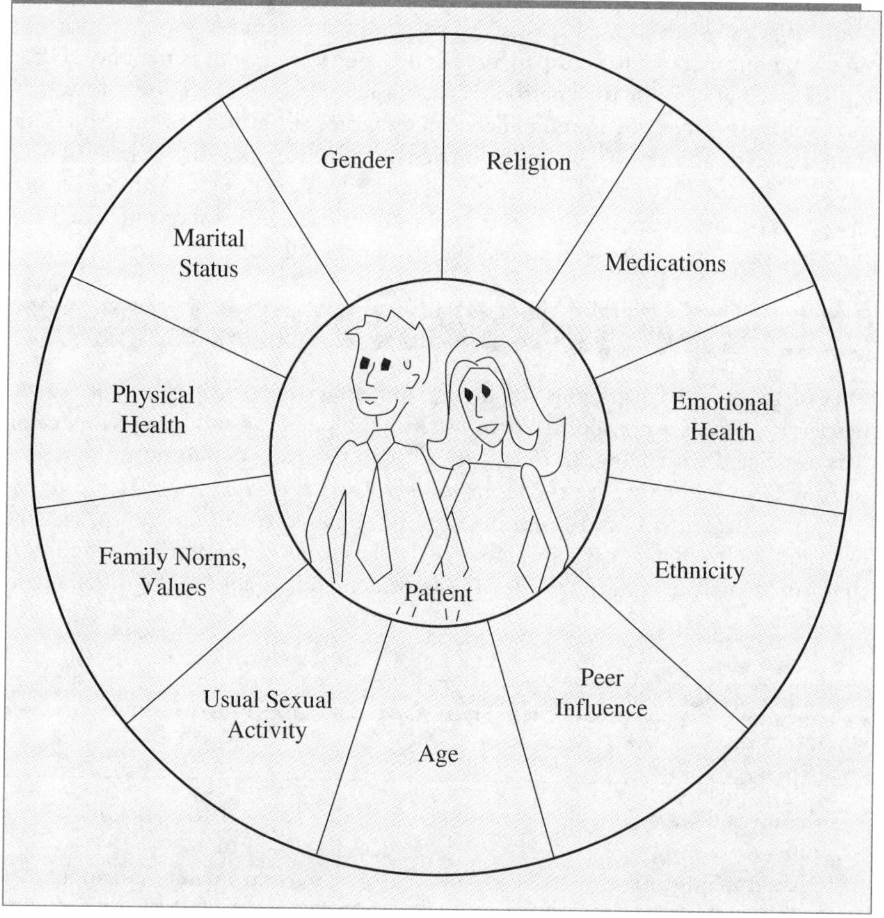

TABLE 18-9	Common Sexuality Issues of the Older Adult

- Vaginal dryness
- Decreased sexual arousal
- Sex and heart problems
- Effects of medication on libido
- Being hugged and touched less by others
- Altered physical appearance
- Impotence
- Fear of revealing that they are not heterosexual

portion of society is now more acceptable. In addition, many types of sexual activities between and among men and women, if not accepted, are tolerated. The oncoming generation of older patients will not be the stereotypical heterosexual.

Despite this change in society, many health care workers ignore, neglect, or refuse to acknowledge sexuality issues. If you find yourself in this group, you are not providing optimal care to your patients nor are you treating your patient holistically. Nurses must look at the total person. For example, assessment and care for two serious problems—acquired immune deficiency syndrome (AIDS) and sexually transmitted diseases (STDs)—may not be carried out. Both are health problems in older adults. You are encouraged, therefore, to take steps to improve care. This may involve expanding your reading on the subject, attending workshops, or discussing the topic with colleagues who are well versed on the subject.

CORE CONCEPTS DEMENTIA AND DELIRIUM

One of the major frustrations for family and caregivers of the elderly is "senile" behavior. *Senile* is a nonspecific term used by the public to indicate mental disorders associated with aging. In today's medical and nursing publications the term is seldom used. Rather, we see the terms *dementia* and *delirium*.

True dementia is an irreversible form of impaired cognition with progressive deterioration in mental capacity. Table 18-10 lists some of the common conditions that can create the clinical manifestations of dementia. Table 18-11 differentiates

TABLE 18-10	Conditions That Can Create Manifestations of Dementia

- Alzheimer's disease	- HIV-related dementia
- Trauma	- Brain tumors
- Huntington's disease	- Multi-infarct dementia

TABLE 18-11	Characteristics of Dementia and Delirium	
Characteristic	**Dementia**	**Delirium**
Other names	• Organic brain syndrome • Often called by the etiology • Old terminology—senility	• Acute confessional state
Common etiologies	• Senile dementia of the Alzheimer type (SDAT) • Multicerebral infarcts • Long-term alcoholism	• Metabolic imbalances • Medication • Massive infection • Prolonged, high fever • Alcohol intoxication and alcohol withdrawal
Onset	• Gradual, insidious; often not noticed until clinical manifestations are severe	• Fast; recognition that individual is not acting normal is readily apparent
Course	• Progressive; almost always irreversible • Aphasia • Anomia	• Reversible with prompt identification and treatment of etiology; "finding words" • Usually rapid speech

between dementia and delirium. Although behaviors associated with dementia and delirium can be very similar, it is important to distinguish between the two. Delirium has etiologies that can be treated, and the impaired cognition, if not completely reversed, can be improved. Understanding the differences in the two conditions will help you in counseling family members and in developing appropriate nursing interventions.

As discussed in the beginning of this chapter, the elderly will be a large portion of all patients in the health care system in the near future. This chapter has presented a few of the major issues associated with gerontological nursing.

STOP ASK YOURSELF

It has been said that "We don't grow old, we become old when we stop growing."

1. How do you interpret this statement?

2. Do you think you will be able to control the way in which you age?

_____

_____

 CYBERLINKS: FLASH CARDS ⎯⎯⎯⎯⎯⎯⎯⎯⎯⎯

Check to see what you now remember by making your own flash cards. Use the CD-ROM that accompanies your textbook to discover how to make flash cards for reviewing and retaining what you have learned.

 CONCEPT MAP WORD BANK ⎯⎯⎯⎯⎯⎯⎯⎯⎯⎯

AGEISM
Definition
Theories
ASSESSMENT
AGE ISSUES

Refer to Concept Maps and Flash Cards on pages viii–ix for an explanation of how to create and use concept maps. In addition, the CD-ROM guides through the construction of concept maps by providing a more detailed introduction, more illustrations of examples, and key steps to follow in designing your own maps.

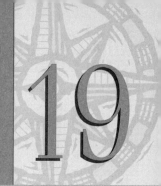

Sexuality

19

ASK YOURSELF

1. Are you comfortable with your own sexuality? Why or why not?

2. Do you think that you would be uncomfortable discussing the patient's sexuality (as it relates to illness) with him or her or with one gender in particular? Why or why not?

CYBERLINKS

Interactive www.thriveonline.com has numerous tools and quizzes that will assist you personally and as a caregiver to deal with some of the complex issues related to sexuality. For example, once at this site, scroll down to sexuality, and click onto tools and quizzes. You can learn about sexually transmitted diseases (STDs), identify which are most common in the place you live, and complete a questionnaire that will help you to understand your own risk.

Supplemental www.LPNresources.com can help enhance your learning by leading you to discover other links with more information about topics you are studying.

We often wonder why it is that nurses can easily ask patients questions about their most intimate bodily functions, but they are unwilling to ask questions of a sexual nature. If we consider such human needs as breathing, eating, and sleeping important, then why isn't sexual functioning (a primary physiologic need) of equal importance? If we are going to practice holistic nursing in which we look at the total being, then we must consider patients' sexuality as part of their complex needs. All of us are sexual beings. All of us wonder how changes in our health status might impact our sexual functioning. Unfortunately, some patients are afraid to ask questions about their sexual health, and as a rule, if the patient doesn't ask, chances are the nurse is not about to bring up the subject. It is equally bothersome to us that many nursing faculties avoid teaching students about sexuality. They may teach the pathophysiology, or even discuss coping with bodily changes, but few require their students to ask patients in-depth questions about sexuality in clinical settings. Is sexuality so taboo a subject that most health care providers refuse to discuss it? Is it more embarrassing than bowel movements and catheters (Figure 19-1)?

CORE CONCEPTS   THE ROLE OF SEXUALITY IN HEALTH CARE

We believe that human sexuality must be incorporated into high-quality health care. Perhaps you are thinking that nurses do discuss sexual health. We did a short, unscientific poll of our colleagues. Seven had had hysterectomies within the last 5 years. Not one of them had been told anything about sexual functioning! They had been told about estrogen therapy, staple and suture removal, and activity level. Not one was told when to resume sexual relations, how sensations might be different, or that lubricants might be needed for vaginal dryness. We find this to be an example of just how poorly informed patients often are about the sexual consequences of their treatment or surgery.

Sexuality is a vital part of our everyday lives. It is important to our relationships, self-esteem, and concept of our maleness or femaleness. Childbearing is also important to the psychological and social identity of many women. How can we ignore such an important part of the lives of our patients?

Figure 19-1 Students Can Be Embarrassed to Ask Questions About Sexuality

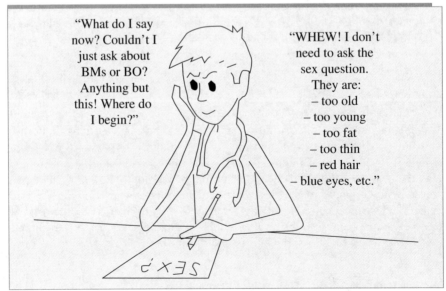

CORE CONCEPTS   **YOUR SEXUAL CONCERNS**

It is quite common for nurses to feel uncomfortable counseling patients with sexual issues. Some concerns include:

- Believing that you do not have the knowledge base or the skills that you need to respond to patients with sexual concerns
- Feeling uncomfortable with your own sexuality and being afraid that you will not be able to handle the concerns of your patient
- Believing that sex is something that you do not openly discuss with anyone

All of these concerns can be dealt with. You need to be willing to work on opening yourself to learning more about sexuality.

ESSENTIAL SKILLS   **GUIDING PATIENTS WITH THEIR SEXUAL CONCERNS**

To guide our patients, we have to ask questions. Don't be afraid to ask questions that relate to sexuality. If you don't ask, you will never know whether your patient has sexual concerns or not, because most patients will not directly bring the subject up themselves. Examples of how you might approach a patient about any sexual concerns are:

- Ask patients whether they have any sexual concerns.
- Ask how their illness has affected their sexuality.
- Ask if any of their medications are interfering with sexual performance.
- Ask if they have any questions or any concerns regarding changes in their sexuality.

To help patients with sexual concerns, you have to ask the questions. Many times patients can read nurses' nonverbal behavior and know that they are not willing to answer their questions about sex. They sometimes test nurses by asking related questions to see how they will respond. They may point out a person on a soap opera and say, "That guy is having trouble satisfying his wife," and then wait for a response. If you say, "So," or, "That's too bad," that will be the end of the exchange. If, however, you say, "That must be difficult for him to deal with," it shows that you acknowledge the difficulty as well as the emotional aspects of the problem. Your patient may go on to discuss a problem that he or she is having.

We will never forget a student nurse who was watching a television show with her patient. The patient welcomed the student and said, "This show is about prostitution." The student responded, "Oh, I don't know how anybody could degrade themselves like that." She overlooked the patient's underlying message—the patient happened to have been a prostitute at one time. The relationship with the student was over. The patient would never ask the student another question because the student was obviously judgmental. Be careful about what you say and how you say it, and what your body says that you are not saying out loud.

Now you know that you need to be willing to ask questions and also examine your own beliefs about sexuality. To feel more comfortable about asking questions, you will need to develop a sexual knowledge base and also formulate a sexual history.

CORE CONCEPTS DEVELOPING A KNOWLEDGE BASE

Most nursing schools will incorporate sexual information into nursing courses. For example, you might learn about taking a sexual history during your family (obstetrics–pediatrics) nursing course. You might learn about breast self-exam during a class on women and cancer. No matter how or where the information is presented, it is essential that you learn the basics of sexual functioning so that you can provide accurate information to your patients. To determine what information your patient needs, you will need to be familiar with the questions on a nursing history that pertain to sexual assessment. In most facilities, the RN will be responsible for the nursing history and admission assessment which will include questions about sexuality, but it helps you to be familiar with the information that is obtained. Table 19-1 lists some guidelines for the interview process. Typically, a nursing history will include information about sexuality. Some questions that you might want to ensure are part of your facility's nursing history are found in Table 19-2. The information in this table will help include basic sexual information during the nursing history. It is also important to include information that is specific to females and males (Table 19-3). There are a number of detailed sexual assessment forms that can be used for patients who are experiencing sexual difficulties. However, individuals trained to deal with sexual problems generally use these assessment tools.

Normal Sexual Response Following a sexual history, it is important for you to understand the basics of the normal sexual response. Although you will probably have learned about normal and abnormal male and female anatomy and physiology, sometimes little is offered about sexual functioning. According to Masters and Johnson (1966), there are four phases to the human sexual response cycle:

1. *Excitement:* When the individual becomes sexually excited by various stimuli. If for some reason the stimuli are withdrawn, then the cycle stops. If the stimulation continues, then the next phase is reached.

2. *Plateau:* When sexual tension increases. This phase may be prolonged if the stimulation continues, or shortened if the stimuli are withdrawn.

3. *Orgasm:* When sexual tension is released. It is important to note that this is entirely an involuntary response and is a total body reaction, even though the most intense sensations are felt in the pelvic area in both males and females.

4. *Resolution:* Occurs following orgasm when the body returns to the preexcitement state.

It is important to note that although males and females both experience the four phases of sexual arousal, they may experience them at different times (Figures

TABLE 19-1	Interviewing to Obtain Sexual Information— Some Do's and Don'ts

Do	Don't
1. Obtain information about all needed areas.	1. Focus only on sexuality.
2. Provide privacy.	2. Obtain information when others are present or take copious notes.
3. Strive for an unhurried atmosphere.	3. Check your watch, tap your foot.
4. Maintain an attitude that is frank, open, warm, objective, empathetic.	4. Project discomfort, become defensive.
5. Use nondirective techniques when possible.	5. Ask many direct questions.
6. Have a prepared introduction to state purpose of interview.	6. Be vague about the purpose of the interview.
7. Use appropriate vocabulary.	7. Use street terms.
8. "Check out" words to ensure patient understands.	8. Assume the patient understands what you're saying.
9. Adjust the order of questions according to client's needs.	9. Follow a rigid format.
10. Give the client time to think and answer questions.	10. Answer question for the patient.
11. Recognize signs of anxiety.	11. Focus on getting information without recognizing patient feeling.
12. Give permission not to do something.	12. Have preset expectations of the patient's sexual activity.
13. Listen in an interested but matter-of-fact way.	13. Overreact or underreact.
14. Identify your attitudes, values, beliefs, and feelings.	14. Project your concerns or problems onto the patient.
15. Identify significant others.	15. Assume that no one else is involved in the patient's sexual concerns.
16. Identify philosophic religious beliefs of patient.	16. Inflict your moral judgments on the patient.
17. Acknowledge when you don't have an answer to a question.	17. Pretend you know when you don't.

Source: Hogan, R. (1985). *Human sexuality: A nursing perspective.* Reprinted by permission of Pearson Education, Inc., Upper Saddle River, NJ 07458.

TABLE 19-2

Data to Be Collected by Nursing History for All Patients

Age	Identifies period in life cycle.	In what year were you born (month, day)?
Gender	Each gender may react differently to life events. Highlight gender identity problems.	[Usually is evident by dress, otherwise:] What sex do you consider yourself to be?
Education, occupation	Sexual practices may be related to education—socioeconomic class; change in occupation may contribute to role disturbances.	How far did you go in school? What do you do for a living? What change has there been in your ability to do your job?
Significant others	Other sources of support, stable or otherwise.	What persons do you consider most helpful right now? In what way? Are they available?
Quality of relationship with significant others	Relationships may be supportive, negative, or punitive, and these affect ability to cope with sexual problems.	Are there any differences in the way you get along with these people since you have been ill or hospitalized (or recently)?
Interests, hobbies	Indicates other support systems and avocational interest that contribute to self-esteem.	What do you do with your free time? What leisure and work activities are important to you? How are these being affected now?
Spritiual/ religious/ philosophical beliefs	Sexual practices may be related to beliefs. Guilt may occur if religious beliefs are compromised. Conflict and anxiety may be experienced by patient if different practices are suggested by nurse.	With what religious denomination are you affiliated? Can you describe any spiritual or other beliefs that are helpful to you now? Do you have or want the support of a clergyman (minister, priest, rabbi)?
Health problems, medical conditions, surgical procedures in past and anticipated in the future; medication therapy	Some medical problems, surgical treatment, or medications result in sexual dysfunction (physiologic changes). Anxiety over outcome or change in body image may lead to functional problems.	What illness and/or surgery have you had in the past? Did they affect your usual way of living or work? Did they affect sexual function? Do you expect this illness/ hospitalization will have effects on your usual way of living or work? In what ways? What medications do you take?

Changes in role relationships and ability to carry out the usual sexual role	Change in ability to carry out what is perceived as the usual sexual role may cause anxiety, depression, and/or sexual dysfunction.	What difference has there been in your functioning in the family? Describe. Can you do your usual tasks or jobs? Describe. Have there been any changes in your relationship (with the way you get along) with others (male, female, significant others)?
Potential changes in ability to carry out usual sexual role	Expectations of problems may cause problems (self-fulfilling prophecy).	What changes do you expect after you get home (or in the future)?
Change in perception of self as male or female due to illness or life events	Anxiety and sexual dysfunction may result from threat to gender identify.	How do you expect this illness (or life event) to affect how you see yourself as a man/woman?
Existing or potential sexual dysfunction	Elicits problems (sexual dysfunction).	Has there been or do you expect to have any changes in sexual functioning (sex life) because of (illness, life events)? Describe.

Source: Hogan, R. (1985). *Human sexuality: A nursing perspective.* Reprinted by permission of Pearson Education, Inc., Upper Saddle River, NJ 07458.

19-2 and 19-3). Note also that there is a refractory period in males. A female can immediately begin another sexual response cycle if adequately stimulated before sexual excitement totally resolves. However, the male requires a refractory period during which he cannot be restimulated. Usually, the length of the resolution period is similar to the length of the excitement phase. Also note that the female typically follows one of the three response cycles (A, B, or C in Figure 19-2). Males have only one (Masters, & Johnson, 1966). In pattern A, the woman experiences multiple orgasms with a very short resolution period. In pattern B, the woman never reaches orgasm but has several peaks during the plateau stage and a prolonged resolution period. In pattern C, the woman experiences an interruption during the excitement phase with an intense orgasm and rapid resolution.

TABLE 19-3	Data to Be Collected About Sexual Function

Female	Male
1. Menstrual history: onset, duration, pain, number of pads, intermenstrual bleeding, discharge. Pregnancies: number of children, miscarriages, contraception, satisfaction with method.	1. Genitourinary problems: infections, penile discharge, pain with urination, difficulty initiating or nocturnal urination.
2. Sexual response: sufficient vaginal lubrication, pain with intercourse, frequency of coitus, achieve orgasm with intercourse or masturbation.	2. Sexual responce: early morning erection, difficulty achieving or maintaining firm erection, change in sexual desire, volume of ejaculate.
3. Satisfaction with sexual response, partner's satisfaction.	3. Satisfaction with sexual response, partner's satisfaction.
4. Infections or venereal disease.	4. Infections or venereal disease.
5. Questions or problems they would like to discuss.	5. Questions or problems they would like to discuss.

Source: Hogan, R. (1985). *Human sexuality: A nursing perspective.* Reprinted by permission of Pearson Education, Inc., Upper Saddle River, NJ 07458.

Figure 19-2 Female Sexual Response Cycle

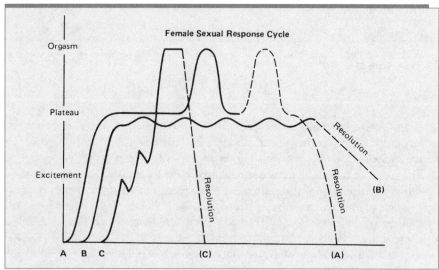

Source: Masters, W. H., & Johnson, V. E. (1966). *Human sexual response.* Boston, MA: Little Brown.

Figure 19-3 Male Sexual Response Cycle

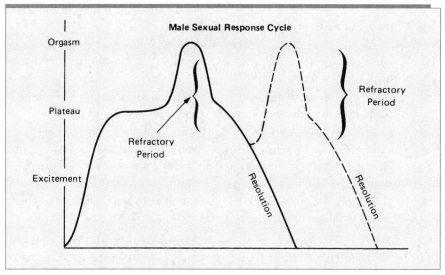

Source: Masters, W. H., & Johnson, V. E. (1966). *Human sexual response.* Boston, MA: Little Brown.

These differences in arousal can lead to sexual difficulty between partners if they are not understood. There have been cases of couples in counseling who were headed for divorce because they believed that if the man and woman do not have simultaneous orgasms, something is wrong with one or the other partner. Although simultaneous orgasms occasionally do occur, it is rare. Other couples have read that unless a woman experiences multiple orgasms, the man is not performing adequately. Although women are capable of having multiple orgasms, some do and some do not. These sexual concerns can lead to anxieties, anger, frustration, and eventually, termination of a relationship.

Illness and Sexuality   It is important for you to realize that there is a strong connection between illness and sexual functioning. Illness may cause a decline in the individual's physical abilities, a change in the individual's sense of maleness or femaleness, or a change in body image. Many chronic illnesses result in sexual difficulties. Some of the more common physical illnesses that cause sexual problems are:

1. *Diabetes:* Can cause impotence in males and frequent vaginal infections or orgasmic dysfunction in females.
2. *Arthritis:* The pain associated with arthritis can cause a decrease in desire for sex due to mobility problems or deformity.
3. *Spinal cord injuries:* The male will experience loss of sensation, but, depending on the level of injury, he may still have an erection reflex. The female will experience a loss of sensation. Both males and females will find

other areas of their bodies that cause sexual responses. Females may be able to get pregnant and carry a fetus to term. Males may benefit from various methods used to treat erectile dysfunction.

4. *Alcoholism:* Can lead to impotence and delayed ejaculation in males. Females can experience problems with sexual arousal and with decreased orgasmic frequency.

5. *Heart disease:* Can interfere with sexual functioning as a result of diminished blood flow, fatigue, or a decreased capacity for activity. Frequently, fear of another heart attack causes anxiety that can lead to sexual dysfunction.

6. *Cancer:* Can cause actual physical changes to sexual organs. Often causes changes in body image that can temporarily cause changes in sexual functioning.

7. *Gastrointestinal (GI) disorders:* Can result in an ostomy, which causes body image problems that cause temporary changes in sexual functioning.

Illnesses may cause specific physical changes, or they may cause a short-term lack of desire for sexual activity. At other times, the actual physical constraints forced on an individual by the environment may cause changes in sexuality. For example, hospitalization, diagnostic testing, and being separated from loved ones may all interfere with a person's normal sexual functioning.

For individuals who must be confined for long periods of time, day passes or other means of providing an outlet for sexual energy are suggested. Most long-term facilities can provide the time and privacy necessary for masturbation or sexual relations. We think that it is essential that we provide patients with an opportunity to maintain a sense of intimacy with their loved ones. Between illness and long-term confinement, we tend to strip all intimacy away. Intimacy is a basic need that we all share.

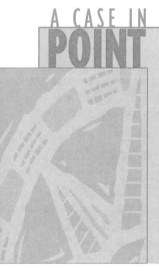

A CASE IN POINT

John and Rita have been married for 41 years. John suffered a lower back injury 6 months ago. His physician told him that he is fully recovered. However, during his last follow-up visit, when he left the examination room to use the restroom and the physician likewise was out of the room, Rita mentioned to the nurse that John is not able to have sexual relations. She says that they haven't discussed the problem. She is upset for him because she knows he must feel awful and is probably embarrassed. They have stopped trying to have relations. Rita tells the nurse that she doesn't know what to do.

CORE CONCEPTS   CARING FOR PATIENTS WITH SEXUAL CONCERNS

You will have many patients who have sexual concerns. Some of these patients will approach you with questions; others will wait for you to question them. Please remember to include at least one question about sexuality in all of your assessments. This will help you to determine if you should follow up with other questions. As stated earlier, your willingness to address sexual issues will enable your patients to confide in you. Nurses are in an excellent position to help most patients deal with sexual problems. Most sexual dysfunctions are the result of a lack of knowledge or inaccurate information. Consider how many of us learn about sexuality from our friends or the media. We are often too embarrassed to discuss sexuality with our parents, and some parents are too embarrassed to discuss sexuality with their children. As a result, many of us reach adulthood with little more than bits and pieces of information that we try to make sense of. Many couples experience anxiety because they fear that they are "not normal." Sometimes, nurses can provide a small amount of seemingly obvious information about sexuality that can provide them with reassurance.

CORE CONCEPTS   MEDICATION AND SEXUAL FUNCTION

Nurses have an opportunity to provide patients with accurate information about medications and sexual functioning. For example, a patient once presented 9 months pregnant even though she "was taking the pill daily." Upon further questioning, we discovered that the patient had inserted her birth control pills vaginally instead of taking them orally. Many patients will be taking medications that interfere with sexual functioning. Again, the nurse is in a unique position to provide patients with information about medications and how they might cause problems.

- It is important for you to know about the effects of medications on sexuality. For example, over-the-counter antihistamines can cause vaginal dryness and subsequent pain during intercourse.
- Many medications cause decreased libido (decreased sex drive) and erectile dysfunction (inability to have an erection). Some cause an increase in libido.
- If you are not sure of how a medication might affect sexual functioning, check your drug book or the *Physician's Desk Reference (PDR)*, or check with a pharmacist.
- Let your patient know what to expect. All too often, a patient stops taking a medication and never informs the doctor of the real reason. How many patients do you know who are noncompliant with blood pressure medications because they cause impotence?
- Patients need to know that other medications are available that may not have the same side effects.

Medications that interfere with sexual functioning are identified and described below.

Anticholinergic Medications Be aware that any medication that causes a dry mouth can cause sexual dysfunction. Most cause erectile failure and inhibit vaginal lubrication that can lead to *dyspareunia* (painful intercourse) and *orgasmic dysfunction* (inability to have an orgasm). Some of those medications include:

- Artane
- Atarax
- Atropine
- Antispas
- Anaspaz
- Benedryl
- Bentyl

- Cytospaz
- Kemedrin
- Norflex
- Pro-Banthine
- Procyclid
- Scopolamine
- THAM or THAM-e

Antihypertensive Medication Antihypertensive drugs frequently cause sexual dysfunction. Most can cause decreased libido, delayed ejaculation or ejaculatory incompetence (inability to ejaculate), and erectile failure. (Note that some patients will experience sexual dysfunction as a result of their hypertension.) All patients taking antihypertensive medications need to be questioned thoroughly about sexual side effects. One of the major problems with hypertension is noncompliance with medications. Although often unwilling to broach the subject, many patients discontinue use due to sexual side effects. If asked, patients will often admit to an inability to have satisfying sexual relations. The patient should be encouraged to speak with the doctor because there are many different medications available. The patient may experience fewer problems on a different drug. Antihypertensive drugs include:

- Aldactone
- Aldomet
- Catapres
- Dibensyline
- Inderal
- Ismelin
- Serpasil

Neuroleptics Most neuroleptic (antipsychotic) medications cause orgasmic dysfunction, ejaculatory incompetence, and erectile failure. Noncompliance with these drugs is common. If possible, patients need to be asked about sexual side effects and whether their noncompliance is due to these effects. Some of the newer medications (Clozaril, Respiradol) may not have the same sexual side effects but further study is needed. Neuroleptics include:

- Haldol
- Mellaril (frequently causes menstrual irregularities, gynecomastia [breast enlargement in males], inhibited ejaculation, and vaginal dryness)

- Prolixin
- Serentil
- Teractin
- Thorazine

Mood Active Drugs Lithium may cause erectile failure and ejaculatory incompetence. Tricyclic antidepressants can cause erectile failure and ejaculatory incompetence. These drugs include:

- Anafranil (may cause spontaneous orgasm in women)
- Elavil
- Norpramin
- Pamelor
- Tofranil

Serotonin reuptake inhibitors (SSRI) have fewer side effects and mild anticholinergic effects. These drugs include:

- Luvox
- Paxil
- Prozac
- Zoloft

Atypical antidepressants have fewer sexual side effects and include:

- Desyrel (Can cause priapism [sustained erection], which is a medical emergency. If not treated immediately, it can result in irreversible impotence.)
- Effexor
- Serzone
- Wellbutrin

Monoamine oxidase inhibitors (MAOIs) cause impotence and ejaculatory difficulties as well as delayed orgasm in women. They include:

- Eutonyl
- Nardil
- Parnate

Tranquilizers impact the central nervous system (CNS). Changes in the CNS will cause changes in sexual functioning. Tranquilizers include:

- Alcohol (causes erectile failure)
- Librium (causes erectile failure and delayed ejaculation or ejaculatory failure)
- Valium (causes decreased libido)

Other Drugs There are many other drugs that can affect sexual functioning. Unfortunately, not many drug books mention sexual side effects. It is always important to assess patients' responses to medication, including any unwanted sexual side effects.

- Baclofen causes erectile failure.
- Clofibrate causes erectile failure.
- Pondiman causes erectile failure and loss of libido.
- Tagamet causes erectile failure that can progress to impotence, which can remain even after the drug is discontinued. Tagamet also causes a decrease in sperm count, which is important information for those concerned about fertility.

Street Drugs   Some street drugs, such as marijuana and heroin, can cause erectile failure.

CORE CONCEPTS | SEVERE SEXUAL PROBLEMS

Occasionally, you will encounter a patient with problems with sexual functioning who needs to be referred for further assessment. Advocate to the physician for referrals in the following circumstances:

- If a patient discloses a problem that is long term or severe, referral should be made to a qualified sex therapist or psychotherapist specializing in relationship disorders.
- Refer patients who may have a physiologic sexual problem.
- Refer patients who are the victims of family violence.
- Refer patients who have long-standing problems related to incest or rape.
- Refer patients to someone else if you are unwilling, or unable, to deal with sexual issues.

Work on developing a comfort level in dealing with questions of a sexual nature. However, if your lack of ability is harmful to the patient, find another nurse who is more comfortable in dealing with sexual concerns. Take the time to observe the other nurse, and learn to handle sexual concerns on your own. Remember when you couldn't catheterize a patient? Remember the fear and feelings of inadequacy? Learning to deal with sexual concerns is like learning any new skill. It all takes practice!

 ASK YOURSELF

1. After reading this chapter, have your concerns related to talking to patients about their sexual problems diminished? If so, why? If not, why not?

_____

_____

2. Imagine yourself confronted with a patient who is struggling to ask a question related to the connection between sexuality and illness: What would you initially say to the patient to put him or her at ease, enabling the patient to more comfortably discuss his or her concern?

_____

_____

 CYBERLINKS: FLASH CARDS —————————

Check to see what you now remember by making your own flash cards. Use the CD-ROM that accompanies your textbook to discover how to make flash cards for reviewing and retaining what you have learned.

 CONCEPT MAP WORD BANK —————————

SEXUALITY
Your concerns
Patient concerns
SEXUAL RESPONSE
Normal
Impact of illness
Impact of medication
SEVERE SEXUAL PROBLEMS

Refer to Concept Maps and Flash Cards on pages viii–ix for an explanation of how to create and use concept maps. In addition, the CD-ROM guides you through the construction of concept maps by providing a more detailed introduction, more illustrations of examples, and key steps to follow in designing your own maps.

20

Culture

 ASK YOURSELF

1. What cultural, ethnic, and racial groups are part of your identity? (Refer to Heritage Assessment on page 211 of this chapter.)

_____

_____

2. What does the phrase *becoming "Americanized"* mean to you?

_____

_____

 CYBERLINKS

<u>Interactive</u> The patient population is becoming ever more diverse. Patients of different cultures who speak different languages usually appreciate any effort the caregiver makes to communicate in their own language. At **www.ipl.org** you can learn to say hello in over thirty languages and find interactive links to resources about the world's cultures and languages.

<u>Supplemental</u> **www.LPNresources.com** can help enhance your learning by leading you to discover other links with more information about the topic you are studying.

Nursing in the twenty-first century will bring with it many challenges not faced by our earlier colleagues. One challenge that we currently must deal with is providing care to individuals from varied cultural backgrounds. The 2000 United States census revealed that more than 280 million Hispanic or Latino individuals now live in this country. Additionally we have 47 million individuals who are of other races, including African American, Native American, Asian, or Pacific Islander. Many of these individuals continue to speak in their native language and maintain the beliefs, values, and traditions of their native culture. Looking at the 1998 data from the United States Immigration and Naturalization Service (INS), we find that in that year, the INS admitted 660,477 immigrants. Although this number varies from year to year, it appears that each year at least 650,000 immigrants will be admitted into this country.

CORE CONCEPTS | **INCORPORATING CULTURAL AWARENESS**

In evaluating the meaning of these figures for health care, it is obvious that nurses will be interacting with patients with varied cultural backgrounds daily. (And this trend toward multiple cultures is not unique to the United States. Countries around the globe are also finding their populations becoming more diverse.) As the number of individuals with varied cultural backgrounds began to increase over the years, nurses have realized that care for one cultural group was not always appropriate for another group. Thus, the idea of transcultural nursing was born. This is an area of nursing that focuses on how cultural values, beliefs, and attitudes influence an individual's health behaviors and, in turn, the delivery of health care. Culture influences how a person views health and illness, as well as how that person will seek health care and interact with health care providers. Giving nursing care in a "culturally competent" manner means that nursing interventions for health promotion, maintenance, restoration, and relief of symptoms are given in a manner that blends with the individual's cultural background.

Initially, health care workers are interested in biologic variations among cultural groups. These include body build and structure, skin color and texture, and enzymatic and genetic variations (Spector, 2000). In addition, different cultural groups are prone to varied specific health problems (Table 20-1).

Although health care workers tend to be aware of biologic differences, they are only vaguely aware of the influence culture has on an individual's response to events along the health–illness continuum. This is another imaginary pathway that demonstrates that there are stages of health, or wellness and illness, ranging all the way from high-level wellness (Dunn, 1961) to death. And in fact, "when there is conflict between the provider's and the client's belief systems, the provider typically is unable to understand the conflict and, hence, usually to find ways of minimizing it" (Spector, 2000). A few of the most prominent areas where culture is often the basis of behaviors include:

- Birth rites
- Death rites
- Dietary beliefs and practices
- Time orientation
- Attitudes toward the elderly
- Personal space
- Infant feeding beliefs and habits
- Gender roles
- Social roles

TABLE 20-1	Examples of Biological Variations Among a Select Number of Ethnic Groups			
African (Black) Americans	Asian/Pacific Islander Americans	American Indians, Aleuts, and Eskimos	Hispanic Americans	European (White) Origin Americans
Sickle-cell anemia	Hypertension	Accidents	Diabetes mellitus	Breast cancer
Hypertension	Liver cancer	Heart disease	Parasites	Heart disease
Cancer of the esophagus	Stomach cancer	Cirrhosis of the liver	Coccidioidomycosis	Diabetes mellitus
Stomach cancer	Coccidioidomycosis	Diabetes mellitus	Lactose intolerance	Thalassemia
Coccidioidomycosis	Lactose intolerance			
Lactose intolerance	Thalassemia			

Source: Adapted from Spector, R. E. (2000). *Cultural care: Guides to heritage assessment and health traditions.* Reprinted by permission of Pearson Education, Inc., Upper Saddle River, NJ 07458.

CORE CONCEPTS **ACCULTURATION AND ASSIMILATION**

Religious and cultural beliefs are often the foundation for the values and practices displayed in many of these behavioral areas. When considering culture, the following two terms come to mind and need to be understood:

1. *Acculturation:* The process of acquiring the behaviors, attitudes, and values of a different culture.
2. *Assimilation:* When an individual, over time, gives up the values, traditions, and traditional ways of their native culture and conforms to the standards and behaviors of the new culture.

You will have patients from foreign countries who will be at various points on the acculturation–assimilation continuum, which is illustrated in Figure 20-1. Note how the two lines overlap. During this overlapping time, individuals are experiencing and living between two cultures.

When you observe a patient from another culture who now accepts practices such as eating common American foods and wearing the latest trendy American clothes, you probably see this as evidence that the patient has adopted the ways of their new culture and is fully assimilated. However, when this patient shows no interest in learning about his or her health needs and self-care, you may become very frustrated. You have failed to realize that in some cultures, health care is centered around one family member. Therefore, the individual has no reason to learn self-care. You have misplaced the client's position on the acculturation–assimilation continuum. Table 20-2 presents examples of health beliefs and practices held by several different cultures.

So, how long does it take for an individual to become "Americanized"? Generally, the process covers two generations and follows this sequence:

- *First generation:* Adult immigrants arrive with a "basket" that is full to the brim with values, beliefs, and attitudes of their home country. Over the years, selected traditional items from the basket are discarded and replaced with the American counterparts as adjustment to the new environment is made.
- *Second generation:* Eventually, these immigrants have a child and the child inherits the basket with its mixed contents. As this child grows, more traditional, cultural items are replaced.

Figure 20-1 Acculturation–Assimilation Continuum

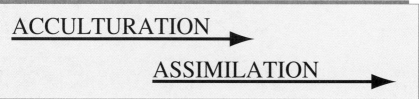

TABLE 20-2 **Comparison of Health Beliefs and Practices of Specific Cultural Groups**

Subculture	Concepts of Health	Origins of Illness	Type of Healer, Prevention, and Healing Practices
African American	Health is measured by one's ability to work. React to poor health only when there is a crisis, such as high fever or bleeding.	Illness may be punishment from God for wrongdoing, or is due to voodoo, spirits, or demons.	Prevention through good diet, rest, cleanliness, and laxatives to clean the system. Wear copper and silver bracelets to prevent illness. Also use some herbs. Some believe in voodoo and religious healing.
Hispanic American	Health is a gift from God, and is also due to good luck. Healthy person has robust appearance and feels well.	Illness may be punishment from God for wrongdoing; or caused by an imbalance between "hot" and "cold" properties of the body.	*Curandero* cures hot illness with cold medicine and vice versa. Illness is prevented by eating well, praying, being good, working, and wearing religious medals.
Asian/ Pacific Island American	Health involves the balance of *yin* and *yang* (negative and positive energy forces). Healthy body is gift from parents and ancestors.	Illness is caused by imbalance of *yin* and *yang*.	Healers include herbalist, spiritual healer, and physician. Food is essential for harmony with nature and is important in cause and treatment of disease. Acupuncture and moxibustion restore balance of yin and yang. Herbal remedies, such as ginseng, are also used.
Native American	Health is harmony between the individual, Earth, and the supernatural, as well as the ability to survive difficult circumstances.	Illness is disharmony and can be caused by violation of taboos, witchcraft, displeasing holy people, annoying the elements, disturbing plant and animal life, neglecting the celestial bodies, or misusing sacred Native American ceremony.	Healer is the medicine man. Illness is prevented through elaborate religious rituals and charms consisting of fetishes and pollen carried in a bag. Medicine and religion are closely related. Do not believe in the germ theory.

Source: Berger, K. J., & Williams, M. B. (1999). *Fundamentals of nursing: Collaborating for optimal health* (2nd ed.). Reprinted by permission of Pearson Education, Inc., Upper Saddle River, NJ 07458.

Personal Care and Family Life	Use of Health Care Delivery System	Health Problems	Death and Dying
African-based family with large extended families, flexible family roles and responsibilities. Strong religious orientation.	May receive inadequate health care. May experience segregation and racism when seeking care. Often use home remedies because of effectiveness and also because they are less expensive.	Hypertension, sickle-cell anemia, some cancers (e.g., lung, oral). High infant–maternal mortality, drug and alcohol abuse, obesity, and AIDS.	Believe in life after death.
Extended family is important. Value helping each other. Patriarchal family, with men making all decisions. Family honor is important. Children are a great source of pride.	Experience barriers to health care because of language (inability to speak English). May seek care from a physician, a folk practitioner, or both. May be late or miss appointments for care because of present time orientation.	Poverty-related diseases, such as tuberculosis, malnutrition, lead poisoning, and drug addiction.	View death and dying as "God's will." Believe in rewards from God in afterlife for good behavior.
Patriarchal family. Women are subservient to men. Ancestor worship and respect and obedience to parents are observed. Divorce is considered a disgrace.	Language barriers may exist: family spokesman may accompany client to Western physician. Prefer physicians from own cultural group if available in the community. May resist painful diagnostic tests. Having to have blood drawn is upsetting.	Respiratory diseases, immunization deficiencies, dental caries, tuberculosis, lactose intolerance.	Believe in reincarnation.
Extended family and tribal ties are strong. Cooperation is emphasized within the family and tribe.	Speak tribal language and may not understand English. Often seek care from medicine man first. General beliefs incompatible with those of health care system. Native Americans living in the eastern United States and most urban areas are not covered by the Indian Health Service.	Cirrhosis of the liver, alcoholism, high infant mortality, shortened life span, suicide, homicide, domestic violence. Leading causes of death are heart disease, accidents, malignant neoplasms, and cirrhosis.	Fear spirits of the dead. Children and family should be with dying person. Many rules and customs surround the dying. Do not believe in life after death.

- *Third generation:* Eventually, the second child has a child whose basket contains mostly American values, beliefs, and attitudes. By the time this child (grandchild of the original immigrants) reaches adulthood, the few remaining traditional cultural patterns have been discarded from the basket, and the individual is functioning fully as an American.

It takes time to adjust to a new and different culture. Many nurses are very surprised to learn that not all individuals believe that illness is due to physical or biologic problems that can be altered by humans. For example, most Americans view a fever, sore throat, and cough as due to some "bug." They go to a physician who gives them a medication that alters the bug in some way and they are better. Andrews and Boyle (1995) point out that in addition to this biomedical–scientific view of health and illness, there are two other major views.

CORE CONCEPTS   **TWO MAJOR VIEWS OF HEALTH AND ILLNESS**

1. *Magicoreligious:* Health and illness are in the control of a force beyond nature such as a god or gods; health is restored as the result of a supernatural agent.

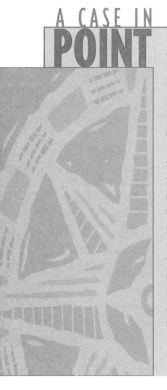

A CASE IN
POINT

Jan, a Jewish practical nurse, is caring for a patient who is of Palestinian descent. Jan is uncomfortably aware of her dislike for this patient, and also of the patient's dislike of her. She discusses her feelings with the nurse in charge, who is also her friend. Her friend asks her the following questions and asks her to think through her responses carefully: What is the source of your dislike? Are you treating the patient differently based on your dislike? Does this patient have any less need for your compassionate care than any other patient? Are you making assumptions about this patient that are fueled only by your own perceptions or misperceptions? Jan reflected on these questions and her thoughts and feelings. She realized that assumptions or real differences had no place in the medical setting. In this setting, she was a nurse, and in that role, the same quality of care is given to everyone.

2. *Holistic:* Health results from a balance and harmony with nature. If this balance is disrupted, the result is illness.

Thus, if nurses were to interact with all patients assuming that they accepted the biomedical view of illness, this would probably result in inadequate nursing interventions for patients who hold another view.

One nursing intervention that frequently offers a great challenge is adjusting an individual's culturally determined dietary practices to conform to a health need. Because food has such significance beyond providing sustenance for the body for all cultures, altering dietary habits to meet health care needs can at times seem like an impossible task. Keithley, Keller, and Vazquez (1996) have provided a unique way to use the Food Guide Pyramid as a foundation for patients with different cultural and ethnic food preferences (Figures 20-2 and 20-3).

Therefore, to give culturally sensitive and competent nursing care, knowledge of many aspects of a particular ethnic group is essential. However, beware of the trap of assuming that because your patient belongs to a specific cultural or ethnic group, they believe and act like the group. The word for this assumption is *stereotyping,* also known as generalizing. If you fall into this trap, you will make some serious errors, and the quality of care to your patients will be inferior to those nurses who choose to become culturally knowledgeable.

Figure 20-2 The Food Guide Pyramid: African American Foods

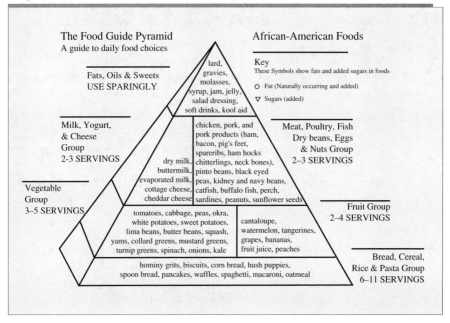

Figure 20-3 The Food Guide Pyramid: Mexican-American Foods

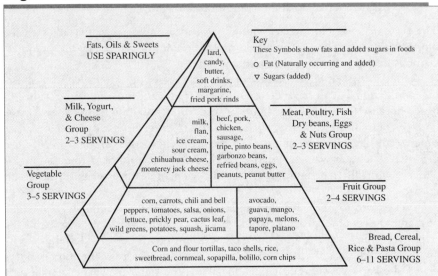

GUIDELINES FOR GIVING CULTURALLY COMPETENT CARE

1. *Learn about your own heritage and culture.* Because you have grown up and have been socialized into a cultural environment, it may seem to you that you do not have a heritage basket. But you do have a basket, and analysis of its current and past contents will expand your horizons.

2. *Recognize that you are also a part of the health care provider culture with its own beliefs and practices.* Table 20-3 provides a brief outline of this culture. The headings are similar to belief and practice headings used to describe cultures in most literature.

3. *Come to terms with ethnocentrism, the belief that some, if not all, of the values and ways of behaving of your culture or ethnic group are better than that of another group.* This can be a destructive force and can interfere with competent care. Yet, it is often an unconscious and persistent force in delivery of health care.

4. *Research information about your patient's cultural background.* This will probably mean that you should add at least one book on transcultural nursing to your personal library (see additional reading list at end of chapter). Remember that often the best source of transcultural information are your patients. Just ask them about their beliefs.

5. *Assess where your individual patient fits on the acculturation–assimilation continuum.* Several formal assessment tools are available to help you do this (Table 20-4 and Figure 20-4). Also, if you are in the patient's home, use your observational skills to pick up on clues about the cultural practices of the members of the household.

6. *Carefully analyze your patient's health behaviors.* Are they truly harmful to the patient's health, or just different from your own or the health care provider culture? This may be a very difficult question to honestly answer because our individual ethnocentric traits often cloud our analysis!

TABLE 20-3	Characteristics of the Health Care Provider's Culture

1. Beliefs
   a. Standardized definitions of health and illness
   b. The omnipotence of technology
2. Practices
   a. The maintenance of health and the protection of health or prevention of disease through such mechanisms as the avoidance of stress and the use of immunizations
   b. Annual physical examinations and diagnostic procedures, such as Pap smears
3. Habits
   a. Charting
   b. Constant use of jargon
   c. Use of a systematic approach and problem-solving methodology
4. Likes
   a. Promptness
   b. Neatness and organization
   c. Compliance
5. Dislikes
   a. Tardiness
   b. Disorderliness and disorganization
6. Customs
   a. Professional deference and adherence to the pecking order found in autocratic and bureaucratic systems
   b. Handwashing
   c. Employment of certain procedures attending birth and death
7. Rituals
   a. Physical examination
   b. Surgical procedure
   c. Limiting visitors and visiting hours

Source: Spector, R. E. (2000). *Cultural diversity in health and illness* (5th ed.). Reprinted by permission of Pearson Education, Inc., Upper Saddle River, NJ 07458.

TABLE 20-4	Cultural Assessment of Health Care Practices

- What has made you ill?
- What do you ordinarily do to keep well or take care of yourself?

    Special diet
    Herbs
    Rituals
    Amulets
    Other

- What drugs, tablets, or foods did you use or are you using? What did you use them for?
- What ceremonies or rituals do you perform to get well?
- Who took care of you when you were sick?
- What did he or she do for you when you were sick?
- When did you last see this person?
- Will you take medication from me today?

Source: Berger, K. J., & Williams, M. B. (1999), *Fundamentals of nursing: Collaborating for optimal health* (2nd ed.). Reprinted by permission of Pearson Education, Inc. Upper Saddle River, NJ 07458.

In addition, you face many challenges when you and your patient speak different languages, both with and without an interpreter. When you converse in English with the patient or interpreter, be very conscious of the words you use. You already know the pitfalls of speaking "Nurse-ese" to patients. But are you aware of your use of idioms and colloquialisms? To English-speaking people, they are natural and immediately placed in context and understood. However, we would like to add a personal experience regarding this type of miscommunication.

One of us participated as an instructor in a literacy project helping adults to speak and read English as a second language. Before class formally began one evening, the instructor said, "Boy, it sure rained cats and dogs yesterday." This made sense to the instructor but not the students! They understood the individual words but not the meaning.

We have hundreds of such phrases in the English language. Based on where your patient is on the acculturation–assimilation continuum, the use of idioms can be very confusing and frustrating to the patient. Humor is an example. Be cautious with its use, as someone who does not speak English fluently can misinterpret it.

If you must use an interpreter in providing nursing care for a patient, use caution. You are better off to use an objective interpreter (e.g., another staff member) than to use a patient's family member. Often, family members will put their own interpretation on what you say before delivering the message. They may "soften the

Figure 20-4 Heritage Assessment Tool

Heritage Assesment Tool

This set of questions can be used to investigate a given client's or your own ethnic, cultural, and religious heritage.

It can help you to perfom a heritage assessment to determine how deeply a given person identifies with a particular tradition. It is most useful in setting the stage for understanding a person's HEALTH traditions. The greater the number of positive responses, the greater the person's identification with a traditional heritage. The one exception to positive answers is the question about family name change. This question may be answered negatively.

1. Where was your mother born? _____
2. Where was your father born? _____
3. Where were your grandparents born?_____
    a. Your mother's mother?_____
    b. Your mother's father? _____
    c. Your father's mother? _____
    d. Your father's father? _____
4. How many brothers _____ and sisters _____ do you have?
5. What setting did you grow up in? Urban _____   Rural_____
    Suburban _____
6. What country did your parents grow up in?
    Father _____
    Mother _____
7. How old were you when you came to the United States? _____
8. How old were your parents when they came to the United States?
    Mother _____
    Father _____
9. When you were growing up, who lived with you?_____
    _____
10. Have you maintained contact with
    a. Aunts, uncles, cousins?   (1) Yes _____   (2) No____
    b. Brothers and sisters?   (1) Yes _____   (2) No____
    c. Parents?   (1) Yes _____   (2) No____
    d. Your own children?   (1) Yes _____   (2) No____
11. Did most of your aunts, uncles, cousins live near your home?
    (1) Yes_____   (2) No _____
12. Approximately how often did you visit your family members who lived outside your home?
    (1) Daily _____   (2) Weekly_____   (3) Monthly_____
    (4) Once a year or less _____   (5) Never _____
13. Was your original family name changed?
    (1) Yes_____   (2) No _____

Figure 20-4 Heritage Assessment Tool (Continued)

14. What is your religious preference?
    (1) Catholic _____   (2) Jewish _____
    (3) Protestant _____   Denomination_____
    (4) Other _____   (5) None_____
15. Is your spouse the same religion as you?
    (1) Yes_____   (2) No _____
16. Is your spouse the same ethnic background as you?
    (1) Yes_____   (2) No _____
17. What kind of school did you go to?
    (1) Public_____   (2) Private _____   (3) Parochial_____
18. As an adult, do you live in a neighborhood where the neighbors are the same religion and ethnic background as yourself?
    (1) Yes_____   (2) No _____
19. Do you belong to a religious institution?
    (1) Yes_____   (2) No _____
20. Would you describe yourself as an active member?
    (1) Yes_____   (2) No _____
21. How often do you attend your religious institution?
    (1) More than once a week _____   (2) Weekly_____
    (3) Monthly_____   (4) Special holidays only _____
    (5) Never _____
22. Do you practice your religion in your home?
    (1) Yes_____   (2) No _____   (if yes, please specify)
    (3) Praying_____   (4) Bible reading _____
    (5) Diet _____   (6) Celebrating religious holidays _____
23. Do you prepare foods of your ethnic background?
    (1) Yes_____   (2) No _____
24. Do you participate in ethnic activities?
    (1) Yes_____   (2) No _____   (if yes, please specify)
    (3) Singing_____   (4) Holiday celebrations _____
    (5) Dancing_____   (6) Festivals _____
    (7) Costumes_____   (8) Other _____
25. Are your friends from the same religious background as you?
    (1) Yes_____   (2) No _____
26. Are your friends from the same ethnic background as you?
    (1) Yes_____   (2) No _____
27. What is your native language? _____
28. Do you speak this language?
    (1) Prefer_____   (2) Occasionally _____   (3) Rarely_____
29. Do you read your native language?
    (1) Yes_____   (2) No _____

Source: Spector, R. E. (2000). *Cultural care guides to heritage assessment and health traditions.* Reprinted by permission of Pearson Education, Inc. Upper Saddle River, NJ 07458

blow" from unpleasant news to protect their loved one. Conversely, they may also give you a softened interpretation of what the family member has said to them.

Another suggestion would be to take a course in another language yourself, so you do not need an interpreter. Many health care facilities actually offer courses in Medical Spanish, for example, so that you at least know how to ask Spanish-speaking patients if they are in pain, need the bedpan, and so on. Take advantage of these opportunities.

Most health care facilities maintain a list of staff members who speak another language, so you will know who is available on your shift to interpret. One of us worked on a unit where we often had elderly Navajo patients who spoke no English. One gentleman would not cooperate with his physical therapist until the physician actually wrote an order for a Navajo-speaking staff member to come in and talk to the patient. A staff member was called, who accompanied the patient to physical therapy and to the orthopedist's office, explaining all along the way what was happening and why. From that day on, the patient was cooperative with his rehabilitation and progressed well enough to return home.

Caring for patients who are culturally diverse is a challenge as well as a wonderful opportunity. It is a chance to demonstrate not only your skill in clinical performance but also your ability to do so in a culturally competent manner. Both are equally important. It requires that you are open-minded and willing to learn about and respect others' cultures. It is part of that holistic care we have been talking about. Your patients' culture will affect how they accept nursing care; your culture will affect how you deliver it. By taking the time to learn about your patients' culture and incorporating that knowledge into your nursing care, you are ensuring success for both you and your patient.

STOP ASK YOURSELF

1. To what extent do you think that you will be engaged in transcultural nursing?

   _____

   _____

2. Given the cultural diversity of the patient population, do you think it would be beneficial to learn a language or languages other than your own? If so, which language, and how would you go about learning it?

   _____

   _____

 ## CYBERLINKS: FLASH CARDS

Check to see what you now remember by making your own flash cards. Use the CD-ROM that accompanies your textbook to discover how to make flash cards for reviewing and retaining what you have learned.

CONCEPT MAP WORD BANK

CULTURE
Definition
Importance in health care
TRANSCULTURAL NURSING
ACCULTURATION
ASSIMILATION
VIEWS OF HEALTH AND ILLNESS

Refer to Concept Maps and Flash Cards on pages viii–ix for an explanation of how to create and use concept maps. In addition, the CD-ROM section guides you through the construction of concept maps by providing a more detailed instruction, more illustrations of examples, and key steps to Follow in designing your own maps.

 BOOKS TO CONSIDER ADDING TO YOUR PERSONAL LIBRARY

Andrews, M. M., & Boyle, J. S. (1999). *Transcultural concepts in nursing care* (3rd ed.). Philadelphia: Lippincott.

Galanti, G.-A. (1997). *Caring for patients from different cultures: Case studies from American hospitals* (2nd ed.). Baltimore: University of Pennsylvania Press.

Geissler, E. M. (1998). *Pocket guide to cultural assessment* (2nd ed.). St. Louis: Mosby.

Spector, R. E. (2001). *Cultural diversity in health and illness* (5th ed.), and companion, *Companion care guides to heritage assessment and health traditions.* Upper Saddle River, NJ: Prentice Hall.

Spirituality

21

ASK YOURSELF

1. Do you agree with the statement that all human beings are spiritual beings? Why or why not?

   _____

   _____

2. What behaviors do you think a patient in spiritual distress might exhibit?

   _____

   _____

CYBERLINKS

Interactive www.healthatoz.com is the site to visit to explore your own mental and spiritual health. Quizzes, tools, and articles are plentiful. Click on Wellness and go to the Mental Health Center.

Supplemental www.LPNresources.com can help enhance your learning by leading you to discover other links with more information about the topic you are studying.

All human beings are spiritual beings. We all have an inborn sense of meaning and understanding about the worth of our being human. Some of us attribute this sense of worth to a higher being and express a belief in God. Others derive this sense of worth from relationships with others and with the environment. Whatever the source of our spirituality, it guides us in our view of the world and interpretation of human values and provides us with structure and meaning as we go about our everyday life. Our developmental age, family and ethnic background, formal religious training, and life events all help to shape the spiritual side of us.

Some of us choose to express our spirituality in a formal manner through an association with a specific religion; others believe that organized religion gets in the way of their spiritual expression. Either way, spiritual well-being is an essential component of well being in general. Spiritual beliefs can help people cope with life stressors and crises as well as provide a sense of purpose. Spiritual beliefs can also help us to develop a sense of inner harmony that allows us to love and trust others and have an abiding sense of peace, hope, and faith. Physical illness forces all of us to face loss, fears, grief, our own mortality, and questions of meaning.

CORE CONCEPTS | **SPIRITUALITY AND HEALTH**

Our knowledge of research in health care has expanded to include the mind's role in the development of illness. Many health problems can be traced to an individual's lifestyle. Therefore, is it so impossible to think that a strong spiritual base can lead individuals toward health, and, in some instances, even a miraculous recovery?

Nurses often have difficulty recognizing and intervening when patients experience *spiritual distress.* Most facility admission assessment forms ask the patient what their religion is, but there is no further assessment of spiritual concerns unless the facility is affiliated with a religious organization. Then, there might be questions on whether or not admission into the hospital will interfere with the patient's ability to practice his or her religious beliefs. New standards from the Joint Commission for Accreditation of Healthcare Organizations (JCAHO) are emphatic about the patient's right to receive care that recognizes both personal dignity and spiritual values. Therefore, nurses must include assessment of a patient's spiritual needs in their holistic approach to patient care.

We believe that there are various reasons why nurses do not intervene in problems that appear to be of a spiritual nature. These are:

- Feelings of discomfort, which may arise from the nurse's failure to come to terms with his or her own spirituality. We must be able to accept our own beliefs and identify those that provide hope, peace, and spiritual well-being in our own lives.
- Inadequate preparation for addressing spiritual issues due to the failure of our nursing schools to place appropriate emphasis on the spiritual aspect of the patient's care.
- The belief that it is inappropriate for nurses to intervene in spiritual matters but should refer all matters of a spiritual nature to a minister, priest, rabbi or other spiritual advisor. Unfortunately, many patients are unable to time their spiritual distress to coincide with a visit from a spiritual advisor.
- The belief that nurses must be of the same religion as the patient to assist them in dealing with spiritual concerns.
- The inability of nurses to confront their own limitations and accept the inevitability of illness, suffering, and death as part of our human condition.

Only after dealing with these issues within ourselves can we begin to help patients experiencing spiritual concerns.

| CORE CONCEPTS | **BEHAVIORS SUGGESTIVE OF SPIRITUAL DISTRESS** |

Individuals will express spiritual distress differently. If the nurse does not specifically ask about spiritual concerns, the patient may not bring them up. There are certain behaviors that may be suggestive of spiritual distress and may require referral to a spiritual leader. According to Murray and Zentner (2001, p. 148), consider referring a patient who exhibits any of the following behavior patterns:

- Withdrawn, sullen, silent, depressed
- Restless, irritable, complaining
- Restless, excitable, garrulous (wants to talk a lot)
- Shows by word or other signs undue curiosity and anxiety about self
- Takes a "turn for the worse," critical, terminal
- Shows conversational interest, curiosity in religious questions, issues; reads religious materials
- Specifically inquires about a chaplain, chapel worship, religious materials
- Has few or no visitors; has no cards or flowers
- Has had, or faces, particularly traumatic or threatening surgical procedure

Many larger hospitals have chaplains who are on duty 24 hours a day. Smaller hospitals may have various pastors within the community who are "on call" to come to the facility as the need arises. Even some long-term care facilities now have a chaplain for at least 8 hours a day. You should familiarize yourself with what spiritual avenues of referral are available at the facility where you are doing your clinicals. Locate the hospital or nursing home chapel, so you can provide that information to patients and their families. Know when services are being held. Consider

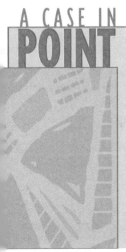

A CASE IN POINT

A patient who is a Seventh-Day Adventist is served stew for dinner. The patient kindly tells the nurse that he doesn't eat stew. The nurse replies that she doesn't like stew either. The patient again tells the nurse that he is unable to eat the stew. The nurse comments that she doesn't blame him. Finally, in exasperation, the patient tells the nurse that he is a Seventh-Day Adventist and doesn't eat meat. The nurse apologizes and resolves to check the notation of religion on the Kardex more carefully and be more sensitive to individual spiritual practices.

contacting someone if the patient is going through any major trauma. Even if the patient doesn't need someone to talk with, the family or friends might. Depending upon the situation, you may need to ask the patient's or family's permission to contact a spiritual advisor for the patient or family and friends. Some people may appreciate the intervention; others may not.

ESSENTIAL SKILLS | QUESTIONS FOR SPIRITUAL ASSESSMENT

To help patients deal with spiritual distress, it is important to first assess what their beliefs are. It is important to determine what spiritual and religious beliefs patients have and how these beliefs relate to their current health situation. There are many spiritual assessment forms available. Murray and Zentner (1997, p. 127) recommend that the following questions be used for spiritual assessment:

1. Who is your God?
   • What is your God like?
2. What is your religion?
   • Tell me about it.
3. Do you believe that a God or someone is concerned for you?
4. Has being sick made any difference in your feelings about your God?
   • In the practice of your faith?
   • If it has, in what way?
5. Do you believe that your faith is helpful to you?
   • If it is, in what way?
   • If it is not, why not?
6. Are there any religious beliefs, practices, or rituals that are important to you now?
   • If there are, could you tell me more about them?
   • May I help you carry them out by showing you where the chapel is?
   • By telling the dietary department about your food preferences?
   • By allowing you specific times for prayer or meditation?
   • By having your loved ones bring any special religious articles from home? (Rosary, prayer beads, Bible, or other religious book, etc.)
7. Is there anything that would make your situation easier?
   • A visit from the minister, priest, rabbi, or chaplain?
   • Someone who could read to you?
   • Time for reading your religious book or praying?
   • Someone to pray with you?
8. Is prayer important to you?
   • If so, how has being sick made a difference in your practice of praying?
   • What happens when you pray?

9. What are your beliefs about illness?
   • About life after death?
10. Is there anything especially frightening or meaningful to you right now?
11. If these questions have not uncovered your source of spiritual support, can you tell me where you do find support?

It is important for you to intervene when patients experience spiritual distress because it allows you to gain deeper insights into your patients' experiences. It can also allow you to share in the awesome life experiences of birth, death, illness, and recovery. Sharing in these life experiences and emotions with your patients will help you further develop your role as patient advocate. You will develop a more accurate perception of exactly what the patient needs and desires. Another reason to intervene in spiritual distress is that you will allow the patient to express spiritual pain that can help in healing that individual's spirit. This healing of the spirit can occur long after the need for technology and physical care has subsided.

Prayer is one of the most significant spiritual experiences for the majority of people. According to a 1997 Gallup survey, over 90% of Americans pray daily and believe that prayer has an effect on their lives (Bacon, 1995; Byrd & Sherrill, 1995; Dossey, 1994; Hughes, 1997). Another poll conducted by *Time*/CNN and *USA Weekend* found that more than 60% of Americans thought that their physicians should discuss faith with their patients and pray with those who request it. A number of research studies have suggested that prayer can speed healing. Praying for and with patients are two of the most direct ways for nurses to be involved in patients' spiritual experiences. Other ways of being involved include reading spiritual books with or to your patient, providing quiet time for meditation and prayer, and being certain that religious articles are close at hand. Remember, your patient may belong to one of the religions listed in Table 21-1, but do not assume that the patient adheres to all of the practices common to that religion.

Occasionally, you may care for patients who follow more nontraditional religions. Native Americans continue to incorporate the use of medicine men, or shamans, in their spiritual lives and healing practices. The word of the medicine man may supercede traditional medical practices but may also be combined with traditional medicine. We have met patients who follow Voodoo practices in the Southeast and Southwest, as well as patients who practice Wiccan and other religions. These religions are not uncommon, and their practitioners have beliefs that could interfere with traditional medical practices. Most of the practitioners believe in spells that can be either good or bad. Illness can be caused by bad spells. For the patient to improve, a healer may be needed to remove the spell. Healers tend to rely on objects, powders, herbs, incantations, and prayer to remove spells. We would encourage you to work with the healer to bring the patient every type of healing possible. Rarely do healers refuse to work with the health care team for the improvement of their patient. Unfortunately, the reverse is not always true. Many health care workers refuse to consider the value of nontraditional forms of healing. For the patient to benefit, you may need to open your heart and mind to new ways of healing. Remember, if your patient believes that the spell can make him or her ill, then

TABLE 21-1	Summary of Major Health Care Implications of Selected Religious Cultures and Subcultures

Religion	Food Preference	Responsibility Related to Patient Belief/Need
Hinduism	Vegetarian; no alcoholic beverages; other restrictions conform to sect doctrine; fasting important part of religious practice, with consequences for person on special diet or with diabetes or other diseases regulated by food	Medical care is last resort; patient considers help will come from own inner resources. Nurse should treat patient with respect and convey sense of dignity. Reinforce need for medical care and explain care measures. Patient may reject help and be stoic. Assess carefully for pain. Provide privacy. Assist to maintain religious practices. Cleanliness and dietary preferences are important. Certain prescribed rites are followed after death. The priest may tie a thread around the neck or wrist to signify blessing; the thread should not be removed. Immediately after death, the priest will pour water into the mouth of the corpse; the family will wash the body. They are particular about who touches their dead. Bodies are cremated. Loss of limb is considered sign of wrongdoing in previous life.
Buddhism Zen, sect of Buddhism Shintoism, Japan's state religion	Vegetarian; no intoxicants; moderation in eating and drinking	Family help care for ill member and give emotional support. Religion discourages use of drugs; assess carefully for pain. Cleanliness important. Question about feelings regarding medical or surgical treatment on holy days. Prepare for death; help patient remain alert, resist confusion or distraction, and remain calm. Last Rite chanting is often practiced at bedside soon after death. Contact the deceased's Buddhist priest or have the family make contact.

TABLE 21-1	Summary of Major Health Care Implications of Selected Religious Cultures and Subcultures (Continued)	

Religion	Food Preference	Responsibility Related to Patient Belief/Need
Islam	No pork or pork-containing products; no intoxicants	Members are excused from religious practices when ill but may still want to pray to Allah and face Mecca. There is no spiritual advisor to call. Family visits are important. Cleanliness is important. After 130 days, fetus is treated as fully developed human. Members maintain a fatalistic view about illness; they are resigned to death, but encourage prolonging life. Patient must confess sins and beg forgiveness before death, and family should be present. The family washes and prepares the body, folds hands, and turns the body to face Mecca. Only relatives or friends may touch the body. Unless required by law, no postmortem or no body part should be removed.
Black Muslim (Nation of Islam)		There is no baptism. Procedure for washing and shrouding dead and performing funeral rites is carefully prescribed. Cleanliness is important.
Judaism	Orthodox eat only kosher (ritually prepared) foods; milk consumed before meat, or meat eaten 6 hours before milk consumed; does not eat pig, horse, shrimp, lobster, crab, oyster, birds of prey if Orthodox. Others may restrict diet. Special utensils and dishes for	There is no infant baptism. Baby boys are circumcised on eighth day if Orthodox. Preventative measures, avoiding illness, are important. Members are concerned about future consequences of illness and medication. They are preoccupied with health; will convey that pain is present and want relief. Nursing measures for pain are important. On Sabbath, Orthodox Jews may refuse freshly

TABLE 21-1	Summary of Major Health Care Implications of Selected Religious Cultures and Subcultures (Continued)	

Religion	Food Preference	Responsibility Related to Patient Belief/Need
Judaism (cont.)	Orthodox. Fasts on Yom Kippur and Tisha Bab; may fast other times but excluded if ill	cooked foods, medicine, treatment, surgery, and use of radio or television. Orthodox male may not shave. Nurse should avoid loss of yamulka, prayer books, or phylacteries. Nurse must arrange for kosher or preferred food; food may be served on paper plates. Check consequences of fasting on person's condition. Visits from family members are important. If patient is without family, notify synagogue so other people may visit. Family or friends should be with dying person. Artificial means should not be used to prolonged life if patient is vegetative. Confession by dying person is like a rite of passage. Human remains are ritually washed following death by members of the Ritual Burial Society. Burial should take place as soon as possible. Cremation is not permitted. All Orthodox Jews and some Conservative Jews are opposed to autopsy. Organs or other tissues should be made available to the family for burial. Parts of the body are not donated to medical science or removed, even during autopsy. Donation or transplantation of organs requires rabbinical consultation. A fetus is to be buried, not discarded.
Christianity		All will wish to see spiritual advisor when ill and to read Bible or other religious literature and follow usual practices.

TABLE 21-1	Summary of Major Health Care Implications of Selected Religious Cultures and Subcultures (Continued)	

Religion	Food Preference	Responsibility Related to Patient Belief/Need
Roman Catholic	Nothing special, except fasting or abstaining from meat on Ash Wednesday and Good Friday; some Catholics may fast every Friday and other holy days	Rosary, Bible, prayer book, crucifix, and medals are important. Infant baptism is mandatory, and especially urgent if prognosis is poor. Baptism is demanded if aborted fetus may not be clinically dead. For baptismal purposes, death is a certainty only if there is obvious evidence of tissue necrosis. Tell priest if you baptize baby; it is done only once. Inquire about dietary preferences and fasting. Members may want information on natural family planning. The Rite for Anointing of the Sick is mandatory. If the prognosis is poor, the patient or his or her family may request it. In sudden death, priest is called to anoint and administer Viaticum, if possible, or special prayers are said. Amputated limb may be buried in consecrated ground; there is no blanket mandate but it may be required within a given diocese. Donation or transplantation of organs is approved providing the recipient's potential benefit is proportionate to the donor's potential harm.
Orthodox Eastern Orthodox (Turkey, Egypt, Syria, Cyprus, Bulgaria, Rumania, Albania, Poland, Czechoslovakia)	Fasting each Wednesday, each Friday, and 40 days before Christmas and Easter; avoid meat, dairy products, and olive oil	Prayer book and icons are important. Infant is baptized if death is imminent. Check consequences of fast days on health; fasting is not necessary when ill. Blessing for the sick (unction) is not Last Rite but a form of healing by prayer. Last Rites are obligatory if death is impending; cremation is discouraged.

	Summary of Major Health Care Implications of Selected Religious Cultures and Subcultures (Continued)
TABLE 21-1	

Religion	Food Preference	Responsibility Related to Patient Belief/Need
Greek	Fasting periods on Wednesday, Friday, and during Lent; avoid meat and dairy products	Prayer book and icons are important. Infant is baptized if death is imminent. Patient prepares by fasting for Holy Communion and Sacrament of Holy Unction. Fasting is not mandatory during illness. Members oppose euthanasia. Every reasonable effort should be made to preserve life until terminated by God. Cremation or autopsies that may cause dismemberment are discouraged. Last Rites are administered for the dying.
Russian Orthodox	Fasting on Wednesday, Friday, and during Lent; no meat or dairy products	Prayer book and icons are important. There is no baptism of infant. Check consequences of fasting on health. Cross necklace is important; it should be replaced immediately when patient returns from surgery. Do not shave male patients except in preparation for surgery. Patients do not believe in autopsies, embalming, or cremation. Traditionally, after death, arms are crossed, and fingers are set in a cross. Clothing at death must be of natural fiber so that the body will change to ashes sooner.
Protestantism (Many denominations and sects)		
Baptist	Some groups condemn coffee and tea; most condemn alcoholic beverages; some groups may fast on Sundays or other special days, especially in Black Baptist churches	There is no infant baptism. Client may be fatalistic; may believe illness is punishment from God, and may be passive about care. Inquire about effect of fasting if client is on special diet, is a diabetic, or has disease dependent on dietary regulation.

TABLE 21-1	Summary of Major Health Care Implications of Selected Religious Cultures and Subcultures (Continued)	

Religion	Food Preference	Responsibility Related to Patient Belief/Need
Brethren (Grace) (Plymouth)	Most abstain from alcohol, tobacco, and illicit drugs	There is no infant baptism. Anointing with oil is done for physical healing and spiritual uplift. There are no Last Rites.
Church of Christ, Scientist (Christian Scientist)	Avoid coffee and alcoholic beverages	There is no infant baptism. If hospitalized or receiving medical treatment, guilt feelings may be intense. Be supportive. Allow practitioner or reader to visit freely as desired. Use nursing measures to alleviate pain. Patient may refuse blood transfusions as well as intravenous fluids and medication. There are no Last Rites or autopsy, unless sudden death.
Church of Christ	Avoid alcoholic beverages	There is no infant baptism. Anointing with oil and laying on of hands are done for healing. There are no Last Rites.
Church of God	Most avoid alcoholic beverages	There is no infant baptism.
Church of Jesus Christ of Latter Day Saints (Mormon)	Eat in moderation; limit meat; avoid coffee and tea; no alcoholic beverages; avoid use of tobacco	There is no infant baptism, but baptism of dead is essential; living person serves as proxy. Laying on of hands is done for healing. White undergarment with special marks at navel and right knee is to remain on; it is considered a safeguard against danger.
Episcopalian	May fast from meat on Friday	Infant baptism is mandatory, but not for aborted fetus or stillbirth. Patient fasts in preparation for Holy Communion, which may be daily; thus, check effects on disease. Rite for Anointing Sick (Last Rites) is not mandatory.

		Summary of Major Health Care Implications
TABLE 21-1		of Selected Religious Cultures and Subcultures (Continued)

Religion	Food Preference	Responsibility Related to Patient Belief/Need
Friends (Quakers)	Moderation in eating; most avoid alcoholic beverages and drugs	There is no infant baptism. Health teaching is important. Give explanations about medical technology used in care. Share information about condition as indicated.
Jehovah's Witnesses	Avoid food to which blood is added, e.g., certain sausages and lunch meats	There is no infant baptism. Members are opposed to blood transfusion. (Hospital administrator or doctor may seek court order to be appointed guardian of child in times of emergency need for blood.) There are no Last Rites.
Mennonite	Most avoid alcoholic beverages	There is no infant baptism. Shock therapy, psychotherapy, and hypnotism conflict with individual will and personality.
Nazarene	Avoid alcoholic beverages	There is no need to baptize infant. Stillborn is buried. Laying on of hands is done for healing. There are no Last Rites.
Pentecostal	Avoid alcoholic beverages	There is no infant baptism. Prayer, anointing with oil, laying on of hands, speaking in tongues, shouting, and singing are important for healing of patient.
Unitarian/ Universalist		Infant baptism is not necessary. Cremation is preferred to burial. Check before calling clergy to visit.
Seventh-Day Adventists	Vegetarian (no meat) or lacto-ovo-vegetarian (may eat milk and eggs but not meat); pork and fish without	There is no infant baptism. Health measures, prevention, and health education are important. Some believe in divine healing and anointing with oil. Avoid admin-

		Summary of Major Health Care Implications
TABLE 21-1		of Selected Religious Cultures and Subcultures (Continued)

Religion	Food Preference	Responsibility Related to Patient Belief/Need
Seventh-Day Adventists (cont.)	fins and scales prohibited; avoid coffee and tea; avoid alcoholic beverages	istering narcotics and stimulants. Use nursing measures for pain; medication is last resort. Check on food preferences. Sabbath is from Friday sundown until Saturday sundown for most groups. Client may refuse medical treatment and use of secular items, such as television, on Sabbath.

Source: Murray, R., & Zentner, J. (2001). *Health promotion strategies through the life span* (7th ed.). Reprinted by permission of Pearson Education, Inc., Upper Saddle River, NJ 07458.

chances are the patient will remain ill regardless of medical intervention. If the patient believes that a healer removes a spell, chances are improvement for whatever reason (healer or medical) will surely follow. There are many things that cannot be explained in our world. Open yourself to new experiences for your own benefit and for your patient's benefit.

People who do not deny but doubt the existence of God because it cannot be proved are agnostics. Atheists deny the existence of a God and reject all religious beliefs. Remember, just because a person says that he or she is an agnostic or an atheist does not mean that he or she has no spiritual beliefs. It is still important for you to consider the patient's spiritual beliefs when providing health care.

It is important for nurses to address a patient's spirituality whether the patient follows a specific religion or not. As nurses, we can provide spiritual comfort and we can see that spiritual resources are available to the patient. We can convey a caring, accepting, nonjudgmental attitude and provide the kind of atmosphere where patients will feel comfortable sharing their spiritual concerns. Remember that spirituality is much more important than checking a box on a required form!

STOP **ASK YOURSELF**

1. Do you think you would be comfortable asking the patient questions related to spirituality? Why or why not?

2. What, if any, new understanding of the role of spirituality in health care have you gained from the reading of this chapter?

_____

_____

 CYBERLINKS: FLASH CARDS ——————————

Check to see what you now remember by making your own flash cards. Use the CD-ROM that accompanies your textbook to discover how to make flash cards for reviewing and retaining what you have learned.

 CONCEPT MAP WORD BANK ——————————

SPIRITUALITY

IMPORTANCE IN HEALTH CARE

SPIRITUAL DISTRESS

SPIRITUAL ASSESSMENT

Refer to Concept Maps and Flash Cards on pages viii–ix for an explanation of how to create and use concept maps. In addition, the CD-ROM guides you through the construction of concept maps by providing a more detailed introduction, more illustrations of examples, and key steps to follow in designing your own maps.

Death and Dying

ASK YOURSELF

1. What fears or concerns do you have related to your own eventual death?

   _____

   _____

2. What fears or concerns do you have related to caring for a dying patient?

   _____

   _____

CYBERLINKS

Interactive **www.healthcentral.com** has cool tools related to the topic of death and dying. For instance, you can estimate your own life expectancy. Once at the site, scroll down to Cool Tools, then to Life and Death, and click on Millennium Life Expectancy.

Supplemental **www.LPNresources.com** can help enhance your learning by leading you to discover other links with more information about the topic you are studying.

Death and dying may or may not be part of your nursing curriculum. If you do learn about death, it will most likely be incorporated into various nursing courses. Whether or not you learn about death and dying in school, we can guarantee that you will be exposed to it during your nursing career.

American society in general would have us believe that death is something to be avoided at all costs. We should not discuss it, we should avoid people who are dying, and most of all, we should not admit that we ourselves will die. Our society is so focused on youth, vitality, and immortality that we often lose sight of the meaningfulness of the dying experience. Other cultures embrace dying people and use the death experience for renewal and growth. As nurses, if we choose to fear death and avoid it, we will treat dying patients in the same manner. If, however, we choose to embrace death and learn from dying patients, we can provide the support, love, and understanding that they need.

| CORE CONCEPTS | **DEATH ACROSS THE LIFE SPAN** |

As stated, all of us will die, and death occurs at all ages and throughout the life span. Although we all have our own individual reaction to death, most of us find it particularly hard to face the death of a child. It is also difficult to face the death of someone close to our own age and the deaths of close relatives and loved ones. Although none of us wants anyone to die, most of us can accept the death of someone who is ill and elderly as being inevitable and probably a relief. Table 22-1 shows how various age groups view and explain death and how society reacts to the death of someone in that age group.

| CORE CONCEPTS | **DEATH AND NURSING** |

All living things will die. It is a fact of nature. Where, when, and how we will die, none of us know. The same holds true for our friends, family, and loved ones. Most of us learn about death at an early age through the loss of a pet, or perhaps a grandparent. Some of us are protected from death and do not experience a death until we are adults. As a nurse, you will definitely experience a patient's death, so you will need to learn to prepare for it and grow from it.

Occasionally, nursing students experience their first death during a clinical rotation. As difficult as it is to lose a patient, it happens to be a good time to experience a death. During your clinical rotation you will have the support of your instructor and fellow students.

Working with the dying can be challenging for nurses. As nurses, we are not immune to death, and we will have to learn how to relate to dying patients.

- Some nurses are very good with dying people; others are not.
- We must learn to show compassion to all patients.
- If you are afraid of dying patients, then take the opportunity to find out why.
- If the dying patient makes you angry, then you need to learn to control your anger.
- If you cannot handle the thought of your own death, then try to come to some understanding of why that is.
- Some nurses need to seek the help of a counselor to come to terms with their feelings about death and dying.

Dying people can teach us many things about ourselves if we leave ourselves open to each learning opportunity.

TABLE 22-1	Death of a Child, Adult, or Elderly Person

Perception of Death	Society's Response

Child

- The very young child (under age 3) has no perception of the permanence of death. By age 3–6, a child understands loss by separation (not permanence). By age 6–9, the child understands that death is permanent. At age 10–12, the child understands death and realizes that it can happen to anyone at anytime (Burgess, 1997).
- Most children are very perceptive and know when they are dying.
- Children may try to protect their parents by not discussing death with them. They need to be encouraged to talk with family members.
- Often children will openly discuss death with other children or with health care givers.

- The death of a child causes much grief and anger.
- Why have they died young?
- How could God take such a young child?
- Ongoing pain for parents and loved ones.
- Loss of continuance of the human race.
- More of a tragedy than the death of someone who has "lived a full life."

Adult

- Young adults are aware of the possibility of death, but rarely think it will happen to them.
- As people age, they become more familiar with death and think about the financial and legal ramifications of an early death.
- A majority of adults face the loss of their parents and, sometimes, siblings and spouses.

- Depends on the age of the individual. Once again, most are more affected by and wonder about the loss of the young adult.
- As people age, they accept that death can occur at any time. Many people believe in the hope of an eternal resting place.

Elderly

- The elderly realize that death is a common event but continue to live their lives to the fullest.

- Our society correlates aging with death.
- People tend to accept the death of an aged person more easily than the death of a child.

| CORE CONCEPTS | **PREPARATION FOR DEATH** |

There are a number of things that must be considered prior to our deaths. Some people are lucky enough and wise enough to attend to all the details of dying. Others die unprepared and leave family or friends to cope with the details of their death.

The Funeral   The majority of individuals in our society will have a funeral or memorial service. The service will depend on the religious affiliation of the deceased as well as personal and family desires. Most nurses are not involved with planning a funeral for patients, but you may need to encourage some patients to consider planning a funeral. Many nurses who work with dying patients have participated in the funeral process. Some things to consider when planning a funeral are:

- Burial or cremation
- Setting of service
- Religious readings or favorite passages
- Who will read or speak
- Music

The Will   A will is an important legal document that helps us to distribute our property upon our deaths.

- A will must comply with the legal statutes in the state in which the person resides.
- Two witnesses who have no beneficiary interest in the estate must sign it.
- If a person dies without a will (intestate), the estate will usually pass to a surviving spouse or children, although this may vary depending on the state in which the person resides, and the estate must pass through the probate process.
- Any person who has specific ideas about the distribution of their property should be encouraged to make a will. A handwritten (holographic) will is acceptable as long as it is witnessed by two people with no beneficiary interest.
- If a patient has no will, a lawyer can be found who will make a hospital visit and complete the document for approval and signatures. The patient must be mentally competent in order to do this and not under the influence of drugs. (Most schools do not recommend that student nurses witness such documents. If a patient wishes to make a will while in the hospital and needs witnesses, refer him or her to the hospital social worker or chaplain.)

| CORE CONCEPTS | **ADVANCE HEALTH CARE DIRECTIVES** |

The federal Patient Self-Determination Act became effective in December of 1991. All federally funded health care institutions are required to provide patients with written information about the right to complete advance health care directives at the time of admission. Most health care facilities present this information to patients or residents upon admission or prior to surgery. Often, the chaplain or social worker will be available to discuss options with patients and their families. These advance directives, if enacted, are placed in the patient's chart on admission. If the patient chooses not to enact them, a signed form stating such should also be included in the chart. All of the advance directives are used to indicate what type of medical care or how much life-sustaining treatment is desired if the patient is no longer physically or mentally able to make those decisions. In most states, these forms must be in writing and are witnessed by two individuals. Sometimes a signature and seal by a notary public are required to certify the signatures of the person directing the advance directives as well as the witnesses.

Students need to be aware that advance directive forms are specific to each state. They are different and may even have different names. Be familiar with the forms that are used in the state where you are going to school or expect to be employed. Figure 22-1 used in this text is a Florida-specific document of a living will. Partnership for Caring (previously Choice in Dying) has all state forms on their Web site at **www.partnershipforcaring.org.** This organization recommends the use of state-specific documents for advance directives. There are several forms of advance directives:

The Living Will

1. The living will allows competent individuals to state how much lifesaving medical intervention they desire if they become unable to make their wishes known.

2. Most living wills state that the individual wishes to be kept pain free, but that extraordinary means of keeping one alive are not desired. Extraordinary means could include the use of the ventilator, insertion of a feeding tube, and so on.

3. The language is often vague. The patient may wish to add in specific information such as:
   - No cardiopulmonary resuscitation (CPR)
   - No respirator
   - No tube feedings
   - No dialysis

4. Living wills require the signatures of two witnesses.

5. There is no legal requirement forcing physicians to follow a living will.

6. There is also no protection from criminal or civil liability for physicians, so many physicians choose to ignore the patient's wishes (Guido, 2001).

The Natural Death Act

1. The natural death act is a living will that is legally recognized and has statutory enforcement (Figure 22-2).

Figure 22-1 Florida Living Will

INSTRUCTIONS	**FLORIDA LIVING WILL**
PRINT THE DATE **PRINT YOUR NAME**	Declaration made this _____ day of _____, _____, *(day)* *(month)* *(year)* I, _____, willfully and voluntarily make known my desire that my dying not be artificially prolonged under the circumstances set forth below, and I do hereby declare that:
PLEASE INITIAL EACH THAT APPLIES	If at any time I am incapacitated and _____ I have a terminal condition, or _____ I have an end-stage condition, or _____ I am in a persistent vegetative state and if my attending or treating physician and another consulting physician have determined that there is no reasonable medical probability of my recovery from such condition, I direct that life-prolonging procedures be withheld or withdrawn when the application of such procedures would serve only to prolong artificially the process of dying, and that I be permitted to die naturally with only the administration of medication or the performance of any medical procedure deemed necessary to provide me with comfort care or to alleviate pain. It is my intention that this declaration be honored by my family and physician as the final expression of my legal right to refuse medical or surgical treatment and to accept the consequences for such refusal. In the event that I have been determined to be unable to provide express and informed consent regarding the withholding, withdrawal, or continuation of life-prolonging procedures, I wish to designate, as my surrogate to carry out the provisions of this declaration:
PRINT THE NAME, HOME ADDRESS AND TELEPHONE NUMBER OF YOUR SURROGATE	Name: _____ Address: _____ _____ Zip Code: _____ Phone: _____
© 2000 **PARTNERSHIP FOR CARING, INC.**	

Source: Reprinted by permission of Partnership for Caring, 1620 Eye Street, NW, Suite 202, Washington, DC 20007, (800) 989-9455.

Figure 22-1 Florida Living Will (Continued)

	FLORIDA LIVING WILL — PAGE 2 OF 2
	I wish to designate the following person as my alternate surrogate, to carry out the provisions of this declaration should my surrogate be unwilling or unable to act on my behalf:
PRINT NAME, HOME ADDRESS AND TELEPHONE NUMBER OF YOUR ALTERNATE SURROGATE	Name: _____ Address: _____ _____ Zip Code: _____ Phone: _____
ADD PERSONAL INSTRUCTIONS (IF ANY)	Additional instructions (optional):
	I understand the full import of this declaration, and I am emotionally and mentally competent to make this declaration.
SIGN THE DOCUMENT	Signed: _____

WITNESSING PROCEDURE
 	
TWO WITNESSES MUST SIGN AND PRINT THEIR ADDRESSES
	Witness 1:
	   Signed: _____
	   Address: _____
	Witness 2:
	   Signed: _____
	   Address: _____

© 2000 PARTNERSHIP FOR CARING, INC.	*Courtesy of* **Partnership for Caring, Inc.** 6/00 1035 30th Street, NW Washington, DC 20007 800-989-9455

Figure 22-2 Declaration of Desire for a Natural Death

DECLARATION OF A DESIRE FOR A NATURAL DEATH

I, _____ being of sound mind, desire that, as specified below, my life not be prolonged by extraordinary means or by artificial nutrition or hydration if my condition is determined to be terminal and incurable or if I am diagnosed as being in a persistent vegetative state. I am aware and understand that this writing authorizes a physician to withhold or discontinue extraordinary means or artificial nutrition or hydration, in accordance with my specifications as set forth below:
(Initial any of the following as desired):

If my condition is determined to be terminal and incurable, I authorize the following:
_____ My physician may withhold or discontinue extraordinary means only.
In addition to withholding or discontinuing extraordinary means if such means are necessary, my physician may withhold or discontinue either artificial nutrition or hydration, or both.
If my physician determines that I am in a persistent vegetative state, I authorize the following:
_____ My physician may withhold or discontinue extraordinary means only.
In addition to withholding or discontinuing extraordinary means if such means are necessary, my physician may withhold or discontinue either artificial nutrition or hydration, or both.
This the _____ day of _____ , 1999.

I hereby state that the Declarant, _____ , being of sound mind, signed the above Declaration in my presence and that I am not related to the Declarant by blood or marriage and that I do not know or have a reasonable expectation that I would be entitled to any portion of the estate of the Declarant under any existing Will or Codicil of the Declarant or as an heir under the Interstate Succession Act if the Declarant died on this date without a Will. I also state that I am not the Declarant's physician, or an employee of any health facility in which the Declarant is a patient, or an employee of a nursing home or any group-care home where the Declarant resides. I further still state that I do not now have any claim against the Declarant.
WITNESS our hands and seals this the _____ day of _____ , 1991.

_____ (SEAL)
Witness

_____ (SEAL)
Witness

CERTIFICATE

I, _____ , Notary Public for _____ , hereby certify that _____ , the Declarant, appeared before me and swore to me and to the witnesses in my presence that this instrument is his/her Declaration of a Desire for a Natural Death, and that he/she had willingly and voluntarily made and executed it as his/her free act and deed for the purposes therein expressed.
I further certify that _____ and _____ , witnesses, appeared before me and swore that they witnessed _____ , the Declarant, sign the attached Declaration, believing him/her to be of sound mind; and also swore that at the time they witnessed the Declaration (i) they were not related within the third degree to the Declarant or to the Declarant's spouse, and (ii) they did not know or have reasonable expectation that they would be entitled to any portion of the estate of the Declarant upon the Declarant's death under any Will of the Declarant or Codicil thereto then existing or under the Interstate Succession Act as it provides at that time, and (iii) they were not a physician attending the Declarant or an employee of an attending physician or an employee of a nursing home or any group-care home where the Declarant resided, and (iv) they did not have a claim against the Declarant. I further certify that I am satisfied as to the genuineness and due execution of the Declarant.
This the _____ day of _____ , 1999.

Notary Public for Mecklenburg
County, North Carolina

(Notary Seal)

My Commission expires: _____

Source: Murray, R. B., & Zentner, J. P. (1997). *Health assessment & promotion strategies through the life span.* (6th ed.). Reprinted by permission of Pearson Education, Inc., Upper Saddle River, NJ 07458.

2. In most states, individuals over the age of 18 are able to sign a natural death act if they are of sound mind and capable of understanding the document.

3. In most states, the document requires the patient's signature and the signature of two witnesses who will not benefit from the patient's death. The witnesses cannot be related to the patient.

4. Some states have a mandatory form that must be filled out; others do not. Be sure that you are familiar with the laws in your state (Guido, 2001).

Durable Power of Attorney for Health Care (DPAHC) or Medical Durable Power of Attorney (MDPA)

1. The DPAHC and MDPA allow a competent person to give decision-making authority about medical interventions to another individual (Figure 22-3).

2. The durable DPAHC and MDPA are only enacted when patients are mentally incapable of making decisions for themselves.

3. This document allows the person who holds the durable power of attorney to do the following:
   - Ask questions
   - Select and remove physicians from the patient's care
   - Assess risks and complications
   - Select treatments and procedures
   - Refuse care and/or life-sustaining procedures
   - Act in full authority as the patient would act if he or she were able to

4. Whoever is given the durable power of attorney is responsible for making medical determinations and does not need to consult with other interested parties.

5. Health care providers are protected from liability if they act in good faith on the agent's decisions (Guido, 1997).

Do Not Resuscitate (DNR) Directives   Some facilities have institutional guidelines regarding do not resuscitate (DNR) or no code orders. Physicians are allowed to place a DNR or no code order in the patient's chart after consultation with the patient or the patient's health care proxy (Guido, 2001). All staff and students caring for the patient should be aware of the patient's wishes concerning a DNR. As a student, that should be one of the first things you educate yourself on before caring for a patient.

Directive to Physicians   Some states recognize a document called a directive to physicians. This document complements the living will and DPAHC (Figure 22-4). The document is directed specifically to physicians and spells out the patient's desires with regard to medical treatment should the individual become incapaci-

Figure 22-3 Florida Designation of Health Care Surrogate

INSTRUCTIONS	**FLORIDA DESIGNATION OF HEALTH CARE SURROGATE**
PRINT YOUR NAME	Name:_____ *(Last)* *(First)* *(Middle Initial)* In the event that I have been determined to be incapacitated to provide informed consent for medical treatment and surgical and diagnostic procedures, I wish to designate as my surrogate for health care decisions:
PRINT THE NAME, HOME ADDRESS AND TELEPHONE NUMBER OF YOUR SURROGATE	Name:_____ Address: _____ _____ Zip Code: _____ Phone: _____ If my surrogate is unwilling or unable to perform his or her duties, I wish to designate as my alternate surrogate:
PRINT THE NAME, HOME ADDRESS AND TELEPHONE NUMBER OF YOUR ALTERNATE SURROGATE	Name: _____ Address: _____ _____ Zip Code: _____ Phone: _____ I fully understand that this designation will permit my designee to make health care decisions and to provide, withhold, or withdraw consent on my behalf; to apply for public benefits to defray the cost of health care; and to authorize my admission to or transfer from a health care facility.
ADD PERSONAL INSTRUCTIONS (IF ANY)	Additional instructions (optional):
© 2000 PARTNERSHIP FOR CARING, INC.	

Source: Reprinted by permission of Partnership for Caring, 1620 Eye Street, NW, Suite 202, Washington, DC 20007, (800) 989-9455.

Figure 22-3 Florida Designation of Health Care Surrogate (Continued)

FLORIDA DESIGNATION OF HEALTH CARE SURROGATE — PAGE 2 OF 2

I further affirm that this designation is not being made as a condition of treatment or admission to a health care facility. I will notify and send a copy of this document to the following persons other than my surrogate, so they may know who my surrogate is:

PRINT THE NAMES AND ADDRESSES OF THOSE WHO YOU WANT TO KEEP COPIES OF THIS DOCUMENT

Name: _____

Address: _____

Name: _____

Address: _____

SIGN AND DATE THE DOCUMENT

Signed: _____

Date: _____

WITNESSING PROCEDURE

TWO WITNESSES MUST SIGN AND PRINT THEIR ADDRESSES

Witness 1:

Signed: _____

Address: _____

Witness 2:

Signed: _____

Address: _____

Courtesy of **Partnership for Caring, Inc.**   10/99
1035 30th Street, NW Washington, DC 20007 800-989-9455

Figure 22-4 Medical Directive

MEDICAL DIRECTIVE

I, _____ , being of sound mind, make this statement as a directive to be followed if I am ever unable to participate in decisions regarding my medical care. Should I become mentally incompetent because of a medical condition like a coma or persistent vegetative state or severe dementia and my doctors do not expect me to recover, I direct the following treatment decisions be made in my behalf. These directions express my legal right to refuse treatment.

	YES	NO	UNSURE
1. CPR: Use drugs, electric shock, and artificial breathing to bring me back to life when my heart stops.	_____	_____	_____
2. Mechanical breathing: Use a machine to do my breathing for me when I cannot breathe unaided.	_____	_____	_____
3. Artificial nutrition: Give me food through a tube in my vein or stomach.	_____	_____	_____
4. Artificial hydration: Give me liquid through a tube in my vein.	_____	_____	_____
5. Hospitalization: Move me from my home or hospice or nursing home to a hospital.	_____	_____	_____
6. Major surgery: Operate on something like a blockage in my stomach or remove my gallbladder.	_____	_____	_____
7. Kidney dialysis: Have a machine do the work of my kidneys—cleansing my blood— when they stop working on their own.	_____	_____	_____
8. Chemotherapy: Give me drugs to fight cancer.	_____	_____	_____
9. Minor surgery: Operate on something minor like an infected toe.	_____	_____	_____
10. Major tests: Do tests like heart catheterization or colonoscopy to see what is wrong inside me.	_____	_____	_____
11. Blood: Transfuse blood or blood products into me if I am in need of them.	_____	_____	_____
12. Antibiotics: Give me drugs to fight diseases like pneumonia or a kidney infection.	_____	_____	_____
13. Minor tests: Do an x-ray or a blood test to see what is wrong with me.	_____	_____	_____
14. Pain medication: Give me enough medication so that I am not in pain.	_____	_____	_____
15. Home: Move me from the hospital so that I can die at home.	_____	_____	_____

16. Other: _____

_____

_____

_____

_____   _____ _____ _____

I provide this directive in addition to my living will.

Signed _____   Date _____

Witness _____

Witness _____

Source: Murray, R. B., & Zentner, J. P. (1997). *Health assessment & promotion strategies through the life span.* (6th ed.). Reprinted by permission of Pearson Education, Inc., Upper Saddle River, NJ 07458.

tated. This document is similar in legality to the living will in that the physician can choose to follow it or not.

Hospice   Hospice is a form of a directive in that it offers terminally ill patients an alternative to dying in a hospital environment with a host of life-sustaining equipment. Hospice also allows the patient to do without signing a living will or other medical directive, as the philosophy behind the hospice movement is that death is a natural part of life. Hospice organizations believe that it is important to offer nursing and medical care to maintain comfort without life-sustaining measures. For example, the patient will not be resuscitated, and other life support systems will not be used when death is near. Hospice personnel provide comfort and support to the family as well as to the individual who is dying. One of the many benefits of hospice care is that it allows the family some relief from caring for the terminally ill individual. After the patient dies, the hospice personnel continue to provide the family with support during their period of grieving.

The objective of hospice care is to keep the patient at home for as long as possible and make the patient's last days as comfortable and meaningful as possible. However, hospice does oversee the care of patients who choose to enter an inpatient hospice bed located in either a progressive care unit of a hospital, in a long-term care facility, or in a total hospice facility. The hospice nurses continue to direct the patient care and visit the patients. This may be done, because the family of the patient can no longer assume the caregiver role or may need some respite from the long months of caregiving.

Most hospices require the patient to be competent to make a decision to choose hospice care. Many also require that the patient be in a terminal condition with a maximum number of months left to live (for example, one hospice treats patients with less than 6 months to live). In 1982, Congress recognized the need for alternative terminal care and authorized Medicare reimbursement for hospice care (Public Law 97-248, 1982). Many hospices are affiliated with hospitals, but there are also a number of hospice home health agencies that may or may not be affiliated with hospitals or other health care facilities.

| CORE CONCEPTS | **REACTIONS OF TERMINALLY ILL PEOPLE** |

Once a person receives a terminal diagnosis, intense emotional reactions are normal. The individual often experiences the following painful feelings:

- Emptiness
- Disbelief
- Rage
- Loss of control
- Fear of pain and suffering
- Isolation
- Alienation

- Fear of abandonment
- Fear of financial ruin

These feelings are quite normal and to be expected (Varcarolis, 1998). The individual usually moves back and forth between feelings and may seem calm one minute and very angry the next. In 1969, Kübler-Ross published a classic text, *On Death and Dying*. Kübler-Ross studied dying patients and learned about the dying process. As a result of this work, Kübler-Ross determined that there are five stages to the dying process:

1. *Denial:* When the patient cannot accept the terminal diagnosis. Denial is healthy and gives the patient time to adjust to the diagnosis.

2. *Anger:* The patient wants to know "why me." Anger may be kept in or it may be displaced onto family, friends, and health care givers.

3. *Bargaining:* The patient usually bargains with God, offering to be a better person or to live a better life.

4. *Depression:* Once the anger and denial have worn off, the patient begins to feel a great sense of loss. Depression occurs when the patient realizes that no amount of medicine, surgery, or alternative therapy can cure his or her illness.

5. *Acceptance:* The patient has finished mourning his or her losses and becomes physically weaker. Often, the patient withdraws and stops communicating with loved ones in preparation for death, although he or she may be comforted by having someone in the room or by someone holding his or her hand.

The nurse needs to intervene with the dying patient depending on which stage the patient is in. In other words, we would not treat a patient in the anger stage in the same way we would treat a patient in the bargaining stage (Table 22-2). It's important to note that often the family of the dying patient will also go through these same stages but may not necessarily be in the same stage as the patient at the same time.

The dying patient has many tasks that need to be accomplished. Some of these tasks are affected by Kübler-Ross's stages of dying, although they are not related. Humphrey (1986) identified the following adaptation tasks:

- Getting affairs in order
- Coping with the loss of both loved ones and self
- Considering future health care needs
- Planning for the time remaining
- Anticipating future pain and physical losses, contributing to a loss of identity
- Considering being a nonperson
- Deciding to speed up or slow down the dying process

TABLE 22-2	Nursing Interventions and Rationales: Working with a Person Who Is Dying

Intervention	Rationale
Stage One: Denial and Isolation	
1. Examine own feelings about death.	1. Personal defenses and fears can be projected onto dying person if not identified and worked out.
2. Encourage the patient's expression of feelings, concerns, and fears: • Sit at bedside. • Actively listen and reflect patient's feelings. • Hold hand or touch shoulder when appropriate.	2. • Provides presence and decreases feelings of abandonment. • Lessens feelings of isolation and keeps channels of communication open. • For some, physical touch provides comfort and demonstrates concern.
3. Provide small amount of information at a time. Encourage questions when patient is ready.	3. Having correct information can decrease anxiety and clarify information.
4. Encourage decisions regarding self-care.	4. Increases feelings of control and encourages functioning at optimum level.
Stage Two: Anger	
1. Acknowledge person's right to be angry.	1. Increases feelings of support and being understood.
2. Understand that anger directed at staff and family is not personal.	2. Feelings of helplessness and loss stimulate anger, which is often projected onto staff and loved ones.
3. Work with patient to rechannel anger into positive channels, eg, making decisions, setting goals, and fighting disease.	3. Can help rechannel energy in ways that help increase self-esteem, feelings of control, and sense of being supported by staff and others.
Stage Three: Bargaining	
1. Offer to contact clergy or rabbi.	1. May assist in dispelling irrational religious beliefs.
2. Encourage discussion of feelings, especially guilt and loss.	2. Decreases feelings of guilt and possible thoughts of being punished for past actions.
3. Encourage patient's positive coping strategies used in the past.	3. Positive reinforcement can strengthen positive behaviors.
4. Encourage periods of time to focus on more satisfying areas of life.	4. Periods of time away from discussion of disease and death helps person put life in broader terms.

TABLE 22-2	Nursing Interventions and Rationales: Working with a Person Who Is Dying (Continued)

Intervention	Rationale
Stage Four: Depression	
1. Focus on daily short-term *obtainable* goals.	1. Emphasizes positive functioning and areas of independence.
2. Continue to spend time with patient on regular basis.	2. Staff awareness of tendency to withdraw can help staff modify own behaviors.
3. Encourage patient to participate in usual activities.	3. Can decrease time spent in brooding and offer broader focus of experience.
4. Encourage patient to participate in support groups.	4. Discussion with others in similar circumstances can decrease feelings of isolation and increase feelings of being understood.
5. Maintain adequate pain control.	5. Physical comfort can increase ability to interact with others and may diminish tendency to withdraw.
Stage Five: Acceptance	
1. Sit with person—even when person does not want to talk.	1. Provides presence and support and decreases feelings of abandonment.
2. Allow appropriate privacy, eg, during toileting and bathing.	2. Maintains sense of dignity.
3. Continue pain control.	3. Provides comfort during final stages of dying.

Source: Varcarolis, E. M. (1998). *Foundations of psychiatric–mental health nursing* (3rd ed). Philadelphia, PA: Saunders.

Most human beings want to feel that their time on earth has not been wasted, and that they will leave something of themselves behind. Dying patients may want to participate in developing an activity to help keep their memories alive for family and friends. For example, they might choose one of the following:

- Writing a journal
- Recording shared times on videotape
- Recording personal messages on audiotape
- Distributing photographs
- Distributing personal possessions to loved ones (Burgess, 1997, p. 248)

CORE CONCEPTS	GRIEF AND GRIEVING

The Individual   Grief begins as soon as a threat of loss occurs. Individuals experience anticipatory grief (grief that occurs as one anticipates loss of self or loved one) at the time of a terminal diagnosis or of a terminal diagnosis of a loved one. Whenever an individual anticipates a loss, or experiences a loss, it is a reminder of all the other losses he or she has ever experienced. Grief is a very private experience. Each individual grieves in his or her own way, depending on background experiences as well as psychological, sociocultural, and spiritual factors. It is important to realize that since we all grieve differently, there is no specific formula for assisting an individual through the grieving process.

The Family   One factor that affects the family is the type of death that has occurred. Some family members have the opportunity to grieve over a longer period of time than others do. For example, a person dying of cancer may live 2 to 3 years; someone else might die unexpectedly in an automobile accident. Either death is traumatic for the family, but if a death is prolonged, the family has the ability to begin working through the grief process while the patient is still living.

Rando (1993) identified six stages of the mourning process. These six stages occur in three phases: avoidance, confrontation, and accommodation (Table 22-3). Rando's phases are similar to Kübler-Ross's stages of dying in that the individual moves back and forth between stages.

The nurse can help the family deal with their grief by developing an awareness of the family's response to dying and death. To help guide a family through the grieving process, you will need to be aware of what the family is experiencing (Table 22-4).

The Child   Children are extremely sensitive to family dynamics and will know when something is wrong. Young children will experience distress when separated from a parent or loved one who is very ill or hospitalized. According to Siegel and colleagues (1992), children experience distress related to the following:

- Increasing limitations of parents' physical or emotional availability
- Loss or separation from parent
- Changes in parents' role functioning
- Changes in family routines
- Changes in family emotional climate
- Decreases in financial resources due to caring for an ill family member

Children need to be made aware of the situation and should be allowed to ask questions. Since children are often very intuitive and sometimes blunt, parents need to be aware that it is not possible to hide their feelings or emotions. Table 22-5 offers some dos and don'ts for discussing death with children.

TABLE 22-3	Rando's Six "R" Processes of Mourning

Avoidance phase
  Recognize the loss
    • Acknowledge the death
    • Understand the death

Confrontation phase
  React to the separation
    • Experience the pain
    • Feel, identify, accept, and give some form of expression to all of the psychological reactions to the loss
    • Identify and mourn secondary losses
  Recollect and reexperience the deceased and the relationship
    • Review and remember the relationship realistically
    • Revive and reexperience the feelings in the relationship
  Reliquish the old attachments to the deceased and the old assumptive world

Accommodation phase
  Readjust to move adaptively into the new world without forgetting the old
    • Revise the assumptive world
    • Develop a new relationship with the deceased
    • Adapt new ways of being in the world
    • Form a new identity
  Reinvest personal energies

Source: Printed with permission from Rando, T. A. (1993, p. 45). *Treatment of complicated mourning.* Champaign, IL: Research Press.

One thing that we have learned through many years of working with suicidal patients is that children have difficulty understanding suicide. The death of a parent is traumatic, but when that death is by suicide, the family is often reluctant to discuss it with a child. Many times, families glorify death by saying things like "Daddy is in heaven," or "Daddy has gone to a wonderful place to be with God," or "Daddy is in a better place and he is happy." Whatever is said, be certain that the child does not think that heaven is a better place to be than earth. We have had very young children decide to join Daddy because heaven sounded much nicer than living. It is difficult to get this concept across to children, but it is important that they know that "Daddy" is dead and that it will be difficult to live without him.

CORE CONCEPTS	DYSFUNCTIONAL GRIEF

In some cases, a surviving family member or friend may experience dysfunctional grief. This is a profound, lasting exaggeration of the grieving process. The survivor becomes dependent on others to make decisions and to get him or her through each day. He or she cannot cope with the activities of daily life and are essentially non-

TABLE 22-4	Family's Response to Dying and Death	
Four Main Stages	**Family Experiences**	**Nurse Can Foster**
Living with Terminal Illness		
Person learns diagnosis, tries to carry on as usual, undergoes treatment	*Impact:* Emotional shock, despair, disorganized behavior	Hope as different treatment methods are used, communication, seeking helpful resources, family cohesiveness
	Functional disruption: Much time spent at hospital (if traditional surgery or treatment chosen), ignoring of home tasks and emotional needs, weakening of family structure, emotional isolation	
	Search for meaning: Questioning why this happened; casting blame on various persons, deity, institutions, habits; realization that "Someday I will die too"	Security
	Informing others (family and friends): Ascent from isolation, with moral and practical support—or feeling of rejection: others do not understand, do not care, or are afraid; possible need to retreat again into emotional isolation	Courage, reliable help, understanding of why some people cannot help
	Engaging emotions: Beginning grieving, fearing loss of emotional control, assumption of roles once carried by dying person	Problem solving; idea that life will change but will be ongoing

TABLE 22-4	Family's Response to Dying and Death (Continued)

Four Main Stages	Family Experiences	Nurse Can Foster
Living–Dying Interval Person ceases to perform family roles, is cared for either at home or in hospital; person needs to come to terms with accomplishments and failures and to find renewed meaning in life	*Reorganization:* Firmer division of family tasks *Framing memories:* Reviewing life of dying person —what he or she has meant and accomplished, new sense of family history, relinquishment of dependency on dying member	Cooperation instead of competition; analysis to see if new role distribution is workable Focus on life review rather than only on what person is now
Bereavement Death occurs	*Separation:* Absorption in loneliness of separation as person becomes unconscious *Mourning:* Guilt, "Could I have done more?"	Intimacy among family members; release of grief as normal
Reestablishment	Expansion of the social network: overcoming feelings of alienation and guilt	Looking back with acceptance and forward to new growth and socialization with a reunited, normally functioning family

Source: Murray, R. B., & Zentner, J. P. (2001). *Health promotion strategies through the life span* (7th ed.). Reprinted by permission of Pearson Education, Inc. Upper Saddle River, NJ 07458.

functional. When grief of this depth persists, professional counseling must be considered. If left untreated, this grief could result in the act of suicide for the survivor.

CORE CONCEPTS | **THE NURSE AND GRIEF**

Everyone grieves, and nurses are no exception. Most nurses believe that they should be able to maintain their "professional demeanor" and not give in to their feelings. When the death of a patient occurs, we have a right to grieve our loss and express our feelings. We also need to comfort other nurses who are grieving. Remember that there is no "right" or "wrong" when it comes to grieving. Grieving as a nurse or a student is especially common in the areas of long-term care and home health, wherein you may care for the same patient for a long period of time. Many facili-

TABLE 22-5	Do's and Don'ts for Discussing Death with Children

Do

- Ask the child what he or she is feeling. Bring up the subject of death naturally in the context of a dead pet, a book character, television show, movie, or news item.
- Help the child have a funeral for a dead pet.
- Help the child realize he or she is not responsible for the death.
- Tell the child what has happened on his or her level (but not in morbid detail).
- Explain the funeral service briefly beforehand; attendance depends on the child's age and wishes.
- Answer questions honestly, with responses geared to the child's age.
- Remember that expressions of pain, anger, loneliness, or aloneness do not constitute symptoms of an illness but are part of a natural process of grieving.
- Help the child realize that the adults are also grieving and feel upset, anger, despair, and guilt.

Do Not

- Admonish the child not to cry; it is a universal way to show grief and anxiety.
- Tell a mystical story about the loss of the person; it could cause confusion and anxiety.
- Give long, exclusively detailed explanations beyond the level of understanding.
- Associate death with sleep, which could result in chronic sleep disturbances.
- Force the child to attend funerals or ignore signs of grieving in the child.

Source: Murray, R. B., & Zentner, J. P. (2001). *Health promotion strategies through the life span* (7th ed.). Reprinted by permission of Pearson Education, Inc. Upper Saddle River, NJ 07458.

ties are beginning to recognize the grief of their staff and are allowing staff members paid time off to attend a funeral service or actually conducting a memorial service within the facility itself to provide an outlet for staff grief.

Be prepared to experience grief as a nurse. Some nurses react to grief by avoidance and refuse to accept their feelings. Other nurses are vulnerable and expose themselves to the grief experience. You will need to learn to experience grief. The most important thing is to put yourself in your patient's shoes. Be empathetic and feel what your patient is feeling. We have cried with parents at the loss of a child and hugged and held the mother of a young man dying of AIDS. For each loss we experience, we know pain, and for the pain we experience, we learn to know joy. Loss is not easy, but just be yourself and offer your heart to the grieving, be they patient or nurse.

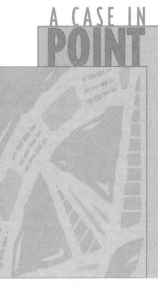

A CASE IN POINT

Jessie was a neonatal nurse who worked in a neonatal intensive care unit (NICU). Jessie was also pregnant and due to deliver her first child in 3 months. At 25 weeks' gestation, Jessie went into premature labor. Despite intervention, she delivered a baby girl with spina bifida by cesarean section. The spinal malformation was severe, and the baby died of sepsis shortly after birth. All of the nurses in the unit who knew Jessie were devastated that the baby had died. No one knew what to do for Jessie. Several nurses felt that Jessie should see and hold the baby, while others felt that she should be spared the sight of her malformed child.

CORE CONCEPTS   **IMPULSIVE SUICIDE**

At some point, you may work with a suicidal patient or even be faced with a suicidal family member, friend, or co-worker. The thought of suicide tends to bring out strong feelings in most people. Some of us believe that suicide is immoral, while others understand that suicide is the result of severe psychological distress. Regardless of your beliefs, suicide happens, and suicide rates in our country continue to rise. Suicide among teenagers and the elderly continue to rise as their numbers also increase (Table 22-6).

Did you ever wonder why it is that the general public often knows the warning signs for cancer, or how to recognize a heart attack, but they have no idea about clues to suicidal behavior? Listed below are some clues to help you recognize a person contemplating suicide:

1. Actual (verbal) clues:
   - "I'm going to kill myself."
   - "I wish I were dead."
   - "My family would be better off without me."
   - "You're going to regret how you've treated me."
   - "I'm tired of living."
   - "Here take this (valued object). I won't be needing it anymore."
   - "I don't need to study for the final exam, I won't be around to take it."

2. Behavior clues:
   - Previous suicide attempt
   - Giving away valued possessions

TABLE 22-6	Summary of Suicide Statistics

- Suicide is the ninth leading cause of death in the United States.
- Suicide is the third cause of death among young people 15–24 years of age.
- The highest suicide rate is for persons over 65 years of age.
- It is estimated that there are about 10 attempted suicides to 1 completion.
- Of *all* suicides, 72% are committed by white males.
- The gender ratio is 4 males to 1 female (4:1).
- Suicide by firearms is the most common method (60% of all suicides).
- Nearly 80% of all firearm suicides are committed by white men.
- Professional persons, including lawyers, dentists, military men, and physicians, have higher-than-average suicide rates.
- Suicide is less frequent among practicing members of most religious groups.

Source: Varcarolis, E. M. (1998, p. 727). *Foundations of psychiatric–mental health nursing* (3rd ed.). Philadelphia, PA: Saunders.

- Drug or alcohol abuse
- Loss of a loved one
- Loss of job/money/prestige
- Prolonged physical illness
- Buying a gun
- Writing a suicide note
- Sudden recovery from a severe depression
- Withdrawal from social activities
- Crying for no apparent reason
- Changes in typical behavior
- Asking others how they would commit suicide if they were going to do it

3. Catastrophic clues (something that is catastrophic for the individual):
   - A student on a football scholarship survives an automobile accident, but is paralyzed from the neck down and unable to play football
   - A young aspiring model breaks her nose and receives several facial scars in a house fire
4. Depressive clues (think of how you feel or act when depressed):
   - Insomnia
   - Anorexia/overeating
   - Sloppiness
   - Inability to concentrate (drop in grades)
   - Feeling worthless
   - Feeling hopeless
   - Loss of self-esteem
   - Rage/anger/hostility

- Preoccupation with death
- Chronic minor illness or accidents

It is important for everyone to be familiar with suicidal clues. An individual who is suicidal will most likely give more than one clue. For example, someone might decide to make a will or plan a funeral after the death of a friend, but that individual is being prudent, not suicidal. However, if the person makes out a will, plans a funeral, says "I wish I were dead," appears depressed, and buys a gun, that person is probably suicidal.

Once it is apparent that the individual may be suicidal, you need to ask, "Are you thinking about harming yourself?" or "Are you considering suicide?" or a similar question. Asking the question does not give the individual the idea to commit suicide. He or she already has the idea. Once you ask the question, the individual will either admit feeling suicidal or deny it. Most people will be honest with you.

Sometimes all it takes is for someone to care enough to ask one tough question. Have you ever had a major problem that you felt you could not share with anyone else? The distress of carrying that burden alone is often very difficult to handle. During that time, did anyone ask you what was wrong? When we are carrying a heavy burden alone and someone cares enough to ask us about it, we are usually able to share the problem. Once you share the problem with someone else, the burden becomes lighter. The same is true of suicidal thoughts. Sometimes when they are shared with someone else, the suicidal individual feels better and may be willing to seek help in sorting out the problem.

ESSENTIAL SKILLS | SUICIDE INTERVENTION DOS AND DON'TS

If the person tells you that they are considering suicide, here are some intervention dos and don'ts.

Do:

- Be direct
- Talk openly
- Be matter of fact about suicide
- Listen attentively
- Allow the person to express feelings
- Accept the person's feelings
- Be nonjudgmental
- Be available
- Offer alternatives (not false reassurances)
- Take action and remove harmful objects if possible
- Get help from someone who specializes in suicide

Don't:

- Dare the person to go through with it
- Leave the person alone

- Tell the person that he or she is being selfish or a coward
- Promise unrealistic things
- Engage in philosophic discussions (you will lose)
- Debate or lecture
- Promise not to tell anyone (you may need to in order to save a life)

Once it is known that a person is considering suicide, you need to determine the seriousness or *lethality* of the plan. The following things need to be considered:

- Does the person have a plan?
- Is the method of suicide (hanging, guns, or pills, etc.) available?
- How deadly is the proposed plan (higher risk of death with guns, automobile accidents, drowning, and electrocution; lower risk with pills, wrist cutting, and carbon monoxide)? Remember that combining two lower-risk methods of suicide, for example taking barbiturates and using carbon monoxide, may place the person at higher risk.

The more serious the suicide plan, the higher the risk of suicide. After determining whether a patient has a plan and how lethal that plan is, it is necessary to develop a plan for dealing with suicidal behavior. Most suicidal individuals need intervention from a crisis center, emergency room, suicide hotline, or mental health provider. Direct the suicidal individual to the closest available site in your area. Accompany him or her to the hospital or crisis center. Encourage him or her to seek help from a suicide or crisis hotline. When suicide is imminent, it is up to you to get help. If in doubt, it is better to err on the side of caution than to wait too long and have someone die.

Even though you intervene in suicidal behavior, it is important to realize that the choice to live or die is left to the suicidal individual. By that we mean that you can intervene, but the person may still commit suicide. Although in health care we talk about a "safe environment," there is no such thing. Patients have committed suicide on locked psychiatric units in padded seclusion rooms. If someone wants to commit suicide badly enough, he or she will eventually succeed.

If you happen to be doing a clinical in an area where suicidal individuals are brought for treatment, be compassionate. In smaller rural hospitals, they may actually be admitted to a medical–surgical floor. We have worked in the emergency department and have seen suicidal patients being treated disrespectfully. If you observe other staff members treating suicidal patients (or for that matter any patient) disrespectfully, report it! We have witnessed doctors requesting oversized nasogastric tubes to insert into the stomach of suicidal patients in order to perform lavage (washing out of the patient's stomach). This was an attempt on the part of the physician to make the treatment so uncomfortable that the patient would not attempt suicide again. All patients deserve to be treated with respect.

If you become angry and frustrated when caring for suicidal patients, you need to determine why. Nurses are not allowed to abuse patients, and verbal abuse is just as harmful as physical abuse. When someone is desperate enough to consider suicide, the health care giver should not add to that distress. As a student, discuss your anger and frustration with your nursing instructor. The instructor may assign you to another patient or help you work through your feelings to be an effective caregiver with the suicidal patient.

ESSENTIAL SKILLS | SUICIDE SURVIVORS

If you have ever experienced a suicide, you know how difficult it is to accept. Survivors of suicide (SOSs) are confronted with the social disgrace that surrounds suicide as well as the loss of a loved one. Most of us find it difficult to comfort someone who is grieving, but we are more uncomfortable when that person has lost someone to suicide. Often, SOSs face their loss alone because they are unsure of how to seek support. Because of the nature of suicide, many survivors end up feeling abandoned and left alone to mourn their loss.

Some points to consider when dealing with SOSs are as follows:

- An SOS experiences a great deal of anger and guilt that is not always associated with the grief process.
- Nurses need to be available and to actively listen to the SOS.
- Do not think about what you should say, but rather listen to what the survivor is telling you.
- Let the survivor come to conclusions about why the individual committed suicide.
- There is no reason for you to try to offer explanations because chances are you do not know why it happened either.
- The death needs to be talked about openly with all family members.
- Sometimes families avoid discussing the suicide because they are afraid to break the silence that follows.
- Often the family is dysfunctional, and silence is the way that they have dealt with other problems.
- To reach all family members, you may need to relate to each one on an individual basis to allow the individuals to express their grief.

SOSs may take longer to heal because of the nature of their loss. Be patient! There are a number of organizations that provide support to the SOS. If the SOS has access to the Internet, these two sites might be of help:

American Foundation for Suicide Prevention: www.afsp.org

Survivors of Suicide: www.members.xoom.com/sos5/

CORE CONCEPTS | TYPES OF SUICIDE

Nonassisted We stated earlier that no matter how you intervene in a suicidal crisis, the decision to live or die remains with the suicidal individual. Some individuals believe in the right to die and believe that they have the right to choose when and how they die. Quality of life, personal dignity, and self-control all lead a person to rational suicide.

When an individual is in a terminal condition and plans for death by his or her own hand, it is called rational suicide. Many suicides occur in this fashion. Most health care givers are not informed prior to a rational suicide because the individual and his or her family do not want any intervention. Another reason is that when a person commits suicide, insurance companies may refuse to pay benefits.

Assisted Suicide   Assisted suicide is similar to rational suicide in that the individual is experiencing a prolonged and terminal illness. With both rational and assisted suicide, individuals consciously choose to die at a time and place that they choose. In rational suicide the individual has the means for suicide at their disposal; in assisted suicide the dying individual requests assistance from a physician who prescribes a lethal dose of a medication. The primary difference between assisted and rational suicide is that, with assisted suicide, the physician is made aware of the patient's desires.

Assisted suicide is illegal in most states, although Oregon passed the Death with Dignity Act in 1994 (Guido, 2001). Dr. Jack Kevorkian and his "death machine" have forced the state of Michigan to consider the issue as well. Initiatives for assisted suicide have been sponsored by the Hemlock Society, Choice in Dying, and Americans against Human Suffering in California and Washington. According to the Oregon Death with Dignity Act, certain provisions must be met prior to writing a prescription for assisted suicide.

To date, most nursing organizations have agreed that nurses should not encourage assisted or rational suicide. Nurses are in a difficult position because they have been taught to be advocates for patient rights, yet to prevent suicide. Many nurses believe that they should be allowed to respect the patient's right to die rather than face a life of disease with pain and unrelieved suffering. Ironically, the patient is more likely to ask a nurse for information about suicide than a physician. Whether or not you sympathize with the patient's request, it is up to you to provide a sounding board for patients who wish to discuss rational suicide. The nurse can deal with these situations by offering to contact resources, request more pain medication, or just spend time with the patient listening to concerns.

Assisted suicide occurs when a patient seeks help to die. Active euthanasia is providing a patient with an easy, painless death with or without the patient's consent. Many disabled people and others with chronic illness fear that the more society approves of assisted suicide, the more likely euthanasia is to follow. No matter how compassionate and ethical our society claims to be, deciding whether or not a person should die and taking that person's life is still murder at this time. There are other countries, however, where active euthanasia is practiced.

Nurses are involved with life and death decisions on a daily basis. You will hear the term "slow code," meaning that a patient is allowed to die before a code is called, or little is done to resuscitate the patient when a code is called. This occurs when some family members wish their loved one to be allowed to die, and others cannot agree. It is also done when the doctor believes that no further intervention will prolong life, and the patient is suffering. This might be described as passive euthanasia. The patient dies because the health care provider does nothing or does something too slowly to be beneficial.

Death is a subject that we are all familiar with but that few people want to discuss. Whether or not we discuss death, it will continue to occur. All of us need support when someone dies, although we all grieve privately and in our own way. It is important for nurses to support dying patients, grieving families, and other nurses when a death occurs.

 ASK YOURSELF

1. Do you think it would be difficult for you to care for a grieving family of a dying patient? What, in particular, would be difficult for you?

   _____

   _____

2. Do you think it would be appropriate or acceptable for you to cry with a dying patient or the grieving family? Why or why not?

   _____

   _____

 CYBERLINKS: FLASH CARDS

Check to see what you now remember by making your flash cards. Use the CD-ROM that accompanies your textbook to discover how to make flash cards for reviewing and retaining what you have learned.

 CONCEPT MAP WORD BANK

DEATH AND DYING

NURSES ROLE

PREPARATION FOR DEATH

GRIEF

SUICIDE

Refer to Concept Maps and Flash Cards on pages viii–ix for an explanation of how to create and use concept maps. In addition, the CD-ROM guides you through the construction of concept maps by providing a more detailed introduction, more illustrations of examples, and key steps to follow in designing your own maps.

Section IV

CLINICAL COMPETENCIES

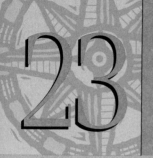

Medication Issues
and Drug Calculations

1. Are medication administration and drug calculation areas of nursing that you would like to better understand? Why or why not?

   _____

   _____

2. What specific areas **of drug** calculations are of greatest concern to you (using conversions, using formulas, etc.)?

   _____

   _____

 CYBERLINKS

<u>Interactive</u> www.healthfinder.com has important information regarding substance abuse. Click on S and then scroll down to Substance Abuse.

<u>Supplemental</u> www.LPNresources.com can help enhance your learning by leading you to discover other links with more information about the topic you are studying.

Regardless of the area of clinical practice, all nursing students, and subsequently many LPN/LVN graduates will administer medications. Medication administration is a grave responsibility, with significant potential for errors that pose serious consequences to patients. Therefore, the guidelines for drug administration cannot be reviewed too often. While this chapter is **not** an in-depth study of clinical calculations, it is meant to supplement what is found in your math textbook or the calculation section of a pharmacology text. Entire courses in clinical calculations or math for medication administration are part of every nursing curriculum. However, the reference provided in this chapter pertains to the core concepts and essential skills most commonly required of LPN/LVNs.

There are five universally accepted rights of medication administration that provide a checklist to guard against error. When administering medication, it is essential that you have the:

1. Right patient
2. Right medication
3. Right dose
4. Right route
5. Right time

As a nursing student, you might hear several more mentioned, including right documentation, but these five are the cardinal rules. Preparing and administering the correct medication dosage is one of your major responsibilities. It often involves the ability to mathematically calculate what that dosage should be. Almost from your first nursing course to your last, faculty will expect you to demonstrate competency in calculating drug doses.

CORE CONCEPTS | **CALCULATION BASICS**

A typical calculation problem nursing faculty will expect you to solve correctly is as follows:

> A patient is to have 100 mg of a medication. The bottle indicates that there is 0.1 g of the medication in one tablet. What do you give the patient?

Faced with this question, students often experience a mild panic attack. Research indicates that many practicing nurses might also have problems solving it correctly, especially if they have been out of school for a while or have not had to do drug calculations. If you follow the basics of medication calculation, you can avoid becoming a member of this group.

Although there are other methods of calculating drug dosages, we will present the two most common ways: formulas and ratio and proportion. Whichever method is used in your school, the use of calculators in your program will be up to the discretion of your instructors. Many schools do not allow the use of calculators. Nursing students may become dependent on them and unable to calculate a drug dosage if they cannot find a calculator to use. We feel that the place of the calculator is to check your answers for accuracy after you have calculated it on paper. This allows you to develop your math skills but still ensure the accuracy of a dosage by confirming the dose with your calculator. Another way to check your calculations is by using both methods (formula and ratio and proportion) to see if you get the same answer.

ESSENTIAL SKILLS | **CALCULATION METHODS**

Whether you are using a formula for calculations or the ratio and proportion method, there are universal abbreviations you need to know:

D = The *desired* strength of the medication, what the patient is to receive or dose.

V = *Vehicle,* or how the medication is packaged, such as the number of pills, number of suppositories, and so on, or the *volume,* such as the amount of liquid involved.

H = On-*hand* strength, the strength that is on the shelf or in the drawer.

X = Amount (number or volume) of the medication that the nurse will actually give to the patient.

Important: X will *always* be how much of the vehicle or volume is to be given to the patient.

Remember: The strength of any medication may be in the metric system, such as milligrams, milliliters, cubic centimeters, kilograms, or grams, or in the apothecary system, such as drams and grains. It may also be in units or milliequivalents. Household measurements might be used in some instances, and these would include units such as teaspoons, tablespoons and ounces. *To be able to calculate many dosages, you must memorize a table of equivalents, so you can go back and forth between the different measurement systems.* Table 23-1 is a simple exchange table that will allow you to convert values from the apothecary system to the metric system and vice versa. If you master these 9 basic values, you can always do ratio and proportion to figure out an equivalent value. Other conversions that will come up often in nursing are:

- 30 mL = 1 oz
- 1 tsp = 5 mL
- 1 Tbsp = 15 mL
- 1 kg = 2.2#

Remember that an exchange table is not a table of exact equivalents but of approximate equivalents. For instance, if the physician's order reads that a patient is to have

TABLE 23-1	**Strength of a Medication**			
Apothecary System		**Metric System**		
Grains	Grams (g)	Milligrams (mg)	Units (U)	Milliequivalents (mEq)
15	1.0	1,000		
7½	0.5	500		
1	0.06	60		

Note: The units and mEq areas are blank. That is because units and mEq are never exchanged into another system of measure. You may, however, have to calculate the amount to give. For example, you are to give 15 mEq and have on hand 30 mEq per 6 cc. Once you place the numbers into the basic drug calculation formula, you will be able to determine that you will need to administer 3 cc.

325 mg of aspirin, and the strength on the aspirin bottle says 5 grains per tablet, you would need to convert the grains to milligrams or vice versa to be able to solve the problem and decide how many tablets of aspirin the patient should receive. According to the table, 60 mg = 1 grain. Using ratio and proportion, 1 gr:60 mg::5 gr:X. This tells us that 5 grains is equivalent to 300 mg. This is the dosage you have on hand. You can solve the problem from there.

ESSENTIAL SKILLS   THE FORMULA METHOD

The following is the most widely used calculation formula for basic calculations, so you might as well let it become part of you.

$$\frac{D \times V}{H} = X$$

To use this formula in the above problem, substitute the numbers for the letters.

D = 325 mg (desired dose)

V = vehicle (number of tablets)

H = 300 mg (dose of the tablets on hand)

X = unknown number of tablets you will give

Therefore:

$$\frac{325 \text{ mg} \times 1 \text{ tab}}{300 \text{ mg}} = 1\frac{1}{2} \text{ tablets}$$

Since you cannot give ½ of a tablet accurately, one tablet would be the correct answer. Although 325 mg does not equal 300 mg, this is an approximate equivalent. Nurses and doctors understand that they are not exact exchanges. Now that you know this, the exact values that pharmaceutical companies put on their labels will not confuse you. Just to be sure, let's do another problem. You need ½ grain of codeine and have on hand 30 milligrams of codeine in 1 tablet. Since grains and milligrams are not the same measure, we must first make them the same by changing grains to milligrams.

$$\frac{1,000 \text{ mg}}{15 \text{ grains}} = \frac{X \text{ mg}}{\frac{1}{2} \text{ grain}}$$

$$\mathbf{X} = 33 \text{ milligrams (33 mg} = \frac{1}{2} \text{ grain)}$$

Again, 33 does not equal 30 but, because we are working with approximates, the ½-grain order is equivalent to the 30-milligram tablet on hand. So, by knowing the nine basic values, you can calculate exchange values.

Important Points to Remember

- The units used to indicate a medication's strength in the metric (grams and milligrams) and apothecary systems (grains) in Table 23-1 do not have an

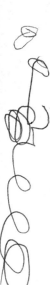

even rate of exchange. That is why you have to convert, or exchange, between the metric system and the apothecary system. (You cannot buy milk in France until you have exchanged your U.S. money for French currency.)

- The two systems listed in Table 23-1 (units and mEq) are two systems unto themselves. They do not and cannot be exchanged into any other system or between each other.
- A medication—in whatever form—has a specific strength in a specific vehicle (package or container).
- The strength of any medication is always in grams, milligrams, micrograms, grains, units, or milliequivalents!
- Everything else—pills, ounces, suppositories, ampoules, milliliters, minims, teaspoons, or tablespoons—is the vehicle package or container for the medication.

Keys to Successful Drug Calculation

- Master the difference between the three parts—D, V, H—and you will always place the right information in its proper formula space!
- Make sure the strength of the desired (D) is the same as the strength on hand (H). Strength desired and strength on hand in the formula must be in the same system.

Now we return to the basic formula and the earlier original problem. The patient is to have 100 mg of a medication. The bottle indicates 0.1 g per tablet. What do you give to the patient? The basic formula:

$$\frac{D \times V}{H} = X$$

Put the numbers into the formula:

D = 100 mg—dose (strength) the patient is to receive

V = 1 tablet—the way the medication is packaged

H = 0.1 g/tablet—dose (strength) of the medication you have available

D and H in this sample are not the same system. One needs to be exchanged for the other.

Now exchange grams for milligrams by using the basic ratio and proportion-type formula used earlier and you find that 0.1 g is the same as 100 mg.

D = 100 mg
V = 1 tablet
H = 100 mg

With the exchange complete, we can now put the numbers in the formula.

$$\frac{[D]\ 100 \times [V]\ 1}{[H]\ 100} = X\ [tablet]$$

$$X = 1$$

The patient should be given 1 tablet.

One more example is given to be sure you have the basics down. The patient is to receive 7½ grains of a medication. The bottle indicates there are 250 mg in each 15 mL. (*Note:* In medication administration, 1 cc and 1 mL have an equal volume. However, mL is becoming the abbreviation used most in print.)

Putting the numbers in their proper places we have:

D = 7½ grains

V = mL

H = 250 mg/15 mL

Again, D and H are not in the same system, so exchange one for the other. In this case, change grains to milligrams. The exchange chart shows that 7½ grains exchanges for 500 mg. So, we can put the numbers in their proper places:

D = 500 mg

V = mL

H = 250 mg/15 mL

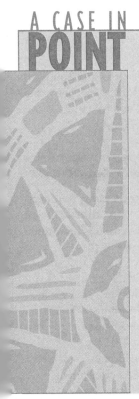

A CASE IN
POINT

A patient is to have 15 mg of medication per kg (kilogram) of body weight. The nurse weighs the patient and finds that he weighs 143 lbs (pounds). The first thing the nurse notices is that kg and lb are not the same units of measurement. She recognizes that in this case, pounds need to be exchanged for kilograms in order to correctly calculate the dose. Her calculations are as follows: The rate of exchange is 2.2 lbs equals 1 kg.

$$\frac{2.2}{1} = \frac{143}{X}$$
$$X = 65$$

This patient weighs 65 kg.

Next:
$$\frac{15 \text{ mg}}{1 \text{ kg}} = \frac{X \text{ mg}}{65 \text{ kg}}$$
$$X = 975 \text{ mg}$$

The nurse concludes that this patient should receive 975 mg of the medication.

The calculation formula now looks like this:

$$\frac{500 \times 15}{250} = X \text{ [mL]}$$

$$X = 30 \text{ mL}$$

When you take 30 mL from the container, you will be giving the patient 7½ grains of the medication.

The above case illustrates a problem which requires the discovery of D (desired) only. Information regarding V and H was not given.

Using the problem presented in the *case in point,* another example of how the formula could be applied is: You know that V is an ampoule (small glass container of medication) containing 2 mL of medication. The ampoule states your on-hand dosage strength to be 750 mg per 2 mL. Now you can solve the rest of the problem. The numbers fit into the formula as follows:

D = 975 mg

V = mL

H = 750 mg/2 mL

D and H are in the same system, so there is no need to exchange. The numbers are ready to put into the formula:

$$\frac{975 \times 2}{750} = 2.6 \text{ mL}$$

To get the ordered strength of 975 mg, you will need one full ampoule (2 mL) and 0.6 mL from a second ampoule. Again, be careful to note that V is mL. You want 2.6 mL, not 2.6 ampoules, which would overdose the patient by 450 mg. You avoid this type of error by always using the vehicle or volume of the on-hand dose and remembering that X will always be in that vehicle.

ESSENTIAL SKILLS | **THE RATIO AND PROPORTION METHOD**

A ratio is the relationship between two numbers, and a proportion shows the equality between two ratios or two fractions. A ratio may be written with the colon between the two numbers, or it may be written as a fraction. For example, we could write 3:5 or ⅗. It means the same thing. We would read the colon or the slash as "is to." Thus, for the above examples, you would say "three is to five." When you are comparing two ratios, the ratios would be divided by a set of double colons. If you are writing them as fractions, there would be an "equal" sign between the two fractions. The double colon or equal sign would be read "as." For instance, "3:5::6:10" would be read "three is to five as six is to ten" to indicate the equality of the two ratios. This could also be written as, ⅗ = ⁶⁄₁₀.

Often in nursing when we are asked to administer a medication, one of the numbers of the ratio is unknown, and we must do a mathematical calculation. Since we know that both sides of the proportion must be equal, this gives us a solid base from which to begin. Remember those initials D, V, H, and X. We will be using them again for the ratio and proportion method. A problem solved in this way would be written out as:

$$H : V :: D : X \quad \textit{or} \quad \frac{H}{V} = \frac{D}{X}$$

Let's look at our previous problem in which the patient needed to receive 975 mg of medication. The medication strength was 750 mg per 2-mL ampoule. First, determine what you *know!* The *known* values usually go on the left side of the equation. Then look at what you need to know, or the *unknown*. Those values go on the right side of the equation. In this case, you know that there are 750 mg of medication in a 2 mL ampoule. What you do not know is how many milliliters it will take to provide 975 mg of medication.

$$\underset{\textit{Known}}{750 \text{ mg } \textit{(on-hand dose)} : 2 \text{ mL } \textit{(vehicle)}} :: \underset{\textit{Unknown}}{975 \text{ mg } \textit{(desired dose)} : X \text{ mL } \textit{(unknown)}}$$

This can also be written as:

$$\frac{750}{2} = \frac{975}{X}$$

Now, you are ready to solve for the value of "X." In solving a ratio and proportion problem, always remember that the *product of the extremes (the two outside numbers) is equal to the product of the means (the two inside numbers).* To then solve the problem:

$$750 \times X = 2 \times 975$$
$$750X = 1950$$
$$\frac{750X}{750} = \frac{1950}{750} \quad \text{(You must divide both sides of the equation by the number to the left of the X.)}$$
$$X = 2.6 \text{ mL}$$

If you are writing both sides of the equation as fractions, you would cross-multiply. Thus, the numerator of one fraction would be multiplied by the denominator of the other fraction. You would still wind up with $750 \times X = 2 \times 975$.

Let's try another example: The physician has ordered a patient to have 35 mg of Demerol. The Demerol comes in a vial that contains 50 mg per 1 mL. How many milliliters would you give to provide the ordered dose?

$$\underset{\textit{Known}}{50 \text{ mg} : 1 \text{ mL}} :: \underset{\textit{Unknown}}{35 \text{ mg} : X \text{ mL}}$$

The product of the extremes equals the product of the means, so:

$$50 \times X = 1 \times 35$$
$$50X = 35$$
$$\frac{50X}{50} = \frac{35}{50}$$
$$X = 0.7 \text{ mL}$$

There are several important points to remember about working a problem in ratio and proportion:

- Any conversions you need to do must be done before setting up the problem. This means that **D** and **H** must be in the same system, just as it was in the formula method.
- The ratios must be stated in the same order on both sides of the equation. For example, if you have written the ratio on the left as milligrams is to milliliters, you must also write milligrams to milliliters on the right. You cannot have "milligrams is to milliliters" on the left and then put "milliliters is to milligrams" on the right. Your answer will never be correct when the measurements are incompatible.
- Before beginning the problem, always ask yourself what information does the problem give you. What do you know? Put that into a ratio on the left. Then ask yourself, what information do you need? Put that information on the right. The problem will usually indicate to you what units you are looking for in the answer. For instance, how many tablets, how many cc, how many mL do you need to give?
- Always assume that if a medication bottle of tablets states milligrams on the label, it is referring to the fact that one tablet contains that many milligrams.
- A vial should have on the label how many milligrams of medication are found in one milliliter of solution. Medication vial labels may have a lot of extra information on them, but look for that one piece that tells you how many milligrams of medication are in one milliliter.
- Decimal fractions should always have a "0" to the left of the decimal if it is less than a whole number. For instance, .7 cc should be written as 0.7 cc. This eliminates any confusion as to whether or not there is actually a decimal point there. Giving 7 cc of a medication is a lot different than giving 0.7 cc of a medication. It is giving 10 times what the doctor ordered and could be fatal!

ESSENTIAL SKILLS | **SIMPLIFIED STEPS FOR MAKING DRUG CALCULATIONS**

Follow these steps for basic drug calculations:

- Find the parts.
  D = the strength of the medication ordered by the physician
  V = the package or form of the strength on hand (pill, liquid, etc.)
  H = the strength of the medication available
- Make sure that D and H are in the same system.
- Place the numbers in the formula and solve, or place them in the ratio proportion format and solve.

Here is a little test. You have an order that reads: "give 4 mL of medication." What part of the calculation formula (D, V, or H) do you have? If you said, "none of the above," you are correct. This order means the physician knows the strength and vehicle of the medication (the H and V in the basic formula), has done the math, and has provided you with X. *Caution:* Good nursing requires that you work backward to determine the strength of the medication in those 4 mL. Why? To be sure that the strength of the medication the patient will receive in those 4 mL is within therapeutic range. Do not assume that because the physician wrote the order, the dose is correct. This could be a very costly assumption.

CORE CONCEPTS	**COMMON ERRORS IN MAKING DRUG CALCULATIONS**

There are two common errors that can be made, especially by inexperienced nurses, when making drug calculations.

1. Errors in basic arithmetic—decimals, fractions, percentages.
2. Overlooking the parts; placing nonrelated material in the formula.

For example, you need 100 mg and the medication label instructions are, "add 5 mL of sterile water to yield 25 mg per 1 mL." This gives us:

D = 100 mg

V = mL

H = 25 mg/mL

Students tend to mistake the 5 mL for V. But, read the label until you find the strength per a specific vehicle or volume! Remember, somewhere on the medication label, the strength per unit will be written.

Ultimately, it is the nurse's responsibility to prevent error. It is the nurse who functions as the final checkpoint before a medication is administered. The physician writes the order, the pharmacist dispenses the medication, and the nurse gives it. This responsibility cannot be taken lightly. It is no secret that nurses make medication errors, which results in various adverse effects to the patient. When analyzed, these errors are almost always due to the nurse skipping one of the basic "rights" (right patient, medication, dose, route, and time). The consequences of such errors for the nurse vary. One may include being sued. In addition, most nurses who have made serious errors have been investigated by their state nursing authority. Up until now, the most severe penalty has been revocation of the nurse's license.

In October 1996, the consequences of medication error took a major turn. In April 1997, a grand jury brought negligent homicide charges against three nurses who, in 1996, were involved in a fatal drug administration to a newborn. This is the first time such charges have ever been made by a government agency. Is this an isolated situation or a coming trend? No one knows. But please remember that safe medication administration requires that you be constantly alert! This is one nursing skill where distractions could lead to fatal errors.

ASK YOURSELF

1. What are the most common errors in drug calculation that you resolve to avoid? What safeguards will you incorporate into the drug administration procedure that will raise your confidence level in the administration of medication?

   _____

   _____

2. What points (that you determine to be key) presented in this chapter do you most want to remember?

   _____

   _____

CYBERLINKS: FLASH CARDS

Check to see what you now remember by making your own flash cards. Use the CD-ROM that accompanies your textbook to discover how to make flash cards for reviewing and retaining what you have learned.

CONCEPT MAP WORD BANK

DRUG ADMINISTRATION
Prevention of error
Rights
DRUG CALCULATION
Formulas

Ratio and proportion
SIMPLIFIED STEPS
COMMON ERRORS

Refer to Concept Maps and Flash Cards on pages viii–ix for an explanation of how to create and use concept maps. In addition, the CD-ROM guides you through the construction of concept maps by providing a more detailed introduction, more illustrations of examples, and key steps to follow in designing your own maps.

Laboratory and Diagnostic Studies

ASK YOURSELF

1. What laboratory or diagnostic tests would you like to know more about?

   _____

   _____

2. What is the nurse's role, in addition to collection (when required) regarding laboratory and diagnostic studies?

   _____

   _____

CYBERLINKS

Interactive Interested in checking your blood IQ or your cholesterol or heart disease IQ? Visit **www.healthfinder.com** to take these quizzes and to learn more about blood and blood safety. Click on the L and scroll down to Lab Tests.

Supplemental **www.LPNresources.com** can help enhance your learning by leading you to discover other links with more information about the topic you are studying.

A complete health and illness assessment has three distinct parts: history, physical, and laboratory and diagnostic studies. This chapter will explore the core concepts and the skills essential for the LPN/LVN to acquire related to laboratory and diagnostic studies. Most students tend to associate laboratory and diagnostic studies with patients who are in the hospital. However, in today's health care environment, these studies are encountered in all health care settings (clinics, long-term care, home health, etc.). In the interest of targeting core and basic concepts, we have chosen to use a question and answer model for ease in presentation and comprehension.

1. **What is the difference between laboratory and diagnostic studies?**

   Laboratory studies:

   • Involve analysis of body fluids collected through basic techniques of blood, urine, and feces samples.
   • May require food, fluid, and/or medication restrictions.
   • The sample collection does not require a separate consent form. (*Note:* The exception in most states is human immunodeficiency virus [HIV] testing, which requires a signed consent before blood can be drawn.)

   Diagnostic studies:

   • Involve analysis of body fluids or tissues collected through invasive techniques.
   • Include viewing of various body structures using special equipment (x-ray, magnetic resonance imaging [MRI], computed tomography [CT] scans, electrocardiogram [ECG], scopes, etc.).
   • Usually require a signed consent form.
   • May require food and fluid restrictions.

   In actuality, although there is a difference between the laboratory studies and diagnostic tests, the terms are frequently interchanged. In the remainder of this chapter, they will be jointly referred to as lab tests.

   Note: Some categories of lab tests are those done to monitor blood levels of medications that have a narrow therapeutic level. That is, the line between a therapeutic and toxic level of the medication is very thin. Some of these tests monitor the effects of medication rather than the blood level of the medication itself. For example, blood levels of heparin are not determined. What is measured, however, is the effectiveness of heparin therapy as determined by activated partial thromboplastin time (APTT) values. On the other hand, serum levels of many drugs are now being monitored. For example, orders to obtain serum levels of many anticonvulsants, antibiotics, and bronchodilators are common. At present there are about 100 medications that are monitored for therapeutic levels, and many lab books now include a chapter on this topic.

2. **How can you learn all of the material about lab tests?** Considering that most of the nursing books about lab tests are often 500 to 700 pages long, you cannot! However, the faculty will expect you to at least be able to do the following:

   • Explain why your patient is having a specific test.
   • Describe the nurse's role for the test—such as what the nurse should teach the client about the test, any special patient preparation, the nurse's role in sample collection, and documentation.
   • Provide normal reference values for the test (normal reference values are almost always included on the test report).
   • Explain the significance of your patient's test results. What implications do the test results have for the nurse?

How can nurses do all that? You will need to do your homework. Once you know your patient is having tests that you are not familiar with, look them up and make notes. Most instructors will allow you to refer to notes when discussing your patient's laboratory and diagnostic tests.

3. **Will you be expected to discuss laboratory tests without notes?** Yes. As you progress in school, you should know that faculty will expect you to discuss common tests without notes. The following are the lab tests you will probably be expected, at some point, to discuss without notes.

   • Urinalysis (U/A)
   • Complete blood count (CBC)
   • Fasting blood sugar (FBS) or routine blood sugars done throughout the shift
   • Electrolytes: sodium, potassium, and chloride
   • Blood urea nitrogen (BUN)
   • Therapeutic drug levels
   • Wound cultures

   Your instructors may have additional lab tests without notes in mind. Be sure to ask.

4. **Where can you find this information about lab tests?** There are two main sources: your course textbook and a lab and diagnostic book. Although required nursing texts will have information about lab tests, a specialty book is recommended. Be sure you select a book that includes information on nursing implications for each test! Most nursing schools will suggest a lab and diagnostic text as an optional book. Many clinical instructors will carry a lab/diagnostic reference book with them, or you might find one on the nursing unit where you are doing clinical. Your school library or reference shelves in the classroom should also provide these books. In addition to the lab books, there are lab cards, which are boxes of index cards with one lab or diagnostic study per card. Since you can take out only the texts of interest, these cards are very convenient for use in clinical training. Again, if you are going to use these boxed sets, be sure the cards contain nursing implications. In addition to these written sources, do not forget that the hospital laboratory performing the laboratory studies will also have information for you regarding specific tests.

5. **Are there some lab tests that are difficult for students to understand?** Yes. There are several tests that students have difficulty with.

   The difference between coagulation tests of PT and APTT:

   • **Prothrombin time (PT):** Used to monitor oral anticoagulant therapy.
   • **Activated partial thromboplastin time (APTT):** Used to monitor heparin therapy.

- One way to remember the difference is PT (two letters) matches the word with few letters (oral), whereas APTT (four letters) matches the word with more letters (injection).
- The **International Normalized Ratio (INR)** will often be given with the PT results. This is an effort to standardize PT results throughout the world.

Drug serum level terms:

- **Steady state:** Indicates whether the plasma level of the drug is being maintained at the desired maintenance level.
- **Peak level:** The time at which a drug is at its highest concentration in the blood. Blood to measure a peak level is drawn at **specific times** related to the drug administration time. The nurse or lab tech should check with the lab for details. The peak level indicates the rate of absorption of the drug.
- **Trough level** (in some labs referred to as "residual level"): The time at which a drug is at its lowest concentration in the blood. Blood for trough levels is usually drawn 5 minutes before the next dose of the drug is to be administered. As with peak levels, the lab should be checked for specifics. The trough level indicates the rate of excretion of the drug.
- The accuracy of drug plasma levels depends on many factors under the nurse's control, including, in many settings, obtaining blood samples for testing. It is essential, therefore, that the nurse or lab tech knows and follows protocol.
- In addition to the timing for drawing the sample, drug plasma levels can be influenced by other factors such as other drugs the patient is receiving. Therefore, as with all lab and diagnostic tests, you need to be cautious when interpreting results.

6. **How have the normal reference values for the various lab tests been determined?** Over the years, data from individuals (usually men) who were considered "healthy" have been gathered and analyzed and a range for each lab test determined. Most lab values have a low and high range. Any values falling within that range are considered normal. It is interesting to note that over the years, most of these ranges remain unchanged. What have changed, however, are the number of new tests and the refinement of many older, established tests.

   When comparing normal ranges between books and between health care facilities, differences are often noted. These occur due to differences in equipment and techniques used to conduct the tests. These differences are usually small and the values all tend to be in the "ballpark" with each other. The values used to report reference numbers, however, can create values that look very different. Older books report most values in mg% (milligram percent), which changed to mg/dL (milligrams per deciliter). With this change, the basic numbers remain the same. For example, a blood glucose of 80 mg% became 80 mg/dL. In an attempt to create more uniformity in reporting on a global basis, the World Health Organization (WHO) is encouraging the adoption of a new system. This system uses the International System of Units (SI). When values are calculated in SI they may or may not look familiar. For example, potassium ranges are 3.5 to 5.3 mEq/L and 3.5 to 5.3 mmol/L (SI). The numbers remain the same while the reporting unit changes. It is different with the hematocrit (Hct). Male values for Hct are generally 40% to 54% while the SI are 0.40 to 0.54. It is anticipated that with time, all values will be reported in SI units. Until then, many labs and books are presenting the current system followed by the SI.

7. **What traps do nurses fall victim to when they are looking at lab results?** Basically, there are two traps.

   - Lab reports are only one part of the picture. They must be evaluated in relation to other assessment data. No interventions should be made based on a lab report alone. A lab value that is outside the normal range, with all other test values inside the normal ranges and assessment findings basically normal, is suspect. Most of the time, the test will be repeated to verify the initial findings.

   - When you find a test result that falls well outside the reference values, you will generally find one or more companion tests that are out of range to some degree. Our physiology is very interconnected and interdependent.

8. **What will be my responsibilities as a graduate in relation to reported lab values?** You will be expected to quickly identify lab values that require immediate intervention. Most institutions have a list of critical lab values and the procedures to be followed when one occurs. The lists often include blood glucose (i.e., values below 40 and above 700 mg/dL), sodium levels, hematocrit, and carbon dioxide combining power. Many hospital labs report critical results directly to the physician, but do not take for granted that this has been done. As a graduate nurse, you must always notify the physician of critical results immediately, and document that you have done so as well as the physician's response. As a student nurse, make sure that the primary nurse in charge of your patient is aware of the lab results. Follow through with what was reported and what was done, so that if you need to make any changes to your patient care, you may do so. For instance, if a patient's potassium level comes back as being high, and the patient is on a potassium supplement, you would want to hold the medication until you receive further orders from the physician via your primary nurse or instructor.

9. **Will I ever have to perform any lab tests?** Yes. Currently, the most common lab test performed by the nurse, often called **point-of-care testing (POC)**, is blood glucose testing. This may also be called a BG chem or a

glucoscan, depending upon the facility. It is anticipated that with advances in lab tests and the advent of simpler, more sophisticated equipment, nurses will be conducting more POC tests.

In addition to this type of test, practical/vocational nursing students are expected to collect urine specimens, both clean catch and catheterized specimens, as well as sputum specimens and stool specimens. You might also be asked to hematest a patient's stool at point-of-care. This requires a special testing kit, which will allow you to see whether or not patients have occult (hidden) blood in their stool.

Labeling specimens correctly is almost as important as the collection process itself.

Errors in labeling can have dire results and lead to wrong diagnoses and treatments.

The label should be checked against the patient's identification band (if in a hospital setting), the patient record, and the patient identified by name. Checking three times helps to prevent error. We can borrow a helpful format from the rules of drug administration: Right patient. Right lab test order. Right time. Right collection procedure. Right label.

Besides participating in the above diagnostic tests, nurses in many settings are collecting blood specimens. However, in some states, practical/vocational nursing students are not allowed to do blood draws. As an LPN/LVN, you might not be able to do a blood draw without special

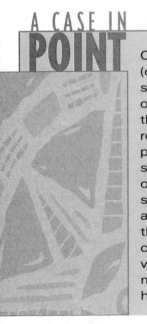

A CASE IN
POINT

One of us (an author) had a funny experience (only in retrospect) that we like to share with the students regarding labeling. We were working on an extended care unit with a patient who had three different physicians. As each one made rounds, he ordered a culture of a different body part or substance: nasal passages, G-tube stoma, and stool. The appropriate labels were ordered from the lab, and were applied to the specimens. It wasn't until the lab tech called us a while after the specimens had been sent to the lab and said, "Please don't tell me that this came out of someone's nose!" that we realized we had put the wrong label on the stool specimen! Fortunately, this mistake was obvious; however, most errors are not.

instructions or as part of your IV certification class. To participate in collecting blood specimens, the nurse should know what diagnostic test is ordered so that proper specimen collection occurs (which includes factors such as collection site and technique, time of collection, labeling, and handling). In addition, blood specimens must be placed in the proper collection tube for test accuracy. Be sure you know the facility policies and procedures concerning blood specimen collections as well as what is in your "scope of practice" within your state.

You can anticipate having many responsibilities in relation to laboratory and diagnostic studies. We have our nursing students spend time in the hospital laboratory to see what happens once the specimens have been collected and sent to the lab. They are always amazed at the number and complexity of the lab tests that can be run. They also come back with a new perspective on how important proper patient preparation and accurate specimen collection and identification are. As a student you should be able to immediately recognize critical values, which you will report to your primary nurse and nursing instructor, so that you and they can respond with appropriate nursing interventions.

 ASK YOURSELF

1. Do you have an easy reference text that lists laboratory and diagnostic tests, the critical values and their meaning? If not, do you plan to acquire one?

   _____

   _____

2. How do you feel about collecting specimens and performing lab and diagnostic tests that are within the parameters of professional practice? Are there any that you like to avoid? Are you concerned about your own health and safety for any of the specimens?

   _____

   _____

 CYBERLINKS: FLASH CARDS

Check to see what you now remember by making your own flash cards. Use the CD-ROM that accompanies your textbook to discover how to make flash cards for reviewing and retaining what you have learned.

 CONCEPT MAP WORD BANK

LAB AND DIAGNOSTIC TESTS
Differences

Information
Difficult tests
Normal reference values
Performance of tests
Collection

Refer to Concept Maps and Flash Cards on pages viii–ix for an explanation of how to create and use concept maps. In addition, the CD-ROM guides you through the construction of concept maps by providing a more detailed introduction, more illustrations of examples, and key steps to follow in designing your own maps.

ECG

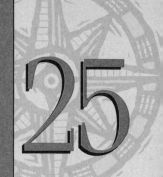

1. What do you already know regarding how the ECG records information about cardiac rhythms?

_____

_____

2. Does the ECG procedure seem complex and daunting to you? Why or why not?

_____

_____

 CYBERLINKS

<u>Interactive</u> Want to hear a heart beating, listen to a healthy heart and a diseased heart beating, view an echocardiogram, and much more? Visit **www.ipl.org** Go to Reference Center and then to Health and Medical Sciences, to Anatomy and Physiology and scroll down to: *The Heart: An Online Exploration.*

<u>Supplemental</u> **www.LPNresources.com** can help enhance your learning by leading you to discover other links with more information about the topic you are studying.

Although many individuals still refer to this diagnostic test as an EKG, the abbreviation currently being used to denote an electrocardiogram is ECG. Not too long ago, the only nurses who performed cardiac monitoring were intensive care and cardiac care nurses. Today, however, cardiac monitoring is a nursing activity in many settings such as telemetry and progressive care units, medical–surgical units, labor and delivery units, postanesthesia units (both in- and outpatient), and oncology units. Occasionally, practical/vocational nursing students may care for a patient who is on telemetry (a continuous monitoring of the patient's heart rhythm) on a medical–surgical floor although the actual cardiac monitor may be located in the intensive care unit. Although the nursing student is not responsible for reading the monitor, we think it is important for the student to comprehend core concepts related to ECGs.

The placement of skin electrodes for an ECG is perhaps the easiest step to learn related to this procedure. The hardest and most complex part of the procedure is being able to interpret the resulting rhythm patterns. Interpretation requires knowledge of cardiac anatomy and physiology and the mechanics of the graphic representations of cardiac rhythm. Many hospitals offer courses in cardiac monitoring to their medical–surgical staff. In some states, practical/vocational nurses are trained especially for telemetry units.

A bare bones understanding related to the ECG is essential for LPN/LVNs regardless of their role in conducting the procedure or identifying abnormalities that require attention.

| CORE CONCEPTS | **ECG FUNDAMENTALS**

Understanding an ECG requires several fundamental pieces of information:

- *Normal blood flow through the heart.* You should be able to trace a drop of blood through the heart. One way to view this blood flow through the heart is to reshape the heart's anatomy into a straight line (Figure 25-1).
- *Heart's electrical conduction system.* Think of this system as starting with a master switch that "turns" cardiac muscles on, rather like turning on the master fuse that all at once turns on all lights in the house. Except that in the heart, the lights come on in sequence, like a set of falling dominos, with the heart's master switch (the SA node) starting the cascade. This cascade is displayed in Figure 25-2.
- *Critical properties unique to heart muscle cells.* These main properties are: automaticity, irritability and excitability, contractility, conductivity, and rhythmicity. The basic definitions follow:
- *Automaticity:* The ability of specific cardiac cells to contract without stimulation by the SA node. For example, by itself, the atrioventricular (AV) node has the capacity to create 40 to 60 cardiac contractions per minute, while the Purkinje and ventricular fibers can independently create 20 to 40 contractions per minute. Beats that occur outside sinoatrial (SA) node stimulation are sometime referred to as **escape beats.**
- *Irritability and excitability:* The ability of cardiac cells to respond when exposed to an electrical stimulus.
- *Contractility:* The ability of cardiac cells to contract—get smaller—when exposed to an electrical stimulus.
- *Conductivity:* The ability of one cardiac cell to pass on an electrical impulse to another cardiac cell.
- *Rhythmicity:* The steady rhythm of normal cardiac cells as they repeat their cycle of stimulation–transmission–contraction–relaxation.

Figure 25-1 Heart Structure in a Straight Line

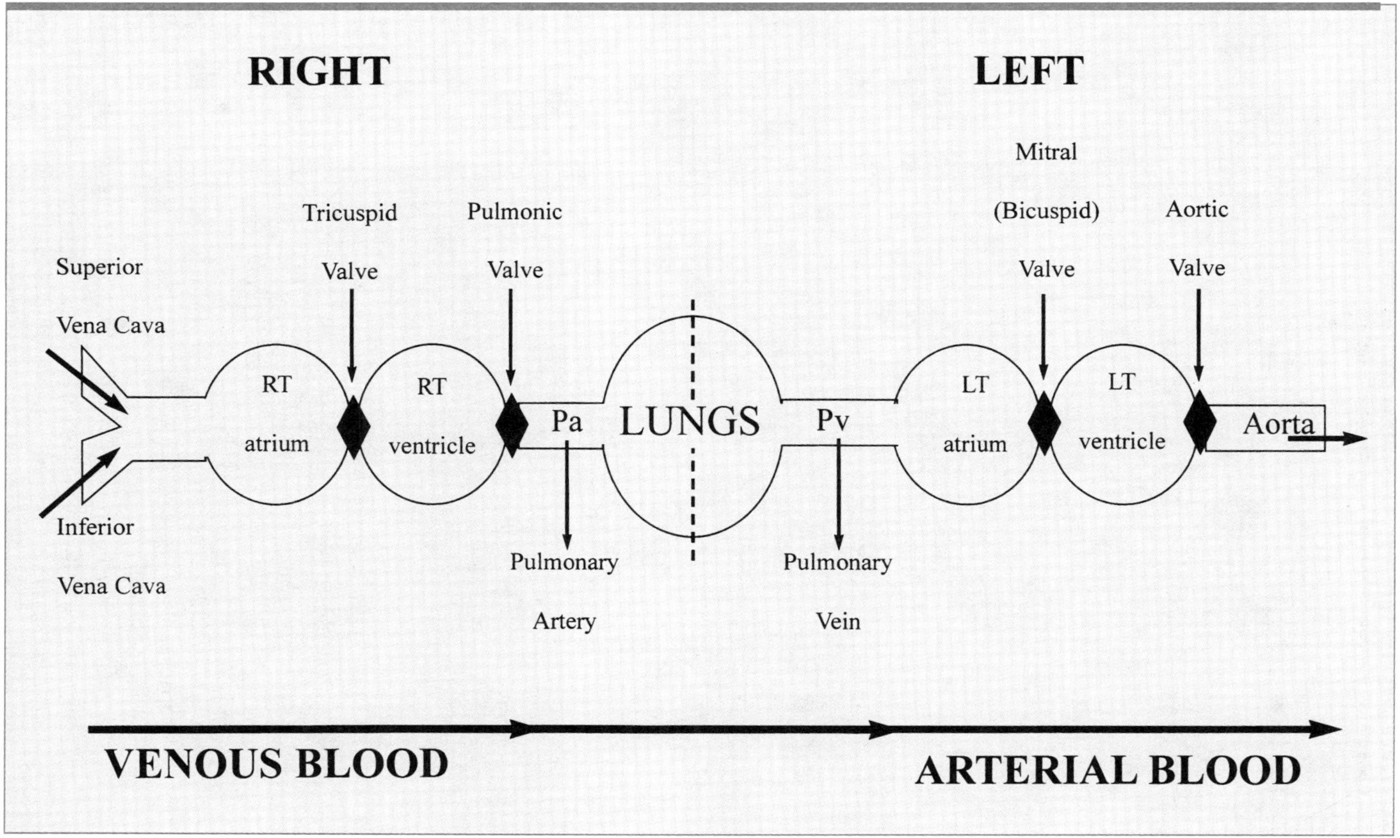

Figure 25-2 Electric Cascade of the Heart

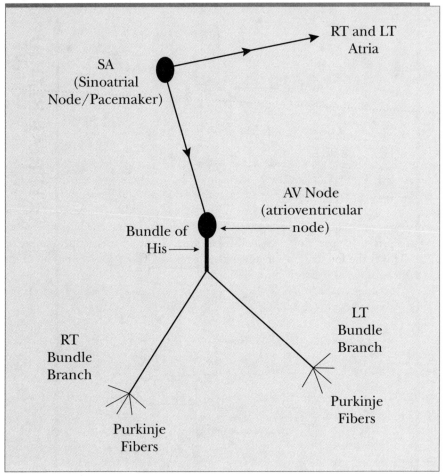

- *Terms associated with the transmission of the impulse along cardiac cells:* polarization, depolarization, repolarization, and refractory period.
  - *Polarization:* Cardiac cells are in a resting state; the outside of the cells is covered with positive particles. The inside of the cells has negative particles.
  - *Depolarization:* The cardiac cells respond to an electrical stimulus and the particles switch so that the cell surface now becomes negative (and the inside positive).
  - *Repolarization:* The process of cardiac cells returning to their original resting state with the cell surfaces containing positive electrical charges.
  - *Refractory period:* The time during which cardiac cells are not ready to respond to a new stimulus; occurs between repolarization and polarization time.

An interesting and proven way for remembering the differences in the transmission of impulses is illustrated below:

Polarization—think P for positive (cell surface is positive and resting)

Depolarization—think D for denial (cell surface becomes negative and active)

Repolarization—think R for return (depolarized cells switch electrical charges and return to the polarized state)

Thus, the sequence is polarization, depolarization, repolarization (P-D-R) over and over again. It is this repetitive sequence of ion exchanges between cell surface and cell interior that moves the electrical stimulus along cardiac cells. When the stimulus has completed the circuit, a heartbeat occurs with the atria contracting followed by the ventricles. One way to think of these terms is an old-fashioned fire line. One person receives the bucket with water (P), turns, passes it on to the next person (D), turns back and gets ready to receive a new bucket (R), gets the new bucket (P), passes it on, and so on. Can you see how the refractory period can influence how many buckets of water any one person can pass along? Or how many times the heart can beat per minute?

This is the foundation for understanding an ECG, which is a record of the electrical impulse as it travels through cardiac cells. The ECG does not directly give any information about the heart's structure. However, analysis of the conduction system through reading the ECG rhythm strip can provide indirect information.

CORE CONCEPTS	**ECG MECHANICS**

An ECG is obtained by placing electrodes on the skin that pick up the electric current that goes through cardiac cells. This current can be recorded on a TV-like monitor, telemetry, or recorded on special paper. In either case, the electrical activity is displayed as a series of waveforms. The wave pattern is analyzed in relation to the ECG paper and expected wave patterns. Figure 25-3 presents a sample of normal size and enlarged ECG paper. As you can see, the standard paper is small. To accurately measure the time intervals, a set of ECG calipers is required (Figure 25-4). However, as technology progresses, there are some computer programs that do pattern interpretation. However, as with all technology, remember that this data must be correlated with the assessment of the patient.

ECGs come in 12 "forms." Although most of the time a single lead is used to analyze the heart's electric conduction system, there are times when the physician needs more information. In that case, a 12-lead ECG will be obtained. This simply means that the electrodes are repositioned several times on the patient to create 12 different views of the heart's electrical system. It is like having your picture taken from 12 different angles at one sitting. You remain sitting in the same chair and do not change your position, yet each frame presents you in a unique view. Thus, a 12-lead ECG views the electrical system of the heart from 12 different angles.

Figure 25-5 shows the basic electrical waveforms, P, QRS (known as the QRS complex), and T, which occur with every cardiac cycle (heartbeat). Note that each

Figure 25-3 Normal Size ECG Tracing Paper

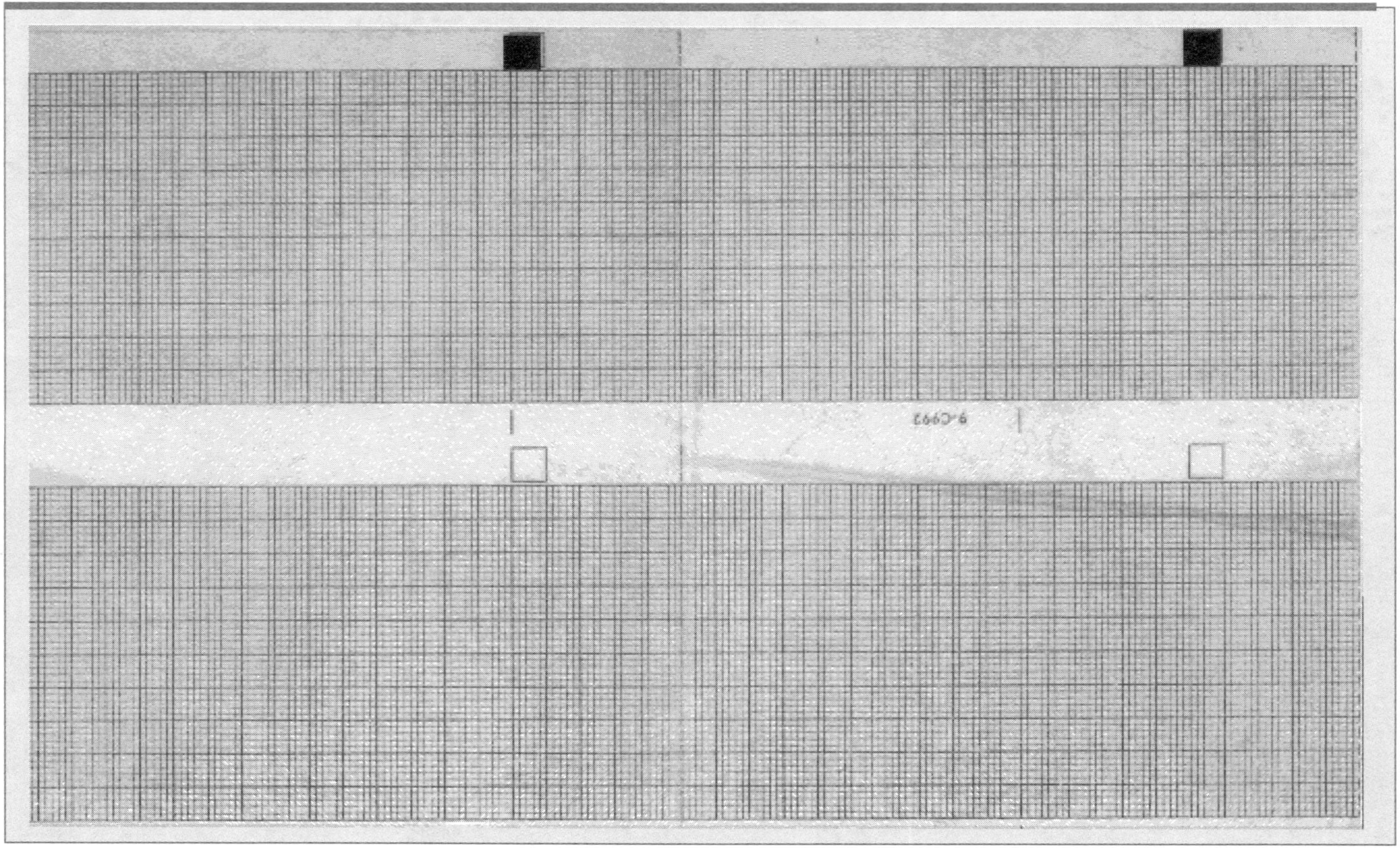

Figure 25-4 Cardiac Calipers

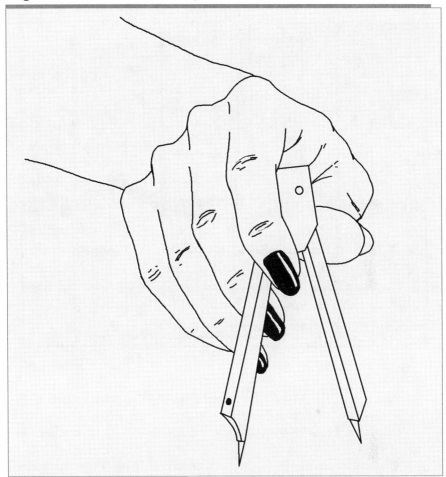

waveform has a time limit. That is, it occupies a specified distance on the grid of the ECG paper, which in turn represents time. Characteristics of the major portions of a normal cardiac cycle are summarized in Table 25-1. When abnormalities are apparent, many other features of the wave formation are analyzed.

Interpreting an ECG rhythm strip requires a systematic approach and additional training. As a rule, cardiac problems that are in tissue above the bundle branches lead to P and PR changes. Pathology in or after the bundle branches leads to abnormalities in the QRS complex.

| CORE CONCEPTS | **ECG DEFINITIONS** |

- *Preload:* Although preload concerns both the right and left ventricles, it mainly refers to the stretching of the left ventricle during filling with blood

Figure 25-5 Normal ECG Patterns with Normal Time Intervals

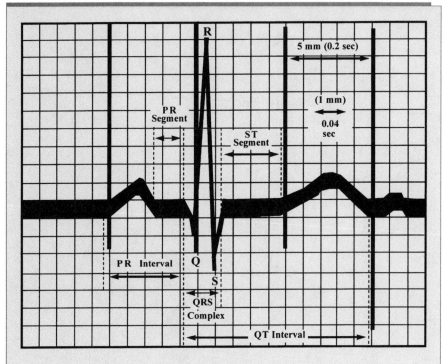

from the left atrium. Like a stretched rubber band has a strong snap when released, the more the left ventricle is stretched with blood, the more force-fully it will eject blood into the aorta on contraction (this is **Starling's law of heart**).

- *Afterload:* Represents the amount of tension or resistance the ventricles must overcome during contraction to open the pulmonic and aortic valves. Afterload for the left ventricle is frequently referred to as **systemic vascular resistance.** Afterload for the right ventricle is referred to as **pulmonary vascular resistance.**

Figure 25-1 will help you visualize the effects of abnormal preload and after-load values. For example, if the muscles of the left ventricle become weak, they will fill with blood, but they will be unable to push the blood out through the aortic valve. Like a rubber band that is constantly overstretched and loses its elasticity, so do overstretched (or damaged) cardiac muscles lose their ejection power. The result is a backup into the left atrium, and eventually the lungs, with development of pul-monary edema. This is a preload problem because the left ventricle is unable to empty completely, becomes overfilled, and blood backs up in the system. The same thing can happen in the right ventricle if it is unable to open the pulmonic valve. Eventually, many things can result from untreated right-sided abnormal preload val-

TABLE 25-1	Normal Cardiac Cycle
Cycle Phase	**Characteristics**
P wave	• Time: < 0.12 sec • Indicates atrial depolarization
PR interval	• Time: < 0.12 to 0.20 sec • Indicates the impulse is traveling through the AV node, bundle of His, and the bundle branches
QRS complex	• Time: < 0.04 to 0.10 sec • Indicates depolarization of the ventricles (remember that once the ventricles depolarize they contract and eject blood, thus creating a heartbeat/pulse)
ST segment	• Time: not usually measured • Should be isoelectric; flat • Indicates ventricular refractory period
T wave	• Time: not measured • Evaluated by how it looks including amplitude (height) • Indicates repolarization of the ventricles

ues, such as edema and increased jugular pressure. Again, Figure 25-1 will help you visualize these events.

Prolonged abnormal afterload, on the other hand, will eventually result in damaged left ventricle muscles. Because the ventricle has to constantly overcome the increased force to open the aortic valve, the ventricle loses its contractility. The afterload problem is the increased systemic force (e.g., high blood pressure) not sick cardiac muscle. Left untreated, the left ventricle can become permanently damaged, leading to a combination of both preload and afterload pathologies.

ESSENTIAL SKILLS   RECOGNIZING ABNORMAL RHYTHM

The last topic which is basic to your understanding of ECGs is life-threatening arrhythmias. An arrhythmia, often called a dysrhythmia, is any rate or rhythm of the heartbeat that is different from a normal one. Although there are some very serious atrial arrhythmias, two abnormal ventricular rhythms require immediate recognition. They are **ventricular tachycardia (V-tach)** and **ventricular fibrillation (V-fib)** (Figures 25-6 and 25-7).

• *Ventricular tachycardia:*
  • Ventricular rate may be as high as 200 beats per minute.
  • The ventricles cannot fill or empty properly, and the result is low cardiac output (the amount of blood that is pumped out of the heart per minute).

Figure 25-6 Ventricular Tachycardia (V-tach)

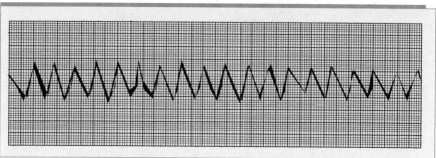

- A variety of consequences, such as weak or absent pulses, hypotension, and congestive heart failure, can result from a low cardiac output.
- *Ventricular fibrillation:*
  - Ventricles are in essence just quivering like a bowl of gelatin.
  - There is no cardiac output.
  - If not treated quickly, death results.

Because these two arrhythmias are so life-threatening, it is essential that you learn what they are. You need to recognize the terms for the rhythms and the urgency with which you should move when told your telemetry patient is in V-tach or V-fib.

Your pharmacology classes will focus on many cardiac drugs for a variety of cardiac conditions, including the arrhythmias just discussed. Knowing something about the anatomy of the heart as well as the electrical conduction that occurs there will help you to understand these drugs more completely. You will become certified in cardiopulmonary resuscitation, if you have not already done so, for any of your patients who suffer cardiac arrest. More technical and extensive nursing interventions for these patients will be the responsibility of the intensive care nurses, although you might be called upon to assist. Today's nurses are responsible for more types of nursing care than nurses in the past ever dreamed could be possible.

This chapter has presented the basic concepts related to ECGs. As a student practical/vocational nurse, you may care for patients with cardiac disorders. The

Figure 25-7 Ventricular Fibrillation

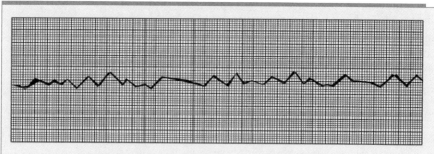

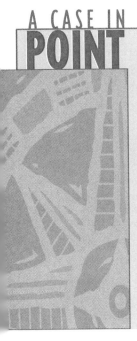

A CASE IN POINT

Sally has been working as an LPN/LVN for over a year. She has recently learned that telemetry machines are being installed on her unit in order for the medical center to expand its ability to care for specific types of cardiac patients. The supervisor tells Sally that she will be involved in the care of the telemetry patients. This news is both exciting and scary to Sally. She has never worked with cardiac patients before and doesn't even remember much about ECGs. She recognizes that she has never been comfortable with ECGs. It is a procedure that has always appeared complex to her. She is comforted, however, when she learns that all staff members on the unit will receive special training in identifying abnormal cardiac rhythms.

information in this chapter provides you with just one more piece of the jigsaw puzzle that makes up the patient's complete health picture. Equipped with the necessary information, you are enabled to give competent, well-integrated nursing care.

STOP ASK YOURSELF

1. Referring to Ask Yourself question 2 at the beginning of this chapter, would your response be different now, after reading this chapter?

   _____

   _____

2. What would you still like to know more about, related to the topics in this chapter? How will you acquire the knowledge and skills you desire?

   _____

   _____

CYBERLINKS: FLASH CARDS

Check to see what you now remember by making your own flash cards. Use the CD-ROM that accompanies your textbook to discover how to make flash cards for reviewing and retaining with you have learned.

CONCEPT MAP WORD BANK —————————

FUNDAMENTALS
Terms
Mechanics
Interpretation
Nursing Role

Refer to Concept Maps and Flash Cards on pages viii–ix for an explanation of how to create and use concept maps. In addition, the CD-ROM guides you through the construction of concept maps by providing a more detailed introduction, more illustrations of examples, and key steps to follow in designing your own maps.

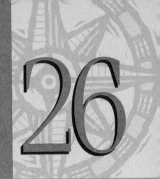

Nutrition

1. How do you regard your own dietary habits—healthy or unhealthy?

   _____

   _____

2. What do you think the nurse's role is in helping patients eat healthily?

   _____

   _____

 CYBERLINKS

Interactive You can calculate your own body mass and check to see if you are a healthy weight at **www.thriveonline.com** Go to Tools and click on Body Mass Index.

Supplemental **www.LPNresources.com** can help enhance your learning by leading you to discover other links with more information about the topic you are studying.

One of nursing's greatest challenges is helping individuals to view dietary habits as having an impact on health and to make changes in their dietary intake accordingly. Although the ultimate function of food is to sustain the body, an individual's background (culture, ethnic group, religion, and knowledge about nutrition, lifestyle, financial situation, and food preferences) has a great influence on what foods are actually ingested. The forces on the individual to maintain the nutritional status quo are great. Therefore, before attempting to change someone's diet, the starting point must be determining the current dietary situation: what, when, and why does the patient eat? The answers to these questions will be the foundation for interventions aimed at creating new dietary patterns that will positively affect their health status.

CORE CONCEPTS | NUTRITIONAL ASSESSMENT

There are many nutrition assessment tools. However, some basic indicators of an individual's nutrition status are:

- General appearance
- Weight and height compared to weight and height tables
- History of recent unplanned weight gain or loss of 10% or more of body weight
- Serum albumin values (normal ranges: 3.5 to 5.0 g/dL)
- H and H (Remember: the first "H" always stands for hemoglobin, Hb, or Hbg, and is reported in g/dL; while the second "H" always stands for hematocrit, Hct, and is reported in percent; normal H and H ranges for men are 13.5 to 17 g/dL and 40 to 45%; for women ranges are 12 to 15 g/dL and 36 to 46%.)

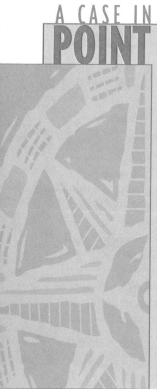

A CASE IN POINT

Mrs. Ulene has recently been diagnosed as a Type 2 diabetic. She is not prescribed insulin or an oral hypoglycemic; instead, the physician is attempting to control her blood sugar levels with diet and exercise. Mrs. Ulene has been instructed to lose weight. She is resisting her new diet regime. The nurse caring for Mrs. Ulene realizes that not only is she not following the prescribed diet, but she has gained weight consistently for the past three weeks. The physician asks the nurse to figure out her problem—why she is noncompliant. The nurse wonders where to begin. She decides she really doesn't have time to "figure it out" and instead tells Mrs. Ulene that she has failed so far to lose weight, she needs to have some will power, and that she had better join a diet program. Mrs. Ulene is dismayed and angry. The conversation was particularly disturbing to the patient because the nurse was also considerably overweight.

CORE CONCEPTS	**SPECIAL AND THERAPEUTIC DIETS**

Currently, the three most common therapeutic diets in use are American Diabetes Association (ADA) diabetic diets, sodium-controlled diets, and fat- and cholesterol-controlled diets. However, there are at least 35 additional types of special diets. Table 26-1 presents a few of these.

As you assist patients adjust to new dietary patterns, one of your interventions will be teaching the patient two key things: the concepts in the Food Guide Pyramid, which in 1992 replaced the four food groups (Figure 26-1); and how to read the nutrition facts panel on food products (Figure 26-2). The material on this panel is established by federal mandate. For foods without labels, such as fruits and vegetables, meats, and fish, the buyer will find the information on a card or sign in the store. If not, the buyer can ask the store manager for the information. Along this same line, nutrition information on any item served in fast-food and regular restaurants must also be available on request. Some fast-food restaurants are beginning to post this information on a bulletin board.

You may also need two other resources for successful intervention. One is a diet manual that lists foods that are allowed and those not allowed on specific therapeutic diets (or has enough information about a specific food for you to determine how the food fits into the patient's therapeutic diet). Your second resource is a registered dietitian. This member of the health care team is essential, especially when dealing with patients who have complex dietary needs. Keep in mind, though, that some facilities require a physician's order for a dietary consult. Some dietitians will answer questions "unofficially" concerning your specific patient.

CORE CONCEPTS	**TRIGLYCERIDES, PHOSPHOLIPIDS, AND STEROLS**

Fats in the diet have really gotten "bad press" to the point that individuals have forgotten the fact that some fats are necessary for health. They are a good source of energy for our bodies, and they are necessary for the transportation of the fat-soluble vitamins of A, D, E, and K throughout our body. The fatty acids are needed for our bodies to manufacture prostaglandins, needed for many bodily functions such as protection of the stomach lining.

TABLE 26-1	A Select Number of Therapeutic Diets

- High or low fiber
- Bland
- Dysphagia
- Renal
- Gastroplasty

- Lactose restricted
- Allergy
- Gluten controlled
- Purine restricted

Figure 26-1 Food Guide Pyramid

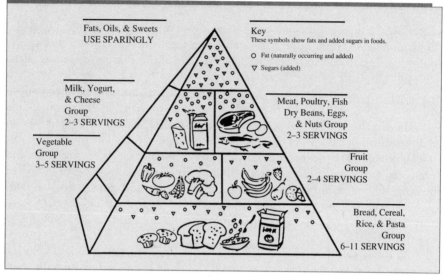

Source: U.S. Department of Health and Human Services.

Fats are divided into 3 categories:

- Triglycerides, the largest class of fats; 3 fatty acids and 1 glycerol molecule
- Phospholipids, of which lecithin is the best known; 2 fatty acids and 1 phosphate group; may be manufactured in the body
- Sterols, of which cholesterol is the best known; contain carbon, hydrogen and oxygen; may be manufactured in the body (Grodner, Anderson, & DeYoung, 1996)

The new recommendation for fat intake is that we take in no more than 20% of our Kcals (kilocalories) daily from fat. Some physicians still hold to the old standard of 30%, while others recommend only 10%. All food labels now tell you what percentage of the total calories from the product come from fat.

High lipid levels in humans have been associated with the development of atherosclerosis, coronary artery disease (CAD), cancer, Type 2 diabetes mellitus, and hypertension. Lipid panels (blood tests for lipid levels) should be done routinely for those over the age of 40 years or those with a family history of hyperlipidemia or high lipid levels. Remember that since phospholipids and cholesterol may be manufactured in the body, not all high cholesterol levels are the result of high-fat diets but may be related to genetics.

Below are listed the different levels of lipids examined in a lipid panel:

- Total triglycerides
- Total cholesterol

Figure 26-2 Standard Nutritional Label

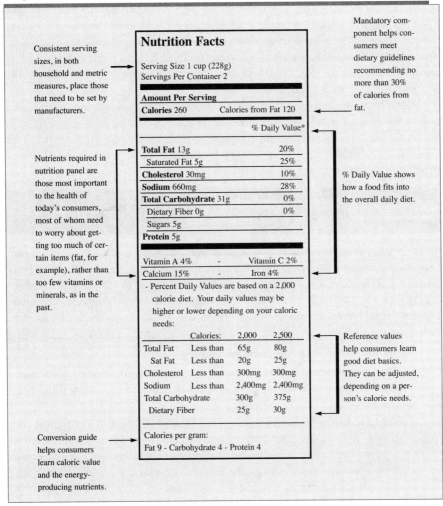

Source: U.S. Department of Health and Human Services.

- HDLs: High-density lipoproteins, which transport fats and cholesterol from the cells to the liver for excretion. These are also called the "good" cholesterol. We refer to them as the "happy" cholesterol in our classes, because they are both "h" words.
- LDLs: Low-density lipoproteins, which carry cholesterol to the cells. These are called the "bad" cholesterol. We refer to them as "lousy," because they are both "l" words.
- VLDLs: Very low-density lipoproteins, which are the largest group of lipoproteins to carry cholesterol to the cells. These are "very lousy."

You may care for patients who have been placed on low-fat diets because of their lipid levels, or because their LDLs were too high and their HDLs were too low. These patients may also be taking lipid-lowering medications, because diet alone has not brought their lipid levels down to normal. Some patients may be taking high doses of vitamin E, which also lowers the lipid level to some extent. Adding oat bran and soy to the diet has also proved effective. Exercise is probably one of the best ways to raise one's HDL level.

As a nursing student, you should certainly do more reading up on this concern of the general public, so you can educate patients and possibly advocate with the physician for a dietary consult for patients with poor lipid panel results. This information can also be beneficial for you. You want to be as healthy as possible and a role model for your patients!

CORE CONCEPTS	**DIETARY-RELATED QUESTIONS ASKED BY STUDENTS**

What is nitrogen balance? Nitrogen is one by-product of protein breakdown. Every 6.25 grams of protein will yield 1 gram of nitrogen that is excreted from the body via urine and feces. So, if in one 24-hour period, urine and feces analysis yields 8 grams of nitrogen, the patient has broken down (catabolized) about 50 grams of protein. There are several terms regarding nitrogen balance with which you need to be familiar:

- **Nitrogen balance** occurs when the amount of protein intake equals the amount of nitrogen lost from the body.
- **Positive nitrogen balance** occurs when protein intake exceeds nitrogen output. This is seen during periods of tissue growth (e.g., infancy and pregnancy).
- **Negative nitrogen balance** occurs when more nitrogen is lost than is consumed in food. It occurs any time that caloric intake is not sufficient to meet energy needs. (Catabolism is greater than anabolism.) A few conditions that can create a negative balance are massive injuries, burns, and infections. In addition, one less obvious situation that creates a negative balance is the inactivity associated with bedridden individuals.

Individuals who are in negative nitrogen balance obviously need to increase their protein intake. The proteins of choice are those proteins with high biologic value (HBV), also known as complete proteins. These foods contain all eight essential amino acids (those the body is unable to manufacture). Remember, there are 20 amino acids: 8 essential and 12 nonessential. It takes all 20 amino acids for the body to make proteins. Therefore, in patients who need to repair damaged tissue (postop, fractures, burns, wounds, decubitus ulcers, etc.), dietary intake of foods with HBV is a must for tissue repair. If the protein is not available, the body will break down body proteins for repair and energy purposes. This is not desirable. Some of the best HBV foods are meats, eggs, cheese, and milk. (Recall that fat does not contain protein; therefore, low-fat or even skimmed milk is an excellent source of protein for individuals with restricted fat intake.)

My patient is a vegetarian. Can he or she get a balanced diet?   Yes. Let's explore the highlights of vegetarians. First, being a vegetarian is not unique to any particular ethnic group; however, it may be associated with certain religions. Second, although there are many variations, there are basically four types of vegetarians based on which nonplant foods are allowed in the diet (Figures 26-3 through 26-6). Those four types are:

- *Semivegetarian:* Included are dairy products, eggs, and fish; excluded are meat and sometimes poultry.
- *Lacto-ovovegetarian:* Included are dairy products and eggs; excluded are meat, poultry, and fish.

Figure 26-3 Food Pyramid Adjusted for a Semivegetarian Diet

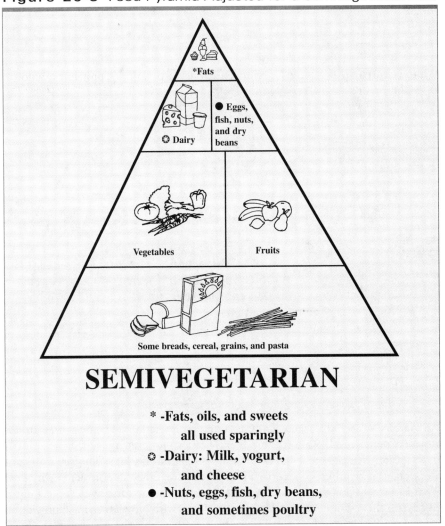

Figure 26-4 Food Pyramid Adjusted for a Lacto-Ovovegetarian Diet

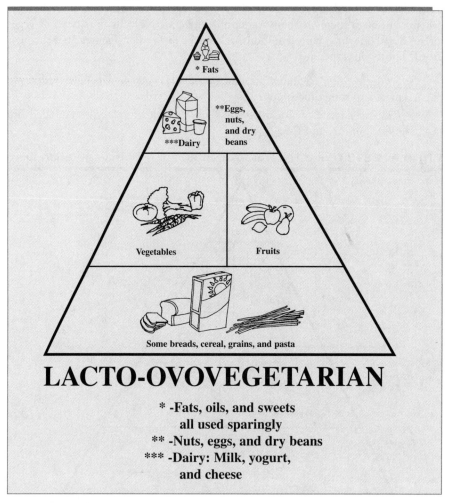

LACTO-OVOVEGETARIAN

* -Fats, oils, and sweets
all used sparingly
** -Nuts, eggs, and dry beans
*** -Dairy: Milk, yogurt,
and cheese

- *Lactovegetarian:* Included are dairy products; excluded are meat, fish, poultry, and eggs.
- *Vegan:* Excluded are all foods of animal origin.

As you can see, being a vegetarian has several interpretations. The first three groups can meet needs for HBV protein foods fairly easily. However, a practicing true vegan has a greater challenge to avoid deficiencies. But it can be done. The key is to consume plants with different essential amino acids so that they complement each other. That is, foods lacking in specific essential amino acids are eaten with foods known to contain them. For example, having baked beans with brown bread will provide all the essential amino acids. This practice requires, however, that the complementary

Figure 26-5   Food Pyramid Adjusted for a Lactovegetarian
Diet

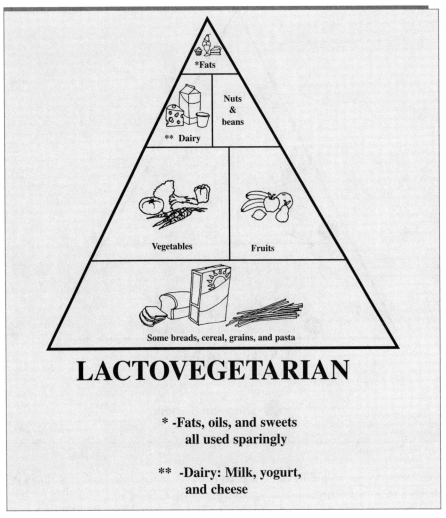

LACTOVEGETARIAN

* -Fats, oils, and sweets
all used sparingly

** -Dairy: Milk, yogurt,
and cheese

foods, if not eaten at the same meals, be eaten throughout the day—every day. A greater challenge is a vegan who has a medical need for a clear liquid diet. Many of the traditional items on this diet have an animal base, including beef and chicken broth and gelatin, which a vegan will not eat. So if your patient has a need for clear liquids much beyond 24 hours, a consultation with a dietitian is essential.

Most vegetarians at any level know a great deal about how to maintain adequate nutrition. Their personal libraries usually include many books on the subject, and there are numerous vegetarian cookbooks. Problems, however, may occur during times of special physiological needs such as pregnancy, lactation, and injury. During these times, some individuals will supplement their vegetarian diets with

Figure 26-6 Food Pyramid Adjusted for a Vegan Diet

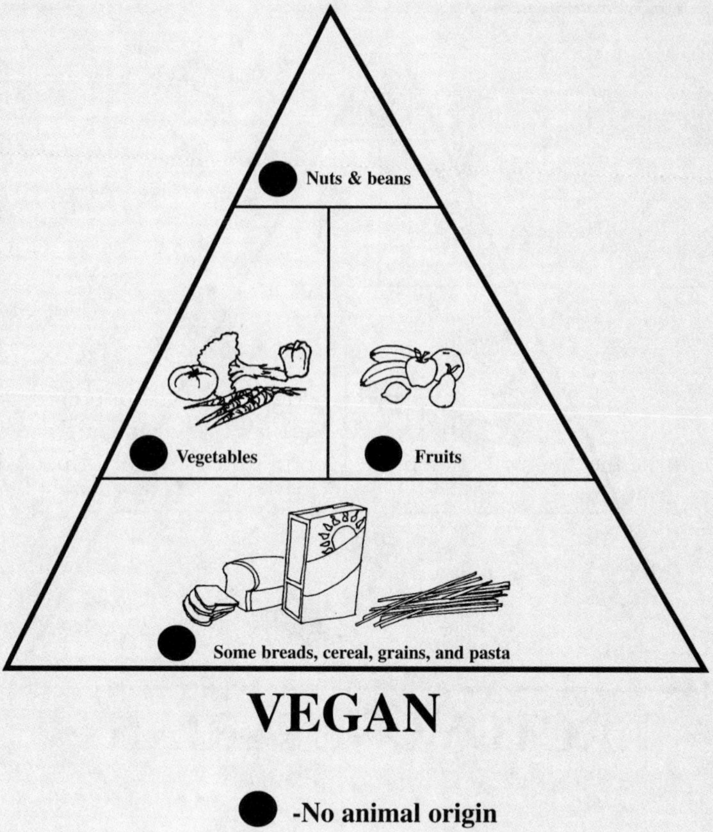

foods they do not ordinarily eat; others will not. Therefore, your task is to do an in-depth dietary assessment and, along with the patient, come to a consensus on how to best meet the increased needs. In addition, it may be necessary for you to increase your knowledge base on vegetarian diets.

What is the glycemic index (GI) value of a food? For many years it was believed that 1 gram of carbohydrate (CHO), regardless of the source, always had the same effect on blood glucose levels. Research since the late 1980s has challenged this belief. The glycemic index represents how quickly 50 grams of CHO in a specific food will change the blood glucose level compared to 50 grams of CHO in white bread, which is used as the standard. Glycemic index values range from 1 to 150. Research indicates that there is a vast difference in the glycemic index of carbohydrate foods. Foods with higher index numbers cause rapid increases in serum glucose; lower numbers cause slow increases.

There are many factors influencing the GI of a food, and much research needs to be done. However, the belief is that not too far down the road, GI information will become part of the dietary control for individuals with diabetes.

What exactly do terms like fat free, organic, and sugar free mean?
Terms used in connection with foods have specific meanings that have been established by the Food and Drug Administration (FDA) as mandated by the Nutritional Labeling and Education Act of 1990. Table 26-2 summarizes the most common terms with their basic FDA definitions. These terms will have the same meaning regardless of which food label they appear on and are based on a single serving of the food.

The following terms have no standard government definition. Therefore, their use in relation to food items is not always clear.

- *Dietetic:* This is a very general term pertaining to diet or proper food. It is sometimes used to indicate foods with low-caloric content. Patients often mistake the dietetic section of the grocery store for diabetic foods. There is no such thing as diabetic foods. With proper guidance, almost any food can be part of a diabetic diet.
- *Natural* or *organic:* Although there is no consensus on this phrase, it generally means that the food (plant or animal) was grown without antibiotics, pesticides, fertilizer, and herbicides. The U.S. Department of Agriculture has developed definitions for the organic food industry, and these can be found on their Web site.

How do I evaluate the many claims made about certain foods and supplements like vitamins and minerals?   Now this is a truly challenging question! Claims that specific foods or substances have remarkable curative or health powers are not new. There are a large number of health claims surrounding specific foods and supplements. More seem to come on the market daily. However, the scientific research supporting many of these claims is usually very limited, since the FDA is not required to approve these supplements. The major task in examining these claims is to separate the wheat from the chaff. Here are a few basic rules to help you do that.

- *Do not take all claims seriously.* This, however, may be difficult, because so many of the products have exaggerated claims that are promoted with very elaborate, sophisticated, glittery promotions. If you are not careful, you may be convinced that this item is the answer to cure all that ails the human body. Therefore, how can companies make these claims if they are not supported by facts? First, the FDA labeling rules have not filled all of the holes. Secondly, some individuals and companies make false claims until they are caught. They may then elect to fight the law several ways, including going to court. Thus, it may take years for issues regarding a product's advertising claims to be settled.

TABLE 26-2	Most Common Food Terms

Fat Terms
- Fat free: Less than 0.5 g of fat
- Saturated fat free: Less than 0.5 g of fat and less than 0.5 g of trans-fatty acids
- Low fat: 3 g or less of fat per serving
- Low saturated fat: 1 g or less per serving and not more than 15% of calories from saturated fatty acids
- Reduced/less fat: At least 25% less fat per serving than the "regular" food
- Reduced/less saturated fat: At least 25% less saturated fat than the "regular" food item
- Cholesterol free: Less than 2 mg of cholesterol and 2 g or less of saturated fats per serving
- Low cholesterol: 20 mg or less and 2 g or less of fat per serving, and, if the serving is 30 mg or less or 2 tablespoons or less, per 50 g of the food
- Reduced/less cholesterol: At least 25% less and 2 g or less of saturated fat per serving than the "regular" food
- Lean (meat, poultry, seafood, game meats): Less than 10 g of fat, 4.5 g or less of saturated fat, and less than 95 mg of cholesterol per serving and per 100 g (3½ oz)
- Extra lean: Less than 5 g of fat, less than 2 g of saturated fat, less than 95 mg of cholesterol per serving and per 100 g (3½ oz)

Sodium Terms
- Sodium free: Less than 5 mg of sodium
- Low sodium: Less than 140 mg of sodium for serving
- Very low sodium: Between 5 and 35 mg of sodium
- Reduced or less sodium: At least 25% less sodium than "regular food"

Sugar Terms
- Sugar free: Less than 0.5 mg of CHO per serving
- No added sugar, without sugar added, no sugar added:
    No sugar added during processing or packing, including ingredients that contain sugars (e.g., fruit juices, applesauce, or dried fruit)
    Processing does not increase the sugar content above the amount naturally present in the ingredients
    The food that it resembles and for which it substitutes normally contains added sugars
    If the food does not meet the requirements for a low- or reduced-calorie food, the product bears a statement that the food is not low calorie or calorie reduced and directs the customers' attention to the nutrition panel for further information on sugars and calorie content
- Reduced sugar: At least 25% less sugar per serving than the "regular" food.

TABLE 26-2	Most Common Food Terms (Continued)

Fiber Terms
- High fiber: 5 g or more per serving (foods making high-fiber claims must meet the definition for low fat, or the level of total fat must appear next to the high-fiber claim)
- Good source of fiber: 2.5 to 4.9 g of fiber per serving
- More or added fiber: At least 2.5 g more per serving than the "regular" food

Lite/Light Terms
- Food contains ⅓ less calories and half the fat of the "regular" food
- The sodium content of a low-calorie, low-fat food reduced by 50%

- *Look for the small print.* Be aware of a claim such as: "These statements have not been evaluated by the FDA. This product is not intended to diagnose, treat, cure, or prevent any disease." This does not automatically mean the claims are false. It only means that the FDA does not have enough research to support or refute the claims.
- *When the advertisement states that the product claims are backed by research, write or call and ask for copies of the research.* If you do not receive any response, be wary. If you do receive a response, use your critical thinking skills to analyze the information. In addition, critically analyze claims that the "established medical community does not want you to know about or use this product because . . ."
- *Currently, the best advice for you and your patient is to accept the dietary information from reputable, known sources until research supports the claim.* A few examples of reliable nutritional information are: registered dietitians, colleges and universities, Federal Food and Drug Administration, and organizations such as the American Cancer Society, the American Diabetes Association, and the American Heart Association. In addition, pharmacists are becoming more literate concerning the use of herbal medications by the general population. There are numerous good publications now on the market that you might want to add to your own library. One such book is the *Professional's Handbook of Complementary and Alternative Medicines,* written by Charles Fetrow and Juan Avila, both pharmacists and professors of pharmacology.

The role of nutrition in maintaining health and preventing and controlling specific health problems is an emerging science. And research may, in time, support many of the claims surrounding current nutrition fads. Until then, be vigilant, and stick with information that you know has a sound research base.

ASK YOURSELF

1. What have you learned or been reminded of in terms of eating healthily that you might want to incorporate into your own dietary regime?

   _____

   _____

2. How would you summarize the ways in which you can best help patients to change their dietary habits when it is part of their prescribed treatment?

   _____

   _____

 CYBERLINKS: FLASH CARDS

Check to see what you now remember by making your own flash cards. Use the CD-ROM that accompanies your textbook to discover how to make flash cards for reviewing and retaining what you have learned.

 CONCEPT MAP WORD BANK

NUTRITION
Purpose
Connection to illness
Assessment
Special diets
FALSE INFORMATION

Refer to Concept Maps and Flash Cards on pages viii–ix for an explanation of how to create and use concept maps. In addition, the CD-ROM guides you through the construction of concept maps by providing a more detailed introduction, more illustrations of examples, and key steps to follow in designing your own maps.

Infection Control

27

 ASK YOURSELF ────────────────────────────────

1. In our recent past, as a country, we have become painfully more aware of the dangers of infection with unfamiliar harmful microorganisms. What is your own level of concern related to the potential for working in an environment where people with infectious diseases are treated?

   _____

   _____

2. What infection prevention measures do you use in your own environment, and what personal habits do you have, in addition to handwashing, that would help prevent the spread of infection?

   _____

   _____

 CYBERLINKS ────────────────────────────────

Interactive Acquired immune deficiency syndrome (AIDS) remains a disease that challenges caregivers from a variety of perspectives. One challenge is educating the public regarding how AIDS is transmitted and how it is treated, and its prognosis in light of new advances. www.thebody.com maintains an interactive question and answer forum on AIDS. It is a valuable resource for patients and caregivers.

Supplemental www.LPNresources.com can help enhance your learning by leading you to discover other links with more information about the topic you are studying.

The prevention and control of infection within the patient environment are important nursing functions, and essential to the care of all patients. Patients who are already ill are much more susceptible to an invasion of disease-causing microorganisms than healthy individuals.

In this chapter, the focus is on core concepts such as the chain of infection and essential skills such as the methods for breaking the chain of infection through the use of aseptic technique. Most educational programs include an introductory skill course that covers infection control. More extensive coverage is included in other courses. However, infection prevention and control are dynamic disciplines. We continue to be bombarded by an ever-growing number of new infectious microorganisms with greater potency and unimaginable danger. Infection prevention and control are areas where the landscape is continually changing. Every nurse must be committed to keeping up with current information related to infection identification, prevention, and control. Knowledge in this instance is the first line of defense.

CORE CONCEPTS | **DEFINITIONS**

To fully understand the concept of infection control, you must be familiar with certain terms:

- A *pathogen* is a disease-producing microorganism; if it is carried within the circulatory system, it is called a *bloodborne pathogen.*
- A *nosocomial infection* is an infection that is acquired while a patient is in a health care facility.
- *Asepsis* is a condition in which there is an absence of disease-causing germs. *Medical asepsis* is the use of clean technique to control and prevent the spread of microorganisms; *surgical asepsis* is the use of sterile technique to control and prevent the spread of microorganisms. In surgical asepsis, all microorganisms are eliminated from the environment.
- *Sterilization* is the process that completely eliminates all microorganisms through various means.
- *Disinfection* is the process that destroys disease-causing microorganisms.

CORE CONCEPTS | **THE CHAIN OF INFECTION**

There are six major factors (links) associated with the spread of communicable diseases. These links form a vicious circle (chain) and are listed as follows:

1. Pathogen or disease-causing agent
2. The agent's reservoir—where it lives and multiplies
3. Portal of exit from the reservoir
4. Mode of transmission away from the reservoir
5. Portal of entry into a new host
6. Susceptible new host

In the control of communicable diseases, the major goal is to break the chain at one of the six links. One of the most important ways to break the chain at any link is thorough hand washing. This means at least a 30-second wash before and after contact with patients or patient items. It should be performed before and after gloving as well. Handwashing is crucial in every area of infection control. It prevents the spread of microorganisms from the agent reservoir, inhibits the exit and transmission of the microorganisms, and protects susceptible new hosts. Other measures to break the chain include immunizations of susceptible populations, which interfere with susceptibility of the new host; sterilization and disinfection, which kills the pathogens; and antibiotics, which interfere with certain physiological functions of an organism preventing it from multiplying. Universal and standard precautions; and maximizing the body's own defense mechanisms by good skin care, promoting good nutrition, and encouraging proper rest and exercise are other effective measures. Figure 27-1 shows in more detail the linking nature of these six factors.

Figure 27-1 Chain of Infection

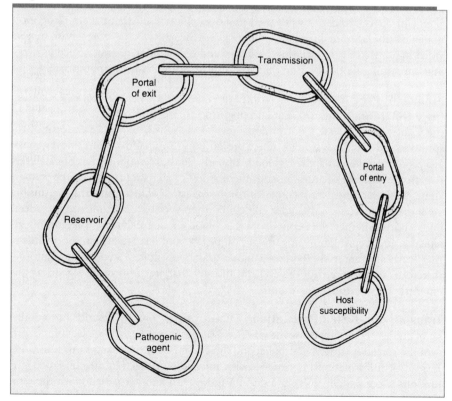

Source: Ball, J., & Bindler, R. (1999). *Pediatric nursing: Caring for children* (2nd ed.). Reprinted by permission of Pearson Education, Inc., Upper Saddle River, NJ 07458.

| ESSENTIAL SKILLS | STANDARD PRECAUTIONS AND UNIVERSAL PRECAUTIONS |

One of the authors of this text has a nurse friend who has taught infection control issues to nursing assistant students for years. She makes a statement to her students, which contains concise wisdom emphasizing the use of standard precautions. Her advice is, "If it's wet, and it isn't yours, wear gloves!"

Universal Precautions   **Universal precautions** is a term developed in 1987 when human immunodeficiency virus (HIV) and an increase in the cases of hepatitis B first gained prominence in health care. Because you do not know which of your patients might be carrying either virus, the practice of universal precautions was developed. This means that, for every single patient you care for, you treat all blood and all body substances containing blood as if they were infectious. *Personal protective equipment* should be available in the workplace. This includes gloves, goggles, masks, and gowns that are resistant to liquid penetration. All health care facilities should provide gloves for you that are of the correct size and material. Since glove usage has significantly increased, there have been many instances of latex allergy or allergy to the powder used in gloves. Most facilities now are using more nonlatex, nonpowdered gloves. Red containers for hazardous wastes should be provided in all health care facilities for sharps and contaminated wastes, such as dressings containing blood. Be sure that you dispose of these wastes appropriately.

Standard Precautions   According to *Taber's Cyclopedic Medical Dictionary* (page 1822, 18th Edition), "standard precautions" are "guidelines recommended by the Centers for Disease Control and Prevention (CDC) to reduce the risk of the spread of infection in hospitals. These precautions (e.g., handwashing, gloves, mask, eye protection, gown) apply to blood, all body fluids, secretions, excretions (except sweat), non-intact skin, and mucous membranes of all patients and are the primary strategy for successful nosocomial infection control." Thus, standard precautions are more inclusive than the older guidelines of universal precautions and include all body fluids whether they contain visible blood or not. Standard precautions are aimed at intercepting transmission at points 3, 4, and 5 on the chain for organisms that leave and enter the body via blood and body fluids. Standard precautions, therefore, do not interrupt the cycle for diseases that are airborne or organisms that enter the body through the mouth.

Transmission-Based Precautions   These precautions are described in another set of guidelines developed by the CDC as a suggestion to health care facilities to prevent the spread of airborne, droplet, and direct contact (wound and skin) infections. Instead of full isolation for patients with infections, these transmission-based precautions allow patients to be placed in a room with another patient with the same infection but no other. The precautions taken are limited to the type of infection the patient has. For instance, if a patient has a contaminated wound, the nurse would wear gown and gloves but would not be required to wear a mask and goggles.

CORE CONCEPTS | COMMUNICABLE DISEASES AND IMMUNITY

One of the main mechanisms for control of many communicable diseases is development of immunity. When considering immunity, it is essential to understand the two major types: active and passive. These terms indicate how the body obtained its immunity. If the body had to work at it, it is known as active immunity. On the other hand, if the body did nothing to get the protection, it is known as passive immunity (Figure 27-2).

Key Terms

- **Immunity:** Protection against an infectious disease as a result of the functioning of a healthy immune system.
- **Antigen:** A substance that the body does not recognize as self. Almost all antigens have a protein component. In the healthy immune system an antigen will cause the body to create a defense against it (called an antibody).
- **Antibody:** A protein created when the body is exposed to an antigen. The antibody makes the antigen incapable of causing harm. Antibodies are specific. That is, they work only when they are paired up with their specific antigen. Antibodies against polio will not protect someone exposed to chickenpox.

The two ways of becoming immune have different characteristics that can be noted in Table 27-1. Let's analyze a few examples and see how they fit into the table.

Figure 27-2 How the Body Acquires Active and Passive Immunity

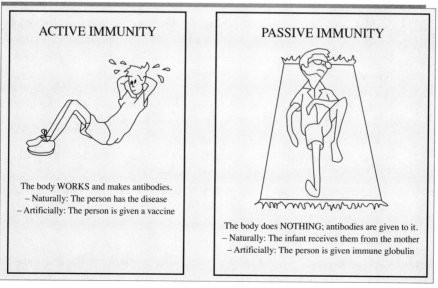

ACTIVE IMMUNITY

The body WORKS and makes antibodies.
– Naturally: The person has the disease
– Artificially: The person is given a vaccine

PASSIVE IMMUNITY

The body does NOTHING; antibodies are given to it.
– Naturally: The infant receives them from the mother
– Artificially: The person is given immune globulin

TABLE 27-1	Two Ways of Developing Immunity	
Terminology	**How the Body Develops Immunity**	**Length of Time the Body Is Protected**
Natural		
Active	Natural contact with the antigen (you are near an individual who has the disease). You develop a clinical or subclinical[a] case of the disease.	Permanent. The individual is considered immune to the specific disease for life.
Passive	Natural contact with the antibody through placenta, colostrum, and/or breastmilk.	Temporary. Protection lasts 6–8 weeks. Then the antibodies are gone and the body no longer has protection.
Artificial		
Active	The body is inoculated with the antigen, called vaccinations.	Premanent. Some diseases require a periodic booster to ensure continued protection.
Passive	The body is injected with a specific antibody, immune globulin (old term: gamma globulin).	Temporary: 6–8 weeks.

[a] Subclinical case occurs when the individual is exposed to small amount of an antigen but, although the body makes antibodies, shows no outward signs of being sick with the disease.

- A child is vaccinated against diphtheria, tetanus, and pertussis (whooping cough). The type of immunity is active, artificial immunity. The child's body has been given antigens (in this example, three specific antigens) and must work to create the corresponding specific antibodies.
- A mother has immunity (antibodies) to measles and is breast-feeding her newborn. The type of immunity is passive, natural immunity. The infant's body is receiving ready-made antibodies from its mother.
- A high school student develops a case of chickenpox. The type of immunity is active, natural immunity. The student's body is exposed to the chickenpox antigen and must work to create antibodies.
- An adult is exposed to hepatitis B and the physician orders an injection of an immune globulin preparation. The type of immunity is passive, artificial immunity. The adult's body is receiving ready-made antibodies in the immune globulin injection.

Understanding the type of immunity an individual possesses influences nursing interventions, especially patient education issues. For example, the CDC recently recommended beginning immunization of all newborns against hepatitis B before the newborn leaves the hospital. This will require that the parent be taught not only the reason for the immunization, but also the importance of following the immunizations schedule after discharge.

Nurses have several major responsibilities in relation to vaccine-preventable diseases.

- *Be sure that the reference vaccine schedule used for children and adults is current.* As of the printing of this book, the recommended immunization schedule for infants and children has been updated for 2002. There is a separate summary of recommendations for adults and adolescents that is dated 2/4/2002. If you are in doubt about the most current immunization schedule, call your local health department or visit the CDC Web page at **www.cdc.gov/nip/acip.**
- *Teach parents the importance of having their children immunized on schedule.*
- *Know and follow specific administration techniques.* For example, in adults, hepatitis B vaccine should be administered in the deltoid muscle.
- *Know the specific vaccine storage and handling requirements.*
- *Be aware of myths associated with vaccinations.* There have been recent concerns in the media regarding the side effects and contraindications for the administration of vaccinations. The CDC has extensive information posted on its Web site pertaining to these topics. Visit **www.cdc.gov/mmwr/preview** so that you have the latest vaccination recommendations and objective findings to share with your clients.
- *Spend time with patients who do not follow vaccination recommendations for infants, children, or adults.* Is their action based on religious or cultural reasons? If so, then attempts to convince them to receive vaccinations may be unethical. If, however, they have other reasons, you may be able to help them realize the benefits of vaccinations. Be cautious with advice to parents that there are no dangers with vaccinations. Although very small in number, problems do occur.
- *As a nursing student, be sure that you follow your school's recommendations for immunizations for yourself.* Remember that, as a nursing student, you could be exposed to communicable diseases. You do not want to be the source of infection for other patients or for your family, nor do you want to get ill and miss out on your classroom or clinical time!

CORE CONCEPTS ■ **EPIDEMIOLOGY**

Epidemiology is the area of study that identifies "causal relationships between health problems and the multitude of etiological factors that initiate them" (Berger & Williams, 1999). The focus of epidemiology is public or community health issues that look at groups of individuals who share a common health problem or specific condition. Often, the common health problem is a communicable disease.

Epidemiologic studies usually play a major role in forming and implementing public health policy.

Epidemiologists are often considered medical detectives. When a problem is identified, they probe every nook and cranny looking for clues that pinpoint a cause and effect relationship. Among the facts gathered are data concerning the time and place of a specific health problem, as well as characteristics of the population affected such as physical, biologic, social, cultural, and behavioral factors. Specifically:

- Epidemiologists study communicable diseases; acute, chronic, and congenital illnesses; and environmental health hazards.
- When analyzing a community health problem, the epidemiologist analyzes it in as much depth as possible by breaking it down into three major areas of investigation:
  1. Host: The individuals involved—age, gender, culture, place of residence, ethnicity, occupation, and so on.
  2. Agent: The cause of the specific health problem; there are two main categories of agents:
     - Infectious agents such as parasites, bacteria, or viruses
     - Noninfectious agents such as smoking, cholesterol, or radiation
  3. Environment: The surrounding conditions:
     - Physical environment includes climate, land, atmospheric conditions, chemicals, or physical agents.
     - Biological environment includes the agent's reservoir, methods of transmission of the agent, and elements in the environment that block the disease development.
     - Social environment includes public policies, housing conditions, cultural habits, and family health practices.

Therefore, the development of a disease or community health problem is the result of many factors interacting, not a single, isolated factor. It is through the analysis of the interplay of these three factors that strategies to control the problem are developed. Although local and state health departments carry out epidemiologic investigations, many investigations are conducted by the Centers for Disease Control and Prevention (CDC), which is a federal agency. The CDC is the leader in epidemiologic studies and, with a knowledgeable and specialized staff, often identifies factors associated with a problem relatively quickly; other times a great deal of time is required. (Note that in 1993, the name of the CDC was expanded to the Centers for Disease Control and Prevention. However, the acronym, CDC, has not changed.)

A few examples of the hundreds of health problems that have been solved or understood as a result of epidemiological research include:

1. Toxic shock syndrome and use of specific tampons
2. Smoking and various health consequences

3. The connection between HIV infection and the development of AIDS
4. Source of a staphylococcal infection in a newborn nursery
5. Connection between fat intake and heart problems
6. Effect of lead ingestion by children and IQ development
7. Legionnaires' disease and air conditioning systems

There are two points that need to be made about the work of epidemiologists. As items numbers 1, 2, 5, and 6 in the previous list indicate, the current scope of investigations goes far beyond traditional communicable diseases. Secondly, epidemiology is not directly concerned with curing or treating a specific disease or condition. However, because epidemiology identifies the interactions of multiple causes, it is often the foundation for actions aimed at treatment or control. The work of epidemiologists was the basis for developing universal and standard precautions.

Nurses who serve as infection control nurses may find themselves doing the work of an epidemiologist in tracing the development of infections within the health care environment. Quite often the staff development coordinator in the long-term care facility is also the infection control nurse. A licensed practical or vocational nurse may fill this role.

The importance of the nurse's role in protecting patients and preventing the spread and development of nosocomial infections cannot be underestimated. Hopefully, from reading this chapter, two issues will stand out as very important to remember: Wash your hands well and often; and use gloves if you are going to be touching anyone else's bodily secretions!

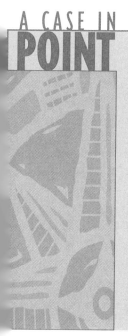

A CASE IN POINT

In the small town of Rosemont, in the last five years, there has been a 20% increase of cases of lung cancer. Health officials and community leaders are aware of the increase and are concerned. An epidemiologist has been consulted. An investigation is conducted. The epidemiologist is focusing the investigation on several factors: during the last five years, more power lines have been installed in the main residential areas, and a chemical plant has opened 10 miles outside the city limits. In addition, the number of individuals who smoke has increased, and a large percentage of the town's population is old. The town's residents want answers immediately but health officials know that the investigation will take a long time since making scientific conclusions is a difficult, painstaking process.

ASK YOURSELF

1. Are the concepts of active and passive immunity clear to you? Would you be able to explain these concepts to patients.

   _____

   _____

2. What concerns do you still have about your own personal safety related to the potential for infection in the work environment? What will you do to alleviate your concerns?

   _____

   _____

 CYBERLINKS: FLASH CARDS

Check to see what you now remember by making your own flash cards. Use the CD-ROM that accompanies your textbook to discover how to make flash cards for reviewing and retaining what you have learned.

 CONCEPT MAP WORD BANK

INFECTION CONTROL
INFECTION PREVENTION
Definitions
Process (Chain)
Precautions
IMMUNITY
EPIDEMIOLOGY

Refer to Concept Maps and Flash Cards on pages viii–ix for an explanation of how to create and use concept maps. In addition, the CD-ROM guides you through the construction of concept maps by providing a more detailed introduction, more illustrations of examples, and key steps to follow in designing your own maps

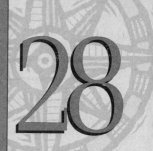

Endocrine Highlights

28

ASK YOURSELF

1. Before reading this chapter, can you identify the organs that make up the endocrine system?

_____

_____

2. What is your understanding of the term *hormone?*

_____

_____

CYBERLINKS

<u>Interactive</u> Diabetes is one of the diseases that you will most often encounter in patients. It is essential that you be not only be knowledgeable regarding diabetes but that you also be able to teach diabetic patients the things they need to know in order to live with the disease. You may be interested in knowing your own risk of developing diabetes. Visit **www.healthfinder.com** to determine your own predisposition. The test is also available in Spanish and is a great resource for patients as well.

<u>Supplemental</u> **www.LPNresources.com** can help enhance your learning by leading you to discover other links with more information about the topic you are studying.

The endocrine system, and more specifically, its malfunction, is singled out (other systems are not discussed in this text) because of the increasing incidence of diabetes. Diabetes presents perplexing problems to health care professionals as the technology associated with treatment and the understanding of the physiology are continuously evolving.

It is essential that nurses keep current regarding all aspects of diabetes as it is likely that a large number of the patients they will care for will have this disease. Therefore, core concepts, which update our understanding of diabetes, are presented.

| CORE CONCEPTS | **STRUCTURE AND FUNCTION OVERVIEW**

The endocrine system consists of organs with secretions, called hormones that go directly into the circulatory system. The main actions of the system center on regulating three body functions: metabolic activity, growth, and reproduction. Fluid and electrolyte balance and blood pressure are also affected by this system. The number of endocrine glands differs for men and women due to the presence of differing reproductive organs. The endocrine glands and hormones they produce are seen in Figure 28-1. Although the number of endocrine glands is small, 50 hormones that they secrete have been identified. Table 28-1 presents an overview of the most commonly seen dysfunctions that occur in the endocrine system.

Students often have difficulty with hypo- and hyperfunction of endocrine glands. Hypofunction of an endocrine glands means too little hormone is being produced and released; hyperfunction means too much hormone is being produced and released. This is one of those times when mastering knowledge of the normal actions of the hormones is well worth the study time.

The production and secretion of hormones from the endocrine glands is controlled by the glands' response to changes in the levels of hormones in the blood or changes in the blood itself. This is referred to as a *negative feedback loop* action. Here's an example:

1. The hormone, calcitonin, is produced by the thyroid gland.
2. The calcitonin blocks the breakdown of bone, preventing calcium from leaving the bone and entering the bloodstream.
3. This lowers the serum calcium (the amount of calcium in the blood).

Figure 28-1 Endocrine Glands

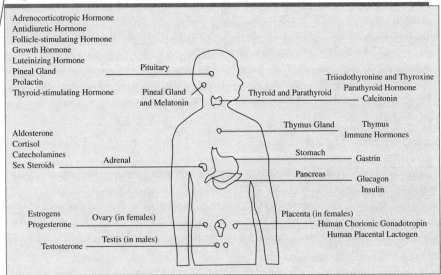

TABLE 28-1	Commonly Seen Endocrine Dysfunctions	
Major Endocrine Gland/Hormone	**Hypofunction Disorder**	**Hyperfunction Disorder**
Pancreas Insulin	Hyperglycemia = diabetes mellitus Based on severity, can be life-threatening	Rare natural occurrence Excess external insulin = hypoglycemia/insulin reaction
Thyroid Thyroxine (T_4); Thyroxine (T_3)	Undetected at birth can lead to cretinism Adult onset leads to myxedema	Graves' disease Severe hyperthyroidism (can be life threatening): thyrotoxicosis, thyroid storm Cushing's disease, a syndrome usually due to excess amounts of glucocorticoids
Adrenal cortex Glucocorticoids (chief one: cortisol, also called hydrocortisone); mineralocorticoids (chief one: aldosterone)	Addison's disease If etiology is at the adrenal cortex, both glucocorticoids and mineralocorticoids are deficient; if etiology is at the pituitary level, glucocorticoids are major deficiency (*note:* If exogenous glucocorticoids are administered for periods of 10–14 days or longer and suddenly stopped [versus dosage being tapered off], adrenal insufficiency[a] may result)	
Growth hormone	Dwarfism (several forms)	In children: gigantism In adults: acromegaly

[a]Adrenal insufficiency from any etiology can be life threatening.

4. If the serum calcium level becomes too low, the thyroid gland is inhibited from releasing any more calcitonin.

5. This allows the serum calcium levels to increase again.

6. This is called *negative* feedback when information fed back to the gland causes it to decrease its secretion of its hormone.

The hypothalamus (considered as part of both the nervous system and endocrine system) and pituitary gland regulate almost all of the glands. The hypothalamus produces and secretes either *releasing factors,* which cause the pituitary to produce and release its hormones, or *inhibiting factors,* which causes it to decrease or temporarily cease production of its hormones. Hormones from the pituitary affect target endocrine glands, so that they, in turn, will release or inhibit their hormone production. The pituitary gland is considered the master gland of the body because of its role in controlling the function of the other endocrine glands. Because of this relationship between the hypothalamus, pituitary and target glands, disorders of an endocrine gland may be due to a problem at any one of these three sites. This disorder may result in an excess or deficiency in a specific hormone.

Two major exceptions to the hypothalamus–pituitary gland and hormone–serum levels loop are the parathyroids and the pancreas. Hormone levels from these two glands respond to serum levels and do not involve the hypothalamus–pituitary loop.

CORE CONCEPTS | **MALFUNCTION OF THE ENDOCRINE SYSTEM**

There are a number of endocrine system diseases or dysfunctions, the two most frequently encountered are hypothyroidism and diabetes mellitus (usually referred to as diabetes). Another type of diabetes is diabetes insipidus, a disorder of the posterior pituitary. When referring to this disease, both words (diabetes and insipidus are always used together).

As mentioned earlier, you will encounter patients with diabetes often both as a nursing student and as a graduate. Notice the vast amount of space devoted to diabetes in most of your nursing texts. Be prepared, therefore, for many classes and test questions on the topic. You will be expected, as a practical/vocational nurse, to have an in-depth knowledge of this condition.

CORE CONCEPTS | **DIABETES**

In this discussion of the disease, we will focus on the most recent information on diabetes classification. Over the years diabetes has had several classification systems. The terms *juvenile onset* and *adult onset* were used until the late 1970s. In 1979, these terms were replaced. Juvenile-onset diabetes became insulin-dependent diabetes mellitus (IDDM), also called Type I diabetes; while adult-onset became non–insulin-dependent diabetes mellitus (NIDDM), also called Type II diabetes.

In 1997, the American Diabetes Association developed a new classification system based on the cause, or etiology, not insulin use. The new system now has four diabetes groups.

1. *Type 1 diabetes:* This type has two categories.
   - *Type 1 immune-mediated:* Individuals in this group have beta-cell destruction (and thus no insulin production) due to an autoimmune response to a viral or environmental stimulus.
   - *Type 1 idiopathic:* Individuals in this group have no evidence of an autoimmune process.

2. *Type 2 diabetes:* In this group are individuals with some insulin production by the pancreas, but the amount is not sufficient to maintain normal blood glucose levels. In addition, insulin receptors on cell surfaces are resistant to letting what insulin is available into the cells for use. Increased glucose production by the liver may also be a factor here as well. Note the change from Roman numerals to Arabic numerals (old Type I and Type II, and new Type 1 and Type 2).

3. *Other specific types:* This category includes individuals whose diabetes is due to such etiologies as drugs or chemicals, genetic defects, pancreatic disease, and pathologies of other endocrine glands that stress the pancreas.

4. *Gestational diabetes:* Diabetes that develops during pregnancy.

As you study this new classification system, it may seem to be the same as the recent Type I and Type II system. As a matter of fact, you may find certain medical professionals still using the old terminology. To help you understand how it is different from the IDDM and NIDDM classification system, we will look at a clinical situation. You are talking to your clinical instructor about your patient who is a Type II diabetic. You proudly tell your instructor that the patient has received her morning dose of long-acting insulin. Your instructor looks at you with a puzzled look and asks, "If she is a Type II diabetic, why is she receiving insulin?" Up to now, this was confusing. Although we know that over time many individuals who have Type II diabetes need exogenous insulin to maintain blood sugar levels, these patients were never reclassified as Type I diabetics.

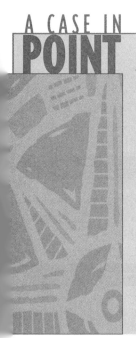

A CASE IN POINT

Mrs. Jones, age 47, has been diagnosed with Type 1 diabetes. She had been noticing excessive thirst, urination, and hunger, and has been rapidly losing weight. When the physician told her that she had Type 1 diabetes and needed insulin, she simply said "Okay." However, when the physician left the room, Mrs. Jones turned to the nurse and cried. She wanted to know what the doctor meant when he said "Type 1." The nurse wondered just where she should begin. What should she explain to Mrs. Jones? Should she lecture her on the 4 types, listing their differences? What did this patient really want to know? The nurse decided to explain to Mrs. Jones that some diabetics needed insulin and some did not. She had the type of diabetes, the nurse explained, that required treatment with insulin.

Because the new terminology is based on the causes for the changes in the pancreas and the insulin receptor sites, it should make understanding this patient easier. This patient would initially be in the new classification system as a Type 2 diabetic. (In the old system she would fit the profile of Type II.) However, as her metabolic needs change, insulin may be added to her health care regime without confusion as to what type she is. The etiology of her condition has not changed; therefore, her classification has not changed. The patient remains a Type 2 diabetic who requires insulin.

This new classification system is the system used in all of the newer texts and journal articles. Realize that if you are reading about diabetes, and the reference is to adult-onset or juvenile-onset diabetes or Type I and Type II, you are reading old material. Textbooks with a copyright of 1999 and later should have the new classification system in use.

In addition to using the most current classification, nurses also need to consistently update their knowledge of the new types of insulin and glucose monitoring equipment continually being introduced on the market. Patients will not only have questions concerning every aspect of their disease, but they will also have questions regarding new products that you need to be able to answer in an informed manner.

 ASK YOURSELF ──────────────────────────────

1. Do you think you could explain the new classification system to another student? If so, what would the key points be? If not, what steps could you take to better understand these concepts?

   _____

   _____

2. What meaning, if any, do you think the diabetic classifications have for patients with diabetes?

   _____

   _____

 CYBERLINKS: FLASH CARDS ──────────────────

Check to see what you now remember by making your own flash cards. Use the CD-ROM that accompanies your textbook to discover how to make flash cards for reviewing and retaining what you have learned.

 CONCEPT MAP WORD BANK ──────────────────

ENDOCRINE SYSTEM
Structure and function

Malfunction
Hypo/Hyperthyroidism
Diabetes
DIABETES CLASSIFICATION

Refer to Concept Maps and Flash Cards on pages viii–ix for an explanation of how to create and use concept maps. In addition, the CD-ROM guides you through the construction of concept maps by providing a more detailed introduction, more illustrations of examples and key steps to follow in designing your own maps.

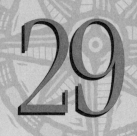

Highlights of Fluids, Electrolytes, and IV Infusions

 ASK YOURSELF

1. What are fluids and electrolytes in the body?

   _____

   _____

2. Do you think that it is essential for you to have a good understanding of the role of fluids and electrolytes in the body? Why or why not?

   _____

   _____

 CYBERLINKS

Interactive **www.family.georgetown.edu** can help you to better understand the importance and nuances of IV fluids.

Supplemental **www.LPNresources.com** can help enhance your learning by leading you to discover other links with even more information about the topic you are studying.

Homeostasis is the term that refers to a state of stability and balance in the body, which must remain constant, despite external environmental factors, in order for the body to function normally. Among the many factors contributing to normal homeostasis of the body are fluid and electrolytes (F/E). This chapter has been divided into three parts each representing core concepts: the basics of fluid balance, the basics of electrolyte balance; and the basics of IV infusions and complications associated with IV therapy. Understanding these somewhat complex concepts is linked to our understanding of such common conditions that are a consequence of imbalance such as ascites, and edema.

CORE CONCEPTS	THE BASICS OF FLUID BALANCE

Water is more necessary to life than food. It is a necessary component of all the fluids in the body as well as being ever-present in most cells. A person's total body water content depends on sex, age, and percentage of body fat. The following percentages of water versus total body weight are averages:

1. Adult male: 60%
2. Adult female: 50%
3. Infant: 70%
4. Newborn: 80%
5. Premature newborn: 90%
6. Elderly (over age 60): fluctuates between 40% and 50%
7. Obese adult: 45%

At times, the newborn will seem like more than 80% water! However, newborns are more prone to fluid imbalances, because they cannot concentrate their urine until at least 3 months of age. Also, the majority of the water of an infant is located in the extracellular fluid compartment (within the vascular system and between cells), so infants are more prone to rapid fluid loss and dehydration than adults. Obese adults are prone to fluid imbalances as well, since fat is essentially water free, which gives them less total water weight than other adults.

Water Compartments   The body has two main fluid compartments (see Figure 29-1).

1. **Intracellular** fluid compartment is the largest compartment; two thirds of the individual's total water volume is in this compartment in an adult.
2. **Extracellular** fluid compartment is the compartment located outside of the cells; one third of the total water volume is in this compartment. This is further divided into:
   • **Intravascular** fluid compartment (located within the blood vessels)
   • **Interstitial** fluid compartment (located between the cells)
3. **Transcellular** fluids are located within the cerebrospinal column, synovial spaces of the joints, within the eyeballs, and within the pleural and abdominal cavities. They do not experience the same fluctuations as the other types of fluids.

Water Movement   Fluid and electrolyte balance within and between these fluid compartments is controlled by many mechanisms. One of the primary control systems is osmosis (Figure 29-2). Three facts associated with osmosis are:

• Osmosis requires a membrane with holes that are big enough to let some particles (solutes) through but not others, thus the term *semipermeable membrane;* cell walls are semipermeable membranes.

Figure 29-1 Major Fluid Compartments

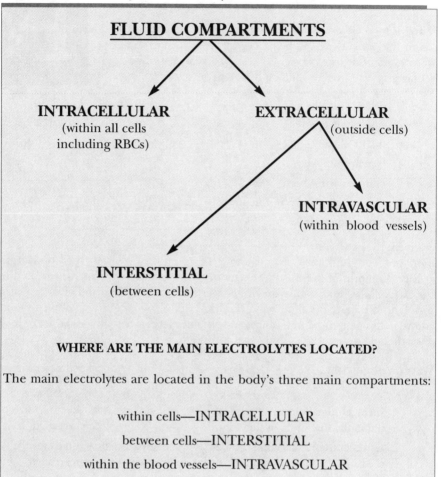

FLUID COMPARTMENTS

INTRACELLULAR
(within all cells
including RBCs)

EXTRACELLULAR
(outside cells)

INTRAVASCULAR
(within blood vessels)

INTERSTITIAL
(between cells)

WHERE ARE THE MAIN ELECTROLYTES LOCATED?

The main electrolytes are located in the body's three main compartments:

within cells—INTRACELLULAR

between cells—INTERSTITIAL

within the blood vessels—INTRAVASCULAR

- In osmosis, it is the water or solvent (what the particles are dissolved in) that moves.
- The water moves through the semipermeable membrane (cell walls) to the compartment with the most particles and solutes; thus, the water moves from an area of lesser concentration to an area of greater concentration.

CORE CONCEPTS | **FLUID IMBALANCES**

There are two basic types of fluid imbalances:

1. Fluid volume excess, or hypervolemia (high volume); also called fluid overload
2. Fluid volume deficit, or hypovolemia (low volume); also called dehydration

Figure 29-2 Moses/Osmosis/Water

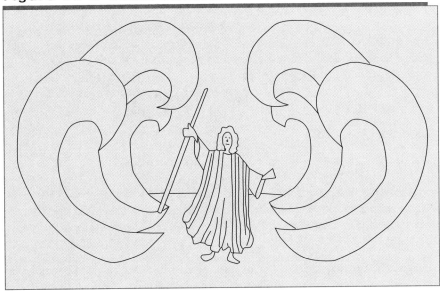

In fluid volume excess, patients have more fluids in their body than the body can effectively handle. This may occur due to some disease conditions such as congestive heart failure or renal disease, or it can be due to excessive fluid intake without adequate fluid excretion. The latter can occur with too many IV fluids. ***Note:*** Any patient receiving intravenous fluids is subject to fluid volume excess, so be alert!

Fluid volume deficit is usually a problem with both deficit of fluids and electrolytes, which will be discussed later in this chapter. This can occur either with inadequate fluid intake or with excessive fluid loss such as might occur with vomiting or diarrhea. You will see more elderly having a medical diagnosis of dehydration than any other fluid and electrolyte imbalance. A lot of that is related to the fact that the elderly do not experience thirst as younger people do and have an inadequate fluid intake. Children and infants are more likely to become dehydrated due to vomiting and diarrhea.

Regardless of which fluid imbalance you are dealing with, an accurate intake and output record will be an essential part of your care.

CORE CONCEPTS THE BASICS OF ELECTROLYTE BALANCE

Electrolytes are a specific group of chemical compounds that separate into **ions** (atoms with an electrical charge) when placed in solution. Ions that carry a positive charge are **cations,** while those that carry a negative charge are called **anions.** The electric charge is necessary for cellular function to occur. The electrolytes are also needed to regulate the movement of water between the fluid compartments. Figure 29-3 illustrates the four most common cations and anions in the human body.

Figure 29-3 The Body's Main Electrolytes

CATIONS	ANIONS
+ CHARGE	– CHARGE
SODIUM ------- Na^+	CHLORIDE ------- Cl^-
POTASSIUM ----- K^+	PHOSPHORUS----- PO_4
CALCIUM ------- Ca^{2+}	BICARBONATE --- HCO_3
MAGNESIUM ---- Mg^{2+}	SULFATE --------- SO_4

Potassium is the major electrolyte of intracellular fluid; sodium is the major electrolyte of the extracellular fluid. Note the concentrations of the electrolytes in each fluid compartment in Figure 29-4.

Measurement and Regulation In the healthy individual, the number of cations equals the number of anions. Electrolytes are often hooked up with a companion (e.g., sodium chloride [NaCl] and magnesium sulfate [$MgSO_4$]). Electrolytes are measured in milliequivalents per liter (mEq/L). A milliequivalent is different than a milligram. Milligrams and milliequivalents are designated dosage measurements. However, milliequivalent is a measure of power; a milligram is a measure of weight. Fluid and electrolyte *balance* is primarily maintained by actions of the kidneys. However, other regulating mechanisms include the antidiuretic hormone (ADH), atrial natriuretic hormone (ANH), renin, angiotensin, aldosterone, and the parathyroid hormone (PTH). When one or more of these regulating mechanisms cannot keep up or malfunctions, indications of fluid and electrolyte imbalance will occur.

Movement There are other factors that cause electrolyte shift. Three of the most common factors are (1) diffusion, (2) active transport, and (3) hydrostatic pressure. Although these are covered in anatomy and physiology texts, here are their basic definitions.

- **Diffusion:** The movement of ions and molecules from areas of high concentration toward areas of low concentration. This is a passive action.
- **Active transport:** The movement of ions and molecules from areas of low concentration to areas of higher concentration. This is not a passive movement; it requires energy. The sodium/potassium pump found within the body is an example of the use of active transport.

Figure 29-4 Location of Major Electrolytes per Fluid Compartment

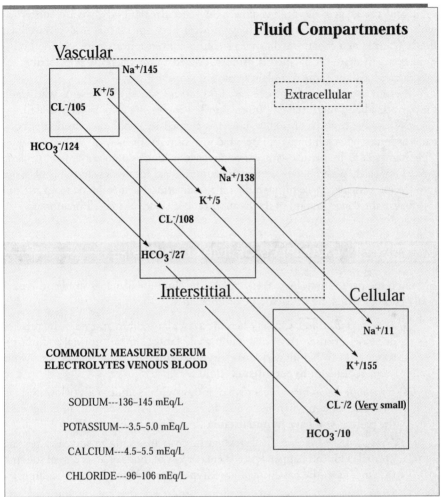

- **Hydrostatic pressure:** The pressure that results when a fluid is in a confining space. It is a "pushing-type" pressure. Capillary blood pressure is a type of hydrostatic pressure.

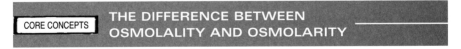

CORE CONCEPTS

THE DIFFERENCE BETWEEN OSMOLALITY AND OSMOLARITY

The concentration of electrolytes and other body substances such as glucose, plasma proteins, and urea create in plasma the phenomenon of **osmolality.** The osmolality of plasma is a measure of its pulling or drawing power on water. The greater the amount of glucose, proteins, and urea in plasma, the higher the serum osmolality value and the greater the pulling power on water. In the body, we are concerned with the solute concentrations (pulling power) between plasma and intracellular fluid. The main mechanism that keeps solute concentrations between the body's fluid compartments in balance is osmosis. When fluids on both sides of the cell membrane have the same osmolality, osmosis stops.

Serum osmolality will be decreased (< 280 mOsm/kg) in patients who are in fluid overload and increased (> 300 mOsm/kg) is patients who are dehydrated.

When the concept of pulling power is applied to a solution outside the body (such as intravenous solutions), it is referred to as osmolarity. As with plasma, solutions with high solute to particle concentration have a high osomolarity value (pulling power) on water. When these solutions are administered intravenously, they pull water into the intravascular space through the cell's semipermeable membrane in an attempt to equalize the concentration of the particles on both sides of the cell membrane.

CORE CONCEPTS | **EXAMPLES OF IMBALANCES**

Although the pathophysiology of electrolyte and fluid imbalance is similar, there are many etiologies that create each type of imbalance.

- *Isotonic imbalances:* Occur when intravascular sodium and water increase or decrease together, thus, maintaining the (approximate) normal sodium-to-water ratio. When they decrease, **hypovolemia** (dehydration) occurs; while increase leads to **hypervolemia** (fluid overload).
- *Hypotonic imbalances:* Occur when intravascular sodium falls below normal. This can happen when there is fluid excess or loss of sodium. In either case, the patient will have **hyponatremia** (low serum sodium).
- *Hypertonic imbalances:* Occur when intravascular sodium increases beyond normal. This can happen when there is a loss of fluids or an excess of sodium. In either case, the patient will have **hypernatremia** (high serum sodium).
- *Drowning:* The effects of aspirating water will depend on the type and amount of fluid aspirated. Salt water is hypertonic compared to the body. When aspirated into the lungs, it will draw fluid into the alveoli, creating pulmonary edema, hypoxemia (low blood oxygen), hypovolemia (low blood volume), and hemoconcentration (or thickened blood). Salt water drowning can also cause **hypernatremia.** Fresh water is hypotonic compared to the body. When aspirated into the lungs, it is absorbed into the bloodstream, creating hemodilution (thin blood), hypervolemia (fluid overload), and hemolysis (destruction of red blood cell membranes).
- *Edema:* Abnormal shift of fluid into interstitial space. Four common causes of edema are osmotic pressure (an overload with hypotonic intravenous fluids); poor lymphatic drainage; increased capillary permeability (as occurs with inflammation, burn trauma, and hypersensitivity reactions); and hypopro-

teinemia, in which plasma proteins create **colloid osmotic pressure** or **oncotic pressure,** which acts like a magnet that keeps fluid in the intravascular space. In hypoproteinemia, plasma proteins are low, pulling power is decreased, and fluid escapes into interstitial space. This is often the basis for edema seen in such conditions as malnutrition, cirrhosis, congestive heart failure, and kidney disease.

· *Third spacing:* An accumulation of abnormal amounts of fluid in body spaces, where it is, in essence, trapped. Since it got there due to malfunction in fluid and electrolyte (F/E) regulation, mechanisms for returning it to normal fluid spaces are also severely hindered. Third spacing can occur in many body areas such as the peritoneal cavity **(ascites),** in intestines proximal to a bowel obstruction, and burns. Third spacing may also be seen within 24 to 48 hours postoperatively, since tissue injury during surgery increases capillary permeability. However, within 48 to 72 hours postoperatively, the fluid may start to move back into the intravascular space. If the patient is also receiving IV fluids, the movement of fluids back into the circulatory system could put the patient into fluid overload!

Table 29-1 is a quick reference for common fluid and electrolyte imbalances.

| CORE CONCEPTS | **THE BASICS OF INTRAVENOUS INFUSIONS** |

Whether or not your state allows practical/vocational nursing students to participate in intravenous fluid therapy, you will be caring for patients receiving IV fluids, and you need to be aware of the types of IV fluids and their effects on your patients.

TABLE 29-1	Quick Reference for Six Common Electrolyte Imbalances

Imbalance	Common Etiologies	Common Assessment Findings
Hypovolemia	Excess IV blood loss, vomiting, diarrhea, excessive sweating, third-space shifting, diabetic ketoacidosis	• Thirst • Tachycardia • Decreasing urinary output • Decreasing mental status • If not identified early may eventually lead to elevated Na, BUN
Hypervolemia	Excess oral fluid intake, renal failure, cirrhosis, fluid shifts following burns	• Tachypnea • Dyspnea • Edema • Weight gain • If not identified early may lead to low hemoglobin and hematocrit, blood urea nitrogen, and sodium levels

TABLE 29-1	Quick Reference for Six Common Electrolyte Imbalances (Continued)

Imbalance	Common Etiologies	Common Assessment Findings
Hyponatremia Serum sodium < 135 mEq/L Results in low serum osmolality	Excess water intake, vomiting, GI suctioning, diarrhea, excessive sweating, diabetic acidosis, renal failure, continuous IV infustion of D_5W	• Low-grade fever • Nausea • Abdominal cramps • Muscle twitching • If untreated and values continue to drop, can lead to changes in mental status as a result of the development of cerebral edema
Hypernatremia Serum sodium > 145 mEq/L Results in increased serum osmolality	Renal failure with decreased sodium excretion, overuse of IV saline solutions, large number of blood trans fusions, severe vomiting or diarrhea, congestive heart failure	• Thirst • Low-grade fever • Restlessness, agitation, weakness, and lethargy, especially when the patient is also hypovolemic • If untreated and sodium levels continue to rise, central nervous system changes will occur including coma and death
Hypokalemia[a] Serum potassium < 3.5 mEq/L Notify physician immediately if values fall near or below 2.5 mEq	Loop diuretics, vomiting, GI suctioning, large number of blood transfusions, severe vomiting or diarrhea, congestive heart failure	• Muscle weakness • Wear, irregular pulse • Anorexia, nausea, vomiting • If untreated and levels fall to critical, it can lead to cardiac and respiratory arrest
Hyperkalemia[a] Serum potassium > 5.3 mEq/L Notify physician immediately if values are near or > 7 mEq	Renal failure (oliguria or anuria), too rapid infusion of IV potassium, initial reaction to massive tissue damage (e.g., trauma, burns, sepsis), metabolic acidosis, receiving potassium-sparing diuretics	• Muscle weakness • Nausea • Abdominal cramping • Diarrhea • Electrocardiographic changes first as T wave abnormalities • If untreated and levels rise to critical, cardiac and respiratory arrest can occur

[a]A few essential notes about potassium:
1. Do not administer potassium IV push.
2. Usual maximum concentration for IV use is 40 mEq/1,000 mL.
3. Usual maximum IV flow rate is ≤ 20 mEq/hr.
4. Current serum potassium levels should be known prior to IV administration of potassium chloride.
5. When administering IV potassium, urinary output should be at least 60 mL/hr.
Many nursing errors have been made (some fatal) in the administration of intravenous potassium.

Groups   Intravenous fluids can be grouped into one of the three tonic groups. These groups are based on normal plasma osmolality of 280 to 300 mOsm/kg. Remember, however, the term for IV solutions is osmolarity. Intravenous solutions are grouped into three groups based on their osmolarity range as follows (osmolarity values can be found on the intravenous solution container).

1. Isotonic: 280–300
2. Hypotonic: Below 180
3. Hypertonic: Above 300

Types of Solutions   As you care for patients who have IVs, it becomes apparent that there are many kinds of solutions that are available and that can be ordered. These solutions can be placed into one of the following three basic groups; each group has a specific osmotic action.

- *Isotonic solution:* This solution has the same concentration of solutes to particles as in another solution. In the body, the comparison is between plasma and normal body cells. Thus, just enough fluid passes in and out of the cells to maintain equilibrium with plasma values, like two children who weigh the same on a teeter-totter. They move just enough to keep the board level. Plasma is 0.9% sodium chloride, or **normal saline (NS).** Cells surrounded by normal saline remain unchanged, like the balanced teeter-totter. Table 29-2 contains common isotonic intravenous solutions with therapeutic uses. There is essentially no change in cell shape or size.
- *Hypotonic solution:* This solution has fewer particles than the cells. When a hypotonic solution surrounds cells, fluid will move into the cells (they have

TABLE 29-2	Common Isotonic Solutions[a]
Solution[b]	**Common Therapeutic Uses**
Sodium chloride	• Fluid loss and rehydration • Hypernatremia • Metabolic alkalosis • Only fluid used with blood transfusions
5% Dextrose in water	• Hydration • Minimal calories
Lactated Ringer's[c]	• Hydration • Burns • Acute blood loss

[a]280–300 mOsm/L, expand the intravascular compartment only.
[b]These fluids, by remaining in the vascular space, can lead to fluid overload. Do careful assessments on patients with increased blood pressure and congestive heart failure.
[c]Has high potassium content. Question if ordered for a pateint with renal failure.

TABLE 29-3 Common Hypotonic Solutions[a]	
Solution[b]	**Common Therapeutic Uses**
0.45% NS (normal saline)	• Cellular hydration • Electrolyte replacement
2.5% D/W (dextrose in water)	• Hydration
5% D (dextrose) in 0.45% NS (normal saline)	• Hydration
Normosol M	• Hydration • Electrolyte replacement

[a]< 280 mOsm/L moves fluid out of intravascular space into intracellular and interstitial compartments.
[b]These fluids, by shifting fluid into cells, can lead to increased intracranial pressure. Use with caution in patients with cerebrovascular accident, head trauma, neurosurgery, as well as those at risk for third-space shifting.

the most particles) in an attempt to make the ratio of fluid to particles the same on both sides of the cell wall. The result is that the cells fill with additional water and swell. Table 29-3 contains common hypotonic intravenous solutions with therapeutic uses.

• *Hypertonic solution:* When this solution surrounds cells, it has more particles than the cells. Again, the key facts with osmosis indicate that fluid will now move out of the cells in an attempt to create concentration equilibrium. The effect on the cells? They shrink. Table 29-4 contains common hypertonic intravenous solutions with therapeutic uses.

TABLE 29-4 Common Hypertonic Solutions[a]	
Solution[b]	**Common Therapeutic Uses**
5% Dextrose in normal saline	• Hydration • Shock until plasma expanders are available
5% Dextrose in 0.45 normal saline	• Progressive treatment of diabetic ketoacidosis
5% Dextrose in lactated Ringer's	• Hydration
5% Dextrose in 0.33 normal saline	• Hydration
10% Dextrose in water	• To provide a small amount of nutritional glucose[c]

[a]> 300 mOsm/L, pull fluid from intracellular and interstitual spaces into the intravascular space.
[b]Because these solutions pull fluids into the vascular space they can lead to expanded intravascular volume. Do careful assessments on patients at risk for circulatory overload.
[c]Remember, it takes 50 g of glucose to create a 5% dextrose solution. Therefore, at 4 calories per gram, 1 liter (1,000 cc) of 5% dextrose provides only 200 calories and a 10% solution will yield only 400 calories. So the belief that an IV is providing the patient with nutrition is incorrect. IVs mainly provide fluid and, based on the solution, various electrolytes.

CORE CONCEPTS	**COMPLICATIONS OF IV THERAPY**

Infiltration occurs when the IV fluid flows into the surrounding tissues instead of into the vein. When this has occurred, the IV site will be cool to the touch, show signs of swelling, and be pale, and the patient will complain of pain or discomfort. This should be reported to the patient's primary nurse immediately. If you are allowed in your state, you may stop the infusion and elevate the extremity before reporting it. **Extravasation** is a much more severe type of infiltration and is caused by the leakage of irritating or damaging medications, such as chemotherapy agents, into the surrounding tissues. This can actually cause tissue necrosis, or tissue death.

- **Infection** may occur because we have penetrated the body's first line of defense, the skin. Signs of infection at the IV site could be redness, warmth, swelling, purulent drainage (pus), and patient complaint of pain. If the infection extends beyond the IV site, the patient may complain of fever and chills. Any evidence of infection needs to be reported immediately, and the policy of the facility followed.

- **Phlebitis** is an inflammation of the vein due to the irritating presence of a foreign object, the IV catheter. If a clot has formed in the area of the inflammation, it is called **thrombophlebitis,** but this is not as common a complication. Signs of phlebitis include pain, redness, warmth, and swelling at the IV site. There might also be a hardness in the vein and a red streak along the length of the vein. Report evidence of phlebitis immediately. Once again, if you are allowed in your state, stop the infusion until the IV

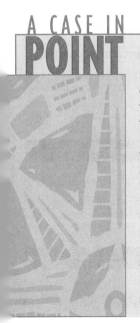

A CASE IN **POINT**

Mr. Ravi is receiving an IV. The nurse caring for Mr. Ravi notices that there is a large soft bump on his arm at the point of the IV needle insertion. Just as she is about to investigate further, the nurse's name is called over the intercom and she is needed in another patient's room. She forgets about Mr. Ravi for some time. In fact, about one hour later, Mr. Ravi rings his call bell. His arm is very painful. When the charge nurse looks at the patient's arm, she is very upset. She leaves the room to look for the nurse who is caring for Mr. Ravi. The charge nurse explains that Mr. Ravi's IV has infiltrated and that this situation requires immediate attention. The nurse learned an important lesson and Mr. Ravi's swollen arm is a sight that she will not forget.

can be removed. Warm soaks will usually be ordered for the site once the IV is discontinued.

- **Fluid overload** may occur. This is more often a problem with the elderly whose veins have lost their elasticity, so that they cannot expand enough to handle the IV fluids. When this occurs, you will note distended neck veins, an increase in blood pressure, and shortness of breath. If you auscultate, or listen to the lungs, you will hear moist breath sounds due to the accumulation of excess fluid in the lungs. If this occurs, notify the primary nurse. You may elevate the head of the bed and start oxygen based on the facility's oxygen protocol. Monitor the vital signs as well.

This chapter has provided basic information concerning interrelated topics: fluids, electrolytes, IV therapy, and the complications of IV therapy. The need to identify patients who are at risk for developing fluid and electrolyte imbalances is extremely important in nursing. Many fluid and electrolyte imbalances have been prevented due to the watchfulness of a knowledgeable nurse. In addition, the need for accurately recording intake and output, weights, and vital signs is extremely important and better understood from the perspective of fluid and electrolyte balance.

 ASK YOURSELF

1. Do you have a better understanding of fluid and electrolytes after reading this chapter? Why or why not?

   _____

   _____

2. Why do you need to be constantly alert for fluid imbalances in patients receiving IVs?

   _____

   _____

 CYBERLINKS: FLASH CARDS

Check to see what you now remember by making your own flash cards. Use the CD-ROM that accompanies your textbook to discover how to make flash cards for reviewing and retaining what you have learned.

 CONCEPT MAP WORD BANK

HOMEOSTASIS
Fluids

Electrolytes
F/E balance
F/E IMBALANCE
IV THERAPY
COMPLICATIONS

Refer to Concept Maps and Flash Cards on pages viii–ix for an explanation of how to create and use concept maps. In addition, the CD-ROM guides you through the construction of concept maps by providing a more detailed introduction, more illustrations of examples, and key steps to follow in designing your own maps.

30

Basics of ABGs

 ASK YOURSELF

1. What are arterial blood gases?

   _____

   _____

2. Do you think that understanding the essentials related to ABGs would be beneficial in helping you competently care for your patients? Why or why not?

   _____

   _____

 CYBERLINKS

Interactive Understanding laboratory results is a continuous challenge for health care professionals. However, at **www.thedoctorsdoctor.com** you can learn just what the normal and abnormal values mean.

Supplemental **www.LPNresources.com** can help enhance your learning by leading you to discover other links with more information about the topic you are studying.

Although arterial blood gases (ABGs) are more commonly ordered on patients in emergency departments and critical care units, they may also be ordered for patients in acute care units where you may be doing clinicals. Many think that ABG value knowledge is not within the scope of practice of the practical/vocational nursing student, but we feel that such knowledge gives you a more complete picture of your patient's health status. You need to be able to recognize any piece of data that is outside of the range of "normal." ABG values provide an objective assessment of arterial blood oxygenation, alveolar ventilation, and acid–base balance. In other words, ABG values will let you know how well your patients are taking in and using oxygen, how well they are getting rid of carbon dioxide, and how well they are balancing acids and bases within the body. In addition to identifying problems, the information is used to monitor the effectiveness of medical and nursing interventions.

CORE CONCEPTS ▮ **ABG BASICS** ────────────────

The core concepts related to ABGs are simplified here and presented in the format of question and answer in order to help you more easily walk through the essentials for understanding ABG results.

1. *What is pH?* This is a value scale used to indicate the acidity or alkalinity of a substance. It actually stands for "parts hydrogen" or "potential of hydrogen" (*Taber's Cyclopedic Medical Dictionary,* 18th Edition, p. 1457). A pH of 7.0 is given to a substance that is neither acid nor alkaline but is neutral. Any substance with a pH less than 7.0 is acid; any substance with a pH greater than 7.0 is alkaline. The more hydrogen ions a substance has, the lower the pH, the more acidic the substance. The fewer hydrogen ions a substance has, the higher the pH, the more alkaline the substance.

2. *Is there one pH for the body?* No. Various body tissues and fluids have their own pH value. For example, saliva has a pH range of 6.6 to 7.5, while urine's pH range is 4.6 to 8.0. However, the value that is crucial to health is pH of arterial blood. Normal arterial blood has a pH range of 7.35 to 7.45. This is a very narrow range, and values outside this range quickly lead to acute illness and if uncorrected, can be fatal. When someone speaks of a patient's pH value, the reference is being made to **arterial blood.**

3. *How does the body achieve this pH value?* The arterial pH depends on the relationship between carbonic acid and bicarbonate within the body. Carbonic acid is made from carbon dioxide (CO_2) combining with water (H_2O); bicarbonate is the most common alkaline substance in the body and comes from the breakdown of carbonic acid and other synthesis activities of the body. As long as there is a **1:20** ratio of carbonic acid to bicarbonate, arterial pH will remain within normal limits (WNL). You should remember some essential facts from chemistry.

   - H_2CO_3 = carbonic acid
   - Carbonic acid can break down into carbon dioxide and water and then go back to carbonic acid.
   - $H_2CO_3 \leftrightarrow CO_2 + H_2O$
   - HCO_3 = bicarbonate
   - Following are the basic combinations for carbon dioxide and bicarbonate (Figures 30-1 through 30-5).
     - Can you see where an imbalance could be due to either too much acid or too little bicarbonate? (Figures 30-2 and 30-3.) In either case, the scale is heavy on the CO_2 side.
     - Can you see where an imbalance could be due to either too much bicarbonate or too little acid? (Figures 30-4 and 30-5.) In either case, the scale is heavy on the HCO_3^- side.
     Note: Once the pH goes *over* 7.45, it is called *alkalosis;* once the pH goes *below* 7.35, it is called *acidosis.*

Figure 30-1 Normal Balance: 7.35 to 7.45; Ratio 1:20

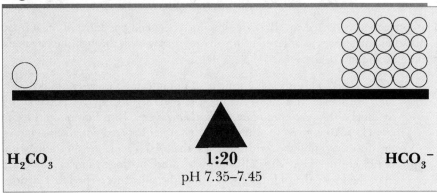

H_2CO_3 **1:20** HCO_3^-
pH 7.35–7.45

4. *How does the body maintain this delicate balance?* Two body organs accomplish the balance between carbonic acid and bicarbonate.
 • The **lungs** control the **carbonic acid** side of the ratio by controlling the body's level of carbon dioxide. (Recall the carbonic acid to carbon dioxide equation is question 3.)
 • The **kidneys** control the **bicarbonate** and H+ ion concentrations by various chemical reactions in the kidney tubules.

 The balance between these controls is reflected in the arterial blood gas values.

5. *What information is indicated in an ABG report?* An ABG report will have at least the following information:
 • **pH:** How acid or alkaline the arterial blood is.

Figure 30-2 Too Much Carbonic Acid: Acidosis

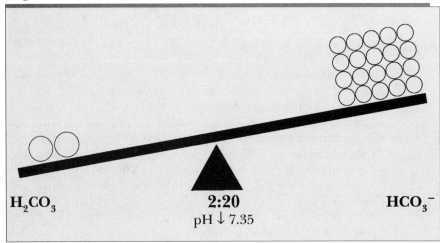

H_2CO_3 **2:20** HCO_3^-
pH ↓ 7.35

Figure 30-3 Too Little Bicarbonate: Acidosis

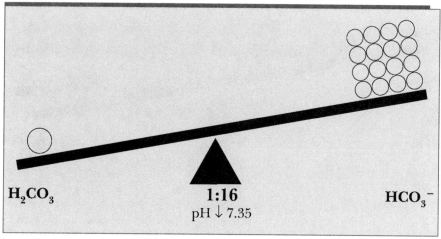

H_2CO_3 **1:16** HCO_3^-
                          pH ↓ 7.35

- **CO_2:** The pressure exerted by the carbon dioxide dissolved in the arterial blood (carbon dioxide tension). Note that carbonic acid is not directly measured. Instead, CO_2, its gaseous state, is measured.
- **HCO_3^-:** The amount of bicarbonate dissolved in the arterial blood.
- **O_2:** The pressure exerted by the oxygen that is dissolved in arterial blood (oxygen tension).
- **SaO_2:** Oxygen saturation, which represents the percentage of hemoglobin that is carrying oxygen.

The oxygen values (O_2 and SaO_2) are essential in evaluating how well the patient's body is being oxygenated. However, these values do not influence the pH value. The pH value is determined by the ratio of carbonic acid to bicarbonate.

Figure 30-4 Too Much Bicarbonate: Alkalosis

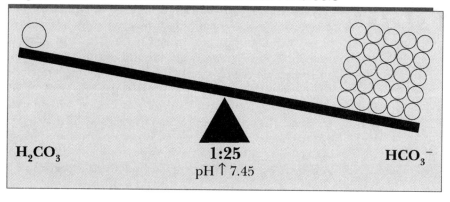

H_2CO_3 **1:25** HCO_3^-
                          pH ↑ 7.45

Figure 30-5 Too Little Carbonic Acid: Alkalosis

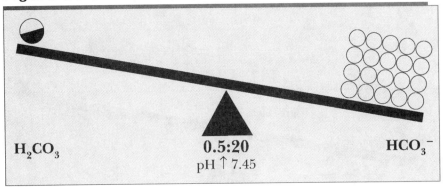

H_2CO_3 **0.5:20** HCO_3^-
pH ↑ 7.45

6. *What are the normal values for ABGs?*
   - pH: 7.35 to 7.45
   - CO_2: 35 to 45 mm Hg
   - HCO_3^-: 24 to 28 mEq/L
   - Remember that the CO_2 and HCO_3^- determine arterial pH. However, ABG reports also include two additional values that evaluate the patient's oxygen status.
   - O_2: 80 to 100 mm Hg
   - SaO_2: 95% to 100%

7. *How do I know if an abnormal pH is due to the lungs (respiratory) or to the kidneys (metabolic)?*
   - Check the pH value. Where is it in comparison to normal—alkaline or acid? Remember that anything below 7.35 is acidosis and anything above 7.45 is alkalosis.

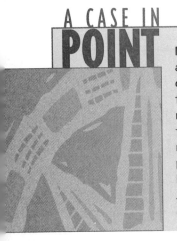

A CASE IN POINT

Nancy, a practical nurse, is assisting the RN with a patient in the intensive care unit. There is concern that the patient may be headed for kidney failure. The physician orders stat ABGs early that morning. The RN is called to another floor to perform a procedure. She instructs the practical nurse to call and get the results of the ABGs and phone the physician if they are abnormal. Fortunately for Nancy, she remembers what ABGs are. Now she must remember what the abnormals would be related to kidney failure.

- Check the CO_2 value. High CO_2 means more of the gas is available for conversion to carbonic acid. Low CO_2 indicates less carbon dioxide is available for conversion to carbonic acid. The CO_2 represents the lungs' side of the balance, **respiratory control.**
- Check the HCO_3^- value. A high value means a large amount of bicarbonate build-up, while a low value indicates bicarbonate loss. The HCO_3^- represents the kidneys' side of the balance, **metabolic control.**
- Determine which value (CO_2 or HCO_3^-) can create the patient's pH. If the CO_2 value is off, then the problem is respiratory; if the HCO_3 value is off, the problem is metabolic. If both values are off, check to see which one is the most off from normal. The value that is most outside of normal indicates whether the problem is more respiratory or more metabolic.
- Here are four examples of laboratory values to illustrate each of the main pH imbalances:

Example 1: pH = 7.31 CO_2 = 50 mm Hg HCO_3^- = 24 mEq/L
—Analysis: pH is less than 7.35, so the condition is acidosis.
            CO_2 is above 45 mm Hg.
            HCO_3^- is normal.

Conclusion: This is an example of **respiratory acidosis.** (*Note:* A pH of 7.31 could not be caused by a bicarbonate value that is within normal limits.)

Example 2: pH = 7.31 CO_2 = 44 mm Hg HCO_3^- = 20 mEq/L
—Analysis: pH is less than 7.35, so the condition is acidosis.
            CO_2 is normal.
            HCO_3^- is less than 24 mEq/L.

Conclusion: This is an example of **metabolic acidosis.** (*Note:* This is the same pH as the first example, but it is due to too little bicarbonate. Refer to Figure 30-3 if you need help visualizing this.)

Example 3: pH = 7.48 CO_2 = 33 mm Hg HCO_3^- = 24 mEq/L
—Analysis: pH is more than 7.45 so the condition is **alkalosis.**
            CO_2 is below 35 mm Hg.
            HCO_3^- is normal.

Conclusion: This is an example of **respiratory alkalosis.** (*Note:* A pH of 7.45 could not be caused by a bicarbonate value that is WNL.)

Example 4: pH = 7.48 CO_2 = 43 mm Hg HCO_3^- = 33 mEq/L
—Analysis: pH is more than 7.45 so the condition is **alkalosis.**
            CO_2 is normal.
            HCO_3^- is above 28 mEq/L.

Conclusion: This is an example of metabolic alkalosis. (*Note:* This is the same pH as the third example, but it is due to too much bicarbonate. Refer to Figure 30-4 if you have difficulty visualizing this.)

8. *Can I tell by looking at an ABG report if the body is attempting to get the pH back into balance?* Yes, but sometimes it is tricky. What you are asking about is called **compensation.** As one system goes out of balance, the other system kicks in to restore and maintain the all-important ratio of 1 part carbonic acid to 20 parts bicarbonate. Generally speaking, the chemical buffering system is activated within seconds of an imbalance. If that is unsuccessful, the respiratory system kicks in to correct the imbalance. The kidneys are the last system to kick in to correct the problem.

   When you look back at the four examples, you see imbalances without evidence that the body is attempting to regain the ratio. These are examples of **uncompensated** situations. The following is an example of a compensated situation.

   $$pH = 7.4 \quad CO_2 = 60 \text{ mm Hg} \quad HCO_3^- = 37 \text{ mEq/L}$$

   Note that the carbon dioxide and bicarbonate values are both abnormal, but the pH is WNL. In this case, the kidneys are retaining bicarbonate to counter the lungs' retention of carbon dioxide, thus keeping the 1 to 20 ratio and a pH that is WNL.

   Compensation can be full or partial. In **full compensation,** the pH is WNL but both carbon dioxide and bicarbonate are abnormal. In **partial compensation,** the pH is still abnormal as well as the carbon dioxide and/or the bicarbonate values. Remember, compensation takes time. Acid–base imbalances with a respiratory cause are generally corrected quicker than imbalances with a metabolic cause.

9. *What is base excess that I see on ABG reports?* **Base excess** (BE) is a value that indicates the sum of the body's buffer **anions**—that is, negative ions. Bicarbonate accounts for only about half of the body's anions. (Total buffer anions are in the range of 45 to 50 mEq/L, while total bicarbonate range is 24 to 28 mEq/L.) Therefore, base excess gives a better view of the **metabolic** side of the acid–base balance.

   Normal values for base excess are −3 to +3 mEq/L. Positive values, those above +3 mEq/L, indicate base excess. Negative values, those below −3 mEq/L, indicate base deficit. The following are two ABG examples that include BE values.

   Example: pH = 7.16 $\quad\quad$ $CO_2 = 57$ mm Hg
   $\quad\quad\quad\quad$ $HCO_3^- = 25$ mEq/L $\quad$ BE = +1

   Both the bicarbonate and BE values are WNL. This is a case of **respiratory acidosis** with no evidence that compensation has begun.

   Example: pH = 7.18 $\quad\quad$ $CO_2 = 41$ mm Hg
   $\quad\quad\quad\quad$ $HCO_3^- = 14$ mEq/L $\quad$ BE = −4

   The respiratory value (carbon dioxide) is WNL, while the bicarbonate is below normal. Note that the base excess is actually a deficit (−4). This value indicates that there is a true deficit of bicarbonate. This example is typical of one that might be seen in an individual with diabetic ketoacidosis. So this represents **metabolic acidosis** where, as yet, there is no compensation by the lungs.

10. *Can you determine the 1:20 ratio from the ABG values?* Yes, but you do not need to. The pH tells you about the CO_2 and HCO_3^- balance. Once the pH is beyond the norm in either direction, the 1:20 ratio has been lost. Although carbonic acid is seldom measured, its normal blood value is 3% of the carbon dioxide value, or 1.05 to 1.35 mEq/L. Remember that normal bicarbonate is 22 to 26 mEq/L. Using these normal ranges, the ratio of carbonic acid to bicarbonate can be calculated. However, although calculating the ratio is possible, it is not practical to do so.

As a student nurse, you should be alert for possible acid–base imbalances. Table 30-1 provides an overview of each of the four basic acid–base imbalances with common etiologies and assessment findings.

When the pH has a metabolic etiology, the pH values and the bicarbonate value go together; that is, high pH plus high HCO_3^- in metabolic alkalosis and low pH plus low HCO_3^- in metabolic acidosis. When the imbalance has a respiratory etiology, the pH value and the carbon dioxide values are opposite; that is, low pH and high CO_2 in respiratory acidosis and high pH and low CO_2 in respiratory alkalosis.

You should now have a solid foundation for understanding ABGs. The next time you look at ABG values, please refer to these guidelines to help you understand what mechanisms are taking place. With practice, the need to refer to this information will become less and less.

TABLE 30-1 | Four Basic Acid–Base Imbalances

Imbalance	Common Etiologies	Assessment Findings
Metabolic acidosis: pH less than 7.35, HCO_3^- will be ↓	Diabetic acidosis, shock, renal failure, intestinal fistulas, lactic buildup as in cardiac arrest	Apathy, disorientation, weakness, stupor, coma, Kussmaul's respiration
Metabolic alkalosis: pH more than 7.45, HCO_3^- will be ↑	Nasogastric (NG) drainage, prolonged vomiting	Shallow and slow respirations, lethargy, irritability, tetany, convulsions
Respiratory acidosis: pH less than 7.35, CO_2 will be ↑	Respiratory depression (drugs, CNS trauma, any condition leading to hypoventilation), COPD, pneumonia	Dyspnea, disorientation, tachycardia, arrhythmias
Respiratory alkalosis: pH more than 7.35, CO_2 will be ↓	Any situation leading to hyperventilation (emotions, pain, respirator overventilation)	Light-headedness, inability to concentrate, numbness and tingling, loss of consciousness

ASK YOURSELF —————————————————————————————

1. What concept(s) in this chapter were most difficult for you to understand?

   _____

   _____

2. Referring to the above question, and assuming you would like to better understand the concept(s), what steps will you take to improve your comprehension?

   _____

   _____

 CYBERLINKS: FLASH CARDS —————————————————————

Check to see what you now remember by making your own flash cards. Use the CD-ROM that accompanies your textbook to discover how to make flash cards for reviewing and retaining what you have learned.

CONCEPT MAP WORD BANK —————————————————————

ARTERIAL BLOOD GASES
Normal values
Abnormal values
Report

Refer to Concept Maps and Flash Cards on pages viii–ix for an explanation of how to create and use concept maps. In addition, the CD-ROM guides you through the construction of concept maps by providing a more detailed introduction, more illustrations of examples, and key steps to follow in designing your own maps.

Section V

MAPPING FOR YOUR CONTINUED SUCCESS

A. REQUIREMENTS OF PROFESSIONAL PRACTICE

B. ADVANCED SKILLS AND OPPORTUNITIES

31

Passing the NCLEX-PN

 ASK YOURSELF

1. What have you heard from other students about the exam? Has the information helped increase or decrease your concerns?

   _____

   _____

2. What do you think you can do for yourself in terms of thinking about the exam that will help you to feel comfortable and confident taking the exam?

   _____

   _____

 CYBERLINKS

Interactive www.nclex-rn.net provides study materials, forms, and links all of which you will want to investigate in preparation for taking the test.

Supplemental www.LPNresources.com can help enhance your learning by leading you to discover other links with more information about the topic you are studying.

If you are interested in reading this chapter, then it is safe to assume that you have been successful in completing or nearly completing nursing school. Congratulations! Now, you are ready for the first of many giant steps in your career. This first leap is a big one. You must successfully pass the National Council Licensure Examination for Practical/Vocational Nurses, called the NCLEX-PN, prepared by the National Council of State Boards of Nursing (NCSBN). This exam has been constructed to measure your knowledge and skills and the use of your critical thinking abilities in providing safe, effective nursing care to a diverse group of patients in a variety of health care settings within the role of the practical/vocational nurse. Whew! That is quite an exam.

As we mentioned in Chapter 3, Study and Test-Taking Skills, you should learn as much about an exam prior to the exam as you are able. This chapter hopes to familiarize you with both the process and the exam itself.

CORE CONCEPTS | APPLICATION

Close to the end of your school year, your instructor will provide you with the applications to qualify you for taking the NCLEX-PN. For most states, there will be two applications. One will go to the Board of Nursing of your state, and one will go to the testing agency currently having a contract with the NCSBN. Some states do not have applicants send applications to the testing agency directly; the state Board of Nursing will provide directions to those students. These applications are to be filled in completely and mailed with the necessary fees to the appropriate agency. The amount of those fees varies in each state. If you are planning to take the NCLEX in another state, be sure you let your instructors know ahead of time, so that they can provide the correct application for you or provide you with a list of addresses for other state Boards of Nursing. The director or coordinator of your nursing program will also be required to submit a list of qualified graduates to the Board of Nursing to validate that you have completed the approved course of study.

CORE CONCEPTS | AUTHORIZATION TO TEST AND WORK PERMITS

Upon receipt of your applications and validation of your graduation, you will receive notification of approval for you to sit for the NCLEX-PN exam. This is called an Authorization to Test and is valid for 60 days. You will make an appointment to take your board exam at that time. We caution students to take the exam as soon after graduation as possible. The sooner you take the exam, the greater are your chances for passing. Even the best students who wait 6 months to take the exam find that it is much more difficult to pass.

Around this same time, you will receive a work permit from your state's Board of Nursing. *You may not work as a graduate practical/vocational nurse until you receive this work permit!* There are some health care facilities so anxious for you to go to work that they may ask you to begin working as a graduate nurse prior to receiving a work permit number. Do not do this, or you jeopardize your chance of being allowed to take the examination. You may go to a general facility orientation and fill out new employee paperwork. You may also go to work as a *nursing assistant* in that facility pending the assignment of a work permit number, but you may not perform duties that are out of the scope of practice for a nursing assistant.

CORE CONCEPTS | DESCRIPTION OF THE EXAM

Remember that the NCLEX exam is designed to test your critical thinking abilities rather than having you regurgitate facts and figures you have learned in your nursing program. It is expected that you will be able to take your classroom knowledge and clinical experiences and apply them to common nursing situations, which will be described in your exam. The construction of the exam is based on the four aspects of the nursing process: data collection, planning, implementation, and evaluation. The writers of the exam have incorporated all of these steps in the nursing process to questions concerning:

- Safe, effective care environment
- Health promotion and maintenance
- Psychosocial integrity
- Physiological integrity

The exam is conducted on a computer. Hopefully, by the time you are ready to take your NCLEX, you have developed a comfort level with a computer. However, the testing center will give you time to become acquainted with the computers for the exam, and you will be given some practice questions before actually beginning. If you find you need assistance with the computer during the exam itself, the testing center staff will provide it. Beginning in 2001, the computers at the testing centers featured a pull-down calculator for students to use for questions requiring mathematical computations.

The NCLEX-PN is written as a series of multiple-choice questions. Each question will give you a description of a typical nursing situation with which a practical/vocational nurse might be faced. There are then four choices of responses for you to decide upon. One of these choices is the **best** answer. It could be that there is only one correct answer, and the others are distractors. However, there could be *more* than one right answer, but there is one *best* answer. This is where your critical thinking abilities will come in. Later in this chapter, we will give you some hints on deciding on the best choice.

The computer, as you are testing, will adjust to how well you answer the questions. This means that no two candidates are taking the same test. If you answer a question correctly, the computer will give you a more difficult question; on the other hand, if you answer a question incorrectly, the computer will give you an easier question. Passing or failing will depend on how you compare to the standards developed by the NCSBN as demonstrating competence in a newly graduated practical/vocational nurse. There will be a time limit of 5 hours in which to take the exam. You may receive a minimum of 85 questions or a maximum of 205 questions. If the computer cuts off at 85, you may have passed the exam very well or flunked it very badly. Many students come out of the exam not knowing which! We have also had students take the entire 205 questions and still pass the exam, so do not let it scare you if you were asked the maximum number of questions. By the way, if you do not pass the exam, you may test again in 91 days. You may test a maximum number of three times in 12 months if necessary. Hopefully, you are not going to need to test more than once.

ESSENTIAL SKILLS   PREPARATION FOR THE EXAM

There are many ways to prepare for the NCLEX exam. You just have to choose the one that is right for you. Most practical/vocational nursing schools will give a practice NCLEX exam prepared by a national testing company to give you an idea of your strengths and weaknesses prior to the actual exam. These are fairly reliable indicators of how you will do. Once the practice exam is given, the company will score the exams and return them to the school, giving you a composite exam score as well as a breakdown score for each individual category that will be covered on the actual NCLEX. In some of these exams, the company will actually give you page numbers in texts that will help you understand the rationales for the correct answers. Your instructor should have a copy of the key, so that you can see which questions you missed and why.

There are numerous NCLEX-PN review books on the market as well. Every major publisher of nursing textbooks produces one. Each one has a CD-ROM with at least 600 questions on it for you to practice for your NCLEX. Your school may even have practice disks at the school in the computer lab. Using other CD-ROM topic reviews that your school has available would also be advisable.

Many nursing programs will offer a review class following graduation to try to "pull it all together" for you. This might be a topic review plus practice test-taking sessions. Tell the instructor of the review class what you feel like the focus needs to be for you. Other students should do the same.

Set up a study schedule for yourself prior to the exam. You may want to meet with the study group you were in during the school year. Ask each other questions. Repetition is the key here. You may get tired of going over and over the same material, but you will find that this helps to take away some of your test anxiety. Create your own nursing situations, perhaps based on real incidents that happened to you throughout the school year, and write out questions to quiz others in your study group. Have them do the same. Think of how you handled a situation, how it

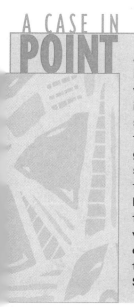

A CASE IN POINT

Jan had felt fairly well prepared weeks before taking the exam. She bought the exam prep books, went over her class notes and texts, and was feeling optimistic. However, days before the exam, she met some friends for drinks to celebrate the fact that she and some of her classmates had just gotten hired by the medical center pending licensure. She overdid it and was sick the day before the exam. Jan also didn't sleep well the night before the exam. The morning of the exam, she felt rushed and couldn't find the things she wanted to take, and hated what she had previously chosen to wear. By the time she got to the test site, she was very anxious and felt nauseous. She hadn't even had time for breakfast.

might have been handled, and how you would handle it differently if you had it to do over again. These types of exercises will stretch your critical thinking abilities.

Preparations for the exam also include being physically ready. Be prepared on the day of the exam, so you do not forget to bring anything. Eat a good breakfast, and dress comfortably. Be sure you leave early enough to allow for any kind of road or traffic delays. Be sure you have everything you need:

- Authorization to Test
- Two forms of ID. The primary ID must bear a picture and your signature; the secondary ID must have your signature.

You will **not** need a calculator or scratch paper. The calculator will be part of the computer program, and the test center will provide scratch paper if you think you need it. A photograph and thumbprint will be taken at the testing center. You will be monitored at all times during the exam, so do not bring anything with you or do anything that would lead anyone to believe you were cheating on the exam.

ESSENTIAL SKILLS TAKING THE EXAM

You might want to review the suggestions in Chapter 3 concerning multiple-choice exams. As with any exam, read the questions closely. Try to answer the question before even looking at the choices. Eliminate the obvious distractors before you begin. Do not read anything into or add anything into the question that is not there. There are no trick questions. They are straightforward. Use only the information that is given to decide on your course of action.

Learn to prioritize. If all of the responses to a situation are correct, how are you going to choose the *best* answer? Our students have told us that this is often the situation with the NCLEX. There are several ways to prioritize. First of all, remember your ABCs:

- Airway
- Breathing
- Circulation

Second, prioritize by reviewing Maslow's Hierarchy of Basic Human Needs:

- Physiological
- Safety and security
- Love and belonging
- Esteem
- Self-actualization

Third, remember the steps of the nursing process, and prioritize your actions by following them.

- Gather data and assess the situation.
- Plan your actions.
- Implement your plan.
- Evaluate the effectiveness of your plan.

If you have questions concerning psychosocial issues, there are two basic steps to follow:

- Validate the patient's feelings (e.g., "I can see you are feeling sad.")
- Try to get more information (e.g., "Tell me why you are feeling sad.")

If you do not honestly know the answer, then make an educated guess. Often, the correct answer will appear more general or be more flexible than the others. If you are still unsure (and this has nothing to do with nursing knowledge), choose an answer that is B or C or is the longest response.

Test Anxiety   Hopefully, you were able to work on this during the school year, but even the most fearless test taker is apt to feel some test anxiety when approaching the NCLEX-PN. Remember, positive self-talk will do wonders for you. You passed a whole year of nursing classes; you can pass the NCLEX! Take your "safe place" with you. Stop the exam if you need to, close your eyes, breathe slowly and deeply, and visualize that safe place. When you feel yourself relaxing, then return to the exam.

Exam Results   Each state will be different in how soon your exam results will be available to you. Many states will allow you to call a 900 number within 48 hours after the exam to receive your unofficial results. Your official results will probably not be available for another 2 weeks. Some states do not provide the results for a whole month, although your license number might be available on your state's Web site within 2 weeks. You will be mailed your license.

STOP   **ASK YOURSELF** ──────────────────────────────

1. After reading this chapter, do you have any new resolve regarding preparing for or taking the exam?

   _____

   _____

2. What psychological preparations will you make for the test? What kinds of things (e.g., prayer, meditation, exercise, breathing exercises, music) can you do in order to calm your concerns? What has worked well for you in the past in terms of decreasing your anxiety?

   _____

   _____

CYBERLINKS: FLASH CARDS ────────────

Check to see what you now remember by making your own flash cards. Use the CD-ROM that accompanies your textbook to discover how to make flash cards for reviewing and retaining what you have learned.

 CONCEPT MAP WORD BANK ────────────

NCLEX EXAM
Application
Test and work permits
Description
EXAM PREPARATION
EXAM RESULTS

Refer to Concept Maps and Flash Cards on pages viii–ix for an explanation of how to create and use concept maps. In addition, the CD-ROM guides you through the construction of concept maps by providing a more detailed introduction, more illustrations of examples, and key steps to follow in designing your own maps.

Job-Seeking Skills

32

ASK YOURSELF

1. What are your employment interests (fields of nursing and clinical settings)?

   _____

   _____

2. What concerns you more: writing a résumé or being interviewed? What is the reason for your response?

   _____

   _____

CYBERLINKS

Interactive www.ipl.org is the site to visit to explore health care employment resources. There are also Internet links at this site specially for job hunting with recruiters and networking opportunities. Go to the Reference Center, then to Health and Medical Sciences, scroll down to Healthcare Management and Policy Resources, and then scroll down to Healthcare Employment Resources.

Supplemental www.LPNresources.com can help enhance your learning by leading you to discover other links with even more information about the topic you are studying.

Another giant step you will take in your nursing career will be to find a job. You may actually begin scouting out the job market prior to graduation. With the current nursing shortage, employers are anxious to begin lining up new graduates to fill job vacancies. However, even though there is a nursing shortage, do not assume that you are guaranteed a job, especially in the locale you want, the specialty area you want, and the shift you want. You must still "sell yourself" to an employer. This chapter has been written to give you some ideas in researching facilities, writing résumés and cover letters, and interviewing techniques.

`CORE CONCEPTS`   **WHERE TO START**

As a new practical/vocational nurse, you may not yet have decided what area of nursing interests you the most. You are entering a field where there are many opportunities for a wide variety of experiences. Consider what health care facilities you liked most during your clinicals as well as which specialty areas within those facilities most appealed to you. Think about health care facilities where you have had no experience, perhaps those in a different location than where you went to school.

First, consider the health care facilities where you had your clinical experiences. What was your impression of the staff? Did you notice a lot of gossip and evidence of discontentment among current employees? If so, there is probably an undercurrent of staff dissatisfaction with management that might make it an uncomfortable place to work at this time. Did you feel welcomed by the staff, or did they treat you as if you were in the way? You can often get the feel of how staff will treat new employees by the way that they treat students. Did the nurses seem to be overworked? Did they get off on time? What was the nurse-to-patient ratio? If the nurses were complimentary of the facility and seemed happy in their surroundings, then this would probably be a good place to work.

If you are looking at facilities where you have had no experience, try to become familiar with them. Many facilities have Web sites with descriptions of their facilities. Of course, there is nothing that compares to actually visiting the facility and talking to current staff. Do your homework before considering a job application to a place that is unfamiliar.

What did you think of the patient care in the facilities where you were as a student? You can often tell a lot about a facility by asking yourself if you would like to be treated there or if you would feel comfortable if a loved one were admitted there. If you had a clinical there, then you probably know the type of care the patients received. That would be very difficult to assess in an unfamiliar facility.

Think about the areas where you had experience as a student. Did you like orthopedics, the newborn nursery, pediatrics, geriatrics, or the surgical suite within the hospital? Did you like the Alzheimer's unit within the long-term care facility? Did you feel most at home in the day care center or making home health visits? Was the dialysis center a good fit for you? Did you enjoy the patient contact within the physician's office? These will all give you clues as to where you might like to work. However, do not rule out anything just because you might have had an unpleasant experience there as a student. It might be entirely different as a graduate nurse. Also, think of your overall goals for yourself as a nurse. What kinds of experiences will contribute to your achieving these goals?

Currently, there are numerous Web sites of job opportunities for practical/vocational nurses. Some of these sites will be listed at the end of this chapter. Research these to see what looks appealing to you. Many Internet sites also give you ideas on writing résumés and cover letters, tips on interviewing and even places to submit your résumé online.

| ESSENTIAL SKILLS | **WRITING A RÉSUMÉ** |

A résumé is a way of introducing yourself on paper. It is a summary of what you will bring to a job, both from an educational standpoint and from an experience standpoint. This may be the first impression that a prospective employer has of you.

Format   Most books on writing résumés suggest that it be printed on white or off-white paper. Beige, ivory, or gray have also been suggested as being appropriate. Pink, lavender, green, and blue are definitely out! Use a clean font that is easy to read. Times New Roman is one of the fonts that would be appropriate. Impact might be used for your name, address, and telephone number at the top of the page or for your headings. Some computer programs have a résumé task wizard as part of the word processing program, with fonts already incorporated into the program. Have at least one-inch margins.

For a new graduate, a one-page résumé is sufficient. An exception to that would be if you had a lot of health care experience in another field, such as respiratory therapy. Then you would want to include that experience as well in your résumé. A résumé should never be longer than two pages. There should be no smudges or white-out used. *Check your spelling and grammar carefully! Proofread, and then have someone else proofread!* Figure 32-1 gives an example of a résumé of a new graduate.

1. *Name, address, and telephone number* should be prominently displayed at the top of the page.
2. Your *career objective* should come next. This should not be specific to a particular job, but should be a broad goal statement that would apply to a variety of health care settings.
3. *Educational background* may be next. Start with your most recent school. Give the name of the school, its location, the dates you attended, and what degree or certificate you achieved.
4. *Employment history or work experience* may follow. Once again, start with the most recent work experience. For each position, list your employer and their address; include your job title and the dates worked. If your job title does not adequately explain your duties, then briefly tell what you did. Do not hesitate to write down experiences that are not health related. A person who has been a waitress has had to deal with similar problems that nurses have had to deal with! Do not go back more than 5 years unless you have no recent job experience. If you have had no recent job experience, you might want to mention why (e.g., "have gone back to school full-time" or "have been a full-time mother for the past five years"). Volunteer experiences could go here, too, in lieu of work experience if you have none.
5. If you received any *awards* in school or any *on-the-job recognition,* place these under a category entitled "Awards" or "Recognition" or "Achievements." You decide what to call it.

Figure 32-1 Résumé of a Recent Graduate

MARY SMITH, LPN
1540 CENTURY LANE
DURANGO, CO 81301
970-000-0000

CAREER OBJECTIVE: To obtain a beginning LPN position in a long-term care nursing facility where quality patient care is a priority, and educational opportunities for nursing staff is promoted and encouraged.

EDUCATION:

2000–2001	Western Slope Community College Ignacio, CO Certificate of Practical Nursing
4/00–5/00	Western Slope Community College Ignacio, CO Certificate of completion of Nurses' Aide Training Program/CPR

EMPLOYMENT:

5/00–present	Certified Nursing Assistant Western Slope Health Care Center Ignacio, CO Provided direct personal care for debilitated elderly residents; assisted with activities of daily living for these residents
12/98–4/00	Dietary Aide Western Slope Health Care Center Ignacio, CO Assisted with food preparation and served meals to elderly residents

AWARDS:

January 2001:	Merit scholarship for second semester in recognition of a 4.0 GPA
August 2000:	Employee of the Month at Western Slope Health Care Center

VOLUNTEER WORK:

12/98–present: Rape Crisis intervention team

STRENGTHS:

Speak English, Spanish, and Navajo
Great people skills
Computer literate
Organized and work well under pressure

REFERENCES AVAILABLE UPON REQUEST

6. If you are a member of any *professional organizations,* you might want to include these as well. As a student, you were eligible to join the National League of Nursing or the state chapter of the National Federation of Licensed Practical Nurses.

7. *Special talents* are not necessary to include but may enhance your résumé. These would be things like the ability to speak another language or to sign, computer literacy, people skills; or volunteer work you have done such as work in a soup kitchen, with a rape crisis team, in a homeless shelter, or in a nursing home.

8. Conclude with *references.* Do not include your reference letters with your résumé. Simply state "references available upon request." If you do list people as your references, be sure you get their permission first, and notify them when you have used their names.

Since you want your résumé to be as clear and concise as possible, there are certain pieces of information that are inappropriate to include. Do not list your age, marital status, number of children, your hobbies, and any other information that is not work related. You also do not want to include work experiences that are more than 5 years old except for the reasons stated above.

ESSENTIAL SKILLS　**WRITING A COVER LETTER** ────────────

A cover letter often accompanies your résumé. The purpose of the cover letter is to introduce you to the reader, state what position you are interested in and why, and state your availability for an interview. Although some graduates choose to send out a generic letter to a number of employers, a better response is received by individualizing your letter for a specific employer. Figure 32-2 gives an example of a cover letter.

Format　The cover letter is less formal than a résumé. It should be between one half and three fourths of a page and never more than one page in length. It should be simple, clear, and concise.

The letter usually begins with an introduction of who you are and what position you are interested in. You might mention how you heard about the job opening—from a colleague, in the newspaper, in a nursing journal, off the Internet, and so on.

The second paragraph is the time to discuss why you would be the perfect candidate for the position. If you did clinicals in that facility, state what you liked about it and why you would like a job there.

The concluding paragraph should request the opportunity for an interview, giving a time that you would be available.

Pointers　Try to get a specific name to address the letter to. Call the facility with the opening to get this information. Spell the name correctly, and use the person's correct title. You may be addressing the letter to a Director of Nursing or to someone in the human resources department. Find out who the appropriate person is. Sign in

Figure 32-2 Cover Letter Example

1540 Century Lane
Durango, CO 81301
August 6, 2001

Ms. Jennifer Jones, RN, BSN
Director of Nursing
Western Slope Health Care Center
Ignacio, CO 81301

Dear Ms. Jones:

I have been employed here at Western Slope Health Care Center since December of 1998 and have worked as both a dietary aide and a certified nursing assistant. As you know, I graduated from Western Slope Community College in May of this year with a practical nursing certificate. I recently passed the NCLEX-PN exam and now am fully licensed as an LPN. I understand that there is a medication nurse position opening up on the skilled care unit, and I would very much like to apply for that position.

As a CNA here, I have been very impressed by the quality of care and by the compassion of the nursing staff for the residents. I feel that I would be continuing that tradition by assuming the role of an LPN. I am already well acquainted with the staff and feel that I have an excellent rapport with them. Of course, I dearly love all of the residents I have helped care for over the years and would like to serve them better in a more professional capacity.

I will be available for an interview between August 13 and August 17. I will call you on Friday to see if any of these days would be convenient for you. Thank you for considering me for this position.

Sincerely,

Mary Smith, LPN

blue or black ink, and keep a copy for your files. *Proofread it before mailing! Make sure your spelling and grammar are correct!* If you have not heard from the employer, follow up your letter and résumé with a telephone call. When one of us was in nursing administration, often the first people we interviewed for a position were those who called regarding their letter and résumé. We knew that they were interested.

ESSENTIAL SKILLS   **THE INTERVIEW**

The interview is your chance to introduce yourself in person, but it is more than that. Look at the interview as having a twofold purpose. The employer may be determining whether or not you are the right person to fill the job opening, but you should also be determining whether or not this is a job you really want to have. Many times what looked good to you before you came loses its attraction as you proceed through the interview.

There are several ways to prepare for a job interview:

- Do some research on the employer. This will prepare you to ask intelligent questions during the interview. You might want to know about staff-to-patient ratios, internships, preceptorships, and orientation programs for new graduates, and educational opportunities.
- Read over your résumé, and see what questions you think the employer might ask based on what they read. Write out the questions, and have a friend ask them of you. You might write out answers, or see how you do by just "playing it by ear." Sample questions to consider are in Figure 32-3.
- Think about what you would be looking for if you were the one doing the hiring; then try to live up to your own expectations.

Interview Tips   When you are invited for an interview, you may be asked to fill out an application first. Be sure you have a copy of your résumé with you. It will certainly help in filling in those dates on the application, or the human resources office might let you just attach your résumé rather than filling in the blanks. Many employers have told us that they make a lot of judgments about the applicant based

Figure 32-3   Interview Questions to Practice

1. Tell me about yourself. A question like this is often asked. You may need to clarify, but most often the employer wants to know about your professional life, not your personal life.
2. Why are you interested in this position?
3. Why do you think you are qualified for this position?
4. What do you like the most about your current job? What do you like the least about your current job?
5. What do you consider to be your greatest strength? What is your greatest weakness?
6. Why did you enter the nursing profession? Why do you stay in nursing?
7. What are your professional goals?
8. How do you see this position as helping you achieve your professional goals?
9. Why should I hire you?

on how they filled out the application. A sloppily filled out application is a sure way to make a poor impression.

Dress neatly and appropriately. Employers are not impressed by prospective employees who show up in shorts and a T-shirt for a job interview. This could indicate a careless attitude. Males or females should wear something conservative—a happy medium between dressy and casual. This is a word to the wise—avoid cologne or after-shave. One of the authors remembers interviewing a nurse who wore so much cologne that it gave her a headache. She cut the interview short and had to open the window to air out the office for an hour afterwards!

Find out where you are going ahead of time, so you will not be late for the interview. Allow for traffic tie-ups and finding a parking space.

If you are a smoker, do not smoke in the car on the way to the interview. Being in a closed environment just makes the smoke smell more pronounced and may be as hard to take as an overabundance of cologne. Using breath mints or chewing gum prior to the interview might be advisable, but do not chew gum during the actual interview.

Greet the prospective employer with a firm handshake, and sit only after you are invited to do so. Make eye contact with the interviewer. Remember the tips from the chapter on communication. Look poised and confident. Ask questions with interest. However, do not start your questions by asking about salary and benefits; that should come up later in the interview. Answer questions clearly and honestly. This is one time to "toot your own horn" by stressing your strengths and what contributions you can make if hired for the position.

There are certain questions that a prospective employer should not ask you; this does not mean they will not ask you these questions. It will be up to you as to whether or not you answer them. Questions about your age, your marital status, whether or not you have children or plan to have children, your height and weight, your race, religion, and disabilities are not permitted. An employer may ask you if you have a disability or illness that would interfere with your performing the job safely and efficiently.

Often, you will be given a tour of the facility at the conclusion of the interview. Use this time to really be observant of the nursing staff and of patient care, especially if you have never been there before.

Sometimes, you will be offered a job on the spot; other times, the prospective employer will tell you they will call you. If you are offered a job, it is up to you whether or not you want to accept it at that time. If you have several job interviews set up, you may want to wait until you have completed all of the interviews before you make a decision. If you do not have other interviews, but you have doubts about the job, then tell the interviewer that you would like to think about it for a few days. If no decision is made before you leave, be sure to clarify expectations. If no job offer has been made, find out if the interviewer will call you or if you should call and when. If you are the one making the decision, tell the interviewer when he or she can expect your decision.

Writing a thank-you note after an interview is optional. Sometimes, people write letters if they were not chosen for a position to thank the interviewer for their time and to ask to be kept in mind if another position becomes available. A last impression may be just as important as a first impression when it comes to getting a job!

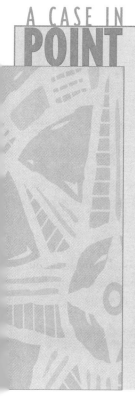

A CASE IN
POINT

Sue has an interview scheduled for a position as an LPN. She has 1 week to prepare. Sue is nervous because she really wants this job, and in the past when she has interviewed or talked to teachers one to one, she has often stumbled over her words and been jittery. She talks to one of her teachers about this. The teacher agrees to send Sue on two mock interviews with other teachers. The teacher will then give her feedback and help her to overcome any problems. Before sending Sue on the mock interviews, the teacher gives her suggestions about how to overcome stumbling on words and being jittery. She tells her to breathe evenly and be conscious of her breaths and to smile when appropriate when the interviewer is talking. The teacher also suggests that Sue hold onto a folder containing her résumé and any other materials so that she will know what to do with her hands and not be so jittery. Sue is grateful for the help and follows the instructions carefully. And happy ending—she gets the job.

ASK YOURSELF

1. Having read this chapter, have your concerns about résumé writing and interviewing diminished? If so, why? If not, why not?

_____

_____

2. What resolve have you formed regarding how to go about finding a job? What skills (résumé and interview) do you still need to improve? How will you do it?

_____

_____

 ## CYBERLINKS: FLASH CARDS

Check to see what you now remember by making your own flash cards. Use the CD-ROM that accompanies your textbook to discover how to make flash cards for reviewing and retaining what you have learned.

CONCEPT MAP WORD BANK ────────────────────

JOB-SEEKING SKILLS
Interests
Résumé
Cover letter
Interview

RÉSUMÉ
Things to do
Things not to do

INTERVIEW
Preparation
Tips

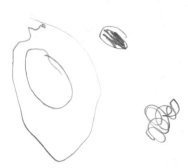

Refer to Concept Maps and Flash Cards on pages viii–ix for an explanation of how to create and use concept maps. In addition, the CD-ROM guides you through the construction of concept maps by providing a more detailed introduction, more illustrations of examples, and key steps to follow in designing your own maps.

 JOB SEARCH ON THE NET ────────────────────────

www.careerbuilder.com
www.emedjobs.com
www.healthcareersonline.com
www.hospitalhub.com
www.hotnursejobs.com
www.jobscience.com
www.medcareers.com
www.medhunters.com
www.nationjob.com
www.nurse-recruiter.com
www.nursingcenter.com
www.nursingspectrum.com
www.vitalcareers.com

Leadership/
Management Skills

33

 ASK YOURSELF

1. What does the term *leadership* mean to you? How do you think leadership differs from management?

   _____

   _____

2. What qualities do you think that a leader should possess?

   _____

   _____

 CYBERLINKS

Interactive **www.nursingworld.com** is a great stopping place to investigate what types of management opportunities exist for nurses. Links to interactive sites exploring leadership topics are also available at this site.

Supplemental **www.LPNresources.com** can help enhance your learning by leading you to discover other links with more information about the topic you are studying.

Another phase of your life beyond nursing school will be to continue to develop your leadership/management skills. Should a newly graduated practical/vocational nurse be expected to have these skills? Think about your nursing class. Did the class elect officers or a class representative to sit on your school's advisory committee? What was so special about the people elected? Students with leadership skills were already emerging even as you were in school. You probably noticed the students who seemed to be drawn to the leadership role in small group activities. Maybe you were one of them; maybe you were not. Think about the traits of the students that you thought of as leaders as you read this chapter. However, do not convince yourself that leaders are only born, not made. Almost everyone has the potential for being a leader or a manager or both. It may take a little longer for these traits to emerge in some people. These individuals need to be nurtured by other leaders and managers. They require more education and experience to build the self-confidence needed to assume the leadership role. This chapter will focus on the need to develop leadership skills, and will discuss leadership styles, challenges to a leader/manager, and styles of conflict management within the leadership role.

CORE CONCEPTS | **LEADER VERSUS MANAGER**

We have been using the term leadership/management together, but they are really different entities, even though they may work hand in hand. A leader may or may not be in the manager role. A manager may or may not be a leader. Think back over different organizations where you have worked. Do you remember leaders who were not managers and managers who were not leaders? A good analogy might be an architect versus a general contractor for a construction project. The architect has the vision for the structure. He or she is able to transfer that dream to paper and lay out a blueprint. The architect is the leader. But it will take a good general contractor to make sure that the structure becomes a reality. He (we will select one gender for the purpose of brevity) will be responsible for coordinating the efforts of many workers, the electricians, plumbers, framers, and the like. He will organize the project and make sure the materials are available and that the correct permits have been obtained. The general contractor is the manager. Periodically, the architect will come by and see the progress. He or she can say, "That's not what I intended" or "Yes, that's exactly the way I wanted it to look." He or she may make suggestions to the manager for changes, or together they might envision something that neither individually had been able to see. This is an example of leaders and managers working hand in hand to achieve a mutual goal. Sometimes, a general contractor may also draw up the house plans. In this way, he becomes a leader and a manager. He has the vision plus the organizational skills to get it done. Hopefully, this helps you visualize the difference between a leader and a manager and how those skills can become intertwined. When you have a manager who is also a leader, you have the best of both worlds. But we also need leaders who are not managers, who are visionaries and who can inspire and motivate the followers by being "down in the trenches" with them. A staff nurse might see a way that patient care could be improved and take her plan to the charge nurse who has the ability to make the changes. Leadership and management—we need both skills in health care.

CORE CONCEPTS | **NEED TO DEVELOP LEADERSHIP SKILLS**

There is still controversy within the nursing profession regarding the placement of LPN/LVNs into leadership or management roles. Many states, such as Florida, feel that a management role is not within the scope of the LPN/LVN and will not allow LPN/LVNs to serve as charge nurses. In other states, LPN/LVNs are daily being asked to manage or lead. They are hired into manager positions such as charge nurse positions within long-term care facilities. They may be hired to supervise a group of home health aides within a home health agency or public health department.

They may be unit managers within a nursing home, supervising other LPN/LVNs. And, on a smaller scale, the LPN/LVN staff nurse is expected to "manage" her or his own patient load. This still requires management skills. The scope of management responsibilities should be defined in your state's nurse practice act. Be sure you are familiar with this act and the extent of managing you will be allowed to do. You should also know under whose authority you fall. Each facility you go to work in should have an organizational chart, which will show you visually where your role lies in the framework of the whole organization. Staff nurses are expected to contribute to the overall quality of patient care by making suggestions for improvement within the unit and working as a team member to achieve this mutual goal. This requires leadership skills. You do not have anything in a nurse practice act to define your role as a leader. It is an expectation in most nursing positions.

CORE CONCEPTS   LEADERSHIP STYLES

You should be familiar with leadership styles, both as a follower and as a leader. We have students spend a day observing charge nurses in a nursing home and then ask them to discuss the leadership style they saw, what made them decide that was the style used, how effective they thought the style was, and how the staff responded to that type of leadership style. After much discussion over the types of leadership styles and their effects on staff, we give the students the opportunity to be team leaders with a group of fellow students and see which style they adopt for their leadership role. Students learn a lot about themselves during this rotation. We have seen very shy, unsure-of-themselves students suddenly blossom into assertive, organized leaders willing to take charge and direct a group effectively.

There are four commonly accepted leadership styles:

1. *Autocratic* leaders make all of the decisions for the group. If you are a parent, you are probably familiar with this style. There are certain times when a child asks "Why?" that you are tempted to say or may actually say "Because I said so, that's why." This is an autocratic leader. They are very task oriented rather than people oriented. They want to get the job done, and they want it done their way. Although this type of leader is not a favorite among staff members, this is the type of leadership style you want to see in an emergency or crisis situation. They take control and direct the rest of the staff in their tasks. People who are new to a job and still unsure of their job responsibilities also appreciate this type of leadership style. The autocratic leader always lets you know where you stand. On the other hand, these leaders do not inspire a lot of loyalty among staff members, and it is difficult to make changes or institute new policies, because the staff has no say in the decision.

2. *Laissez-faire* leaders are on the other end of the spectrum. These leaders do not supervise or manage or give any kind of direction to the workers on their unit. The workers are basically in charge and decide what they will and will not do. Consequently, the work may or may not get done.

Although the goal of most laissez-faire leaders is to be well liked by their staff, they usually wind up being resented by a staff who would like some direction and encouragement. We have seen this type of charge nurse. Certified nursing assistants basically run the unit. They receive no guidance throughout the shift. They just "do their own thing," which does not necessarily mean that all of the work has been done. They rarely communicate with the charge nurse. As you can imagine, working for this style of leader would totally intimidate a new, inexperienced employee. Chaos might result if there are a lot of new employees. This leadership style certainly empowers experienced staff by making them autonomous, but teamwork may be lacking.

3. *Democratic* leaders run their units as democracies. They allow staff members to have input into the way the unit is run and the decisions that must be made. They know their staff and show appreciation for the qualities of each. This type of leadership encourages teamwork and loyalty to the organization. Staff members feel as if they have "ownership" of decisions and are more likely to comply with changes. This type of leadership is very time consuming, and staff needs to be willing to be available to be part of the group process. An obvious drawback to this style of leadership would be in an emergency or crisis situation where decisions must be made immediately, and there is no time for a group consensus.

4. *Multicratic leaders* are leaders who base their leadership style on the situation. They are usually a combination of autocratic and democratic. They are able to critically think, so that they know which leadership style to use at any given time, which will provide the best environment for both staff and patients. They may ask for input from staff with guidelines, but then issue the final decision based upon a thorough investigation of facts, feelings, and comments.

Some business leaders have identified and defined other types of leadership styles, but we think these are the primary styles you will see in health care. Read through these again, and identify which style you think you will use as a leader. Also, consider the one you would like to see being used on the unit where you might be working as a staff nurse.

CORE CONCEPTS CHALLENGES FOR THE CHARGE NURSE

Being in charge, or being a manager, will provide you with a sense of accomplishment as well as frustration. You will feel a sense of accomplishment when things are going smoothly; patient care is being provided in a caring, efficient way; staff is getting along well; attendance problems are at a minimum; there are no conflicts with management or other departments; and there are no new policies that need to be developed or implemented. How long do you think this ideal scenario will last? Frustrations are bound to develop when any of the above situations change. Duties include:

- Administrative:
  1. Hiring and firing of personnel
  2. Counseling personnel when there are problems
  3. Maintaining a close relationship with management to keep the lines of communication open
  4. Conducting regular staff meetings to keep the lines of communication open with your staff as well
  5. Writing and implementing new policies as the need arises
  6. Maintaining a good relationship with other departments
  7. Scheduling the staff for your unit
- Management of patient care:
  1. Assessing the needs of the unit for the day
  2. Organizing the assignments to accomplish the tasks to be done
  3. Making rounds on all patients
  4. Assisting staff nurses with daily routines
  5. Ensuring that equipment and supplies are available for staff to get the work done
  6. Motivating staff
  7. Communicating with physicians, other departments, and administration as the need arises

Of course, this is a limited list, as there is much more involved in the charge nurse position, but this will give you an idea of the breadth of duties with which you might be faced. Most job descriptions will also include an "other duties as assigned," which gives your employer a lot of leeway in what is expected of you. "It's not in my job description" is difficult to use as an excuse for not doing something when you have generic "duties"!

Motivation   An important part of your job will be to motivate your employees to do their job and to do it well. Employees need to be praised and often, both for exceptional jobs and for little things. The nursing assistant who spends extra time applying makeup to the residents should receive praise as much as the nursing assistant who suggests ways that the baths can be done more timely and efficiently. Another motivator for staff is to see you willing to work side by side with them. If all of your staff is busy, and a patient light comes on, then answer it. You will really earn respect from those you are supervising. Staff needs to also see that policies are followed to the letter and not just applied to some staff members. Showing favoritism is a poor motivator for other staff. Using disciplinary measures when they are called for indicate to staff that you are fair and objective. It is very disheartening to staff members when they see the same staff nurse drag in 15 minutes late every morning without anyone ever addressing the problem.

Discipline and Counseling   When a problem like the one mentioned above occurs, counseling and disciplinary action are in order. The cardinal rule here is that you *never* question or discipline an employee in front of other employees. Always seek a private place to investigate the problem. Employees need to know that you respect them as a person even though they are having a problem. Get to the source of the problem, point out the facility policy on the problem, and give the employee a correction plan. This usually involves telling them what they have to do and giving them a time frame in which it must be done. The correction plan should also state the consequence if the plan is not followed.

Encouraging Teamwork   The old saying "two heads are better than one" really applies in health care. Two bodies are better than one is also true. When you are a democratic or autocratic leader, you are naturally encouraging teamwork among your staff members. The work gets done much more quickly and efficiently when two people are working together. Praise all efforts at teamwork.

Time Management   When you are managing a unit, you must also manage your time. The key to managing time effectively and efficiently is to POP: prepare,

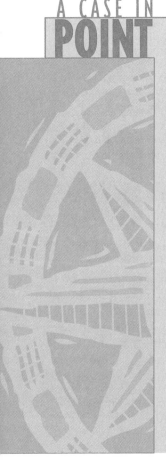

A CASE IN
POINT

Pat is the charge nurse on a skilled nursing unit in the nursing home. Pat arrived at 6:45 and is getting report for the day shift. Pat is given the following information: Mrs. Jones has a doctor's appointment at 8 A.M. and needs to eat breakfast early. Mr. Smith fell during the night. However, there are no apparent injuries according to the night nurse, but he doesn't want to get up this morning. Mrs. Brown is running a fever of 102 orally. The doctor and family have not been notified, since this is a new occurrence and just started at 6 A.M. She has no other symptoms. The lab technician is coming in at 7:30 for the monthly blood draw, but the list cannot be found. The CNAs Pat will be working with have come up to the desk during report and tell her that she needs to come look at the "mess" the previous shift left for them to clean up. There is a blood glucose test that needs to be done at 7:30 A.M. on a diabetic resident. Pat is supervising another LPN as the treatment nurse. She arrived late because she had a fight with her husband and has obviously been crying. The medication pass needs to begin by 8 A.M. At first, Pat is overwhelmed. She pauses a moment and remembers POP. She immediately begins to prioritize the day.

organize, and prioritize. Know what you can assign to others and what you must take care of yourself.

| CORE CONCEPTS | **CONFLICT RESOLUTION** |

It has been found that managers spend an equivalent of 1 month a year on solving conflicts among their staff. Conflicts are bound to arise, and there are some common methods of resolving them. Keep in mind that conflicts are not always bad things, and if handled appropriately, good things may emerge. We will briefly describe commonly accepted conflict management techniques and then give you a scenario of a conflict that might occur on your nursing unit.

Conflict Resolution Styles

1. In *avoidance,* the manager simply ignores the conflict and hopes that it will go away. In some instances, this may be true, but the conflict may return at some time in the future, because the root causes of it were never resolved.

2. The *authoritarian* style of conflict management is usually the one chosen by the autocratic leader. The manager simply states how things will be settled, and that's the way it is. There is no arguing about it. This style does work in certain instances, especially if it is viewed as a temporary measure because of the time factor involved. However, if the manager never gets back to the original issue for a more permanent solution, the conflict may arise again, because there was no discussion involved in the decision.

3. In the *accommodation* style, one party simply gives in to the other party involved. This may work when the outcome of the resolution is more important to one party than to the other one, and it is easier to give in than to argue about it. This is not really satisfactory when it is the same party giving in all of the time. Initiative and motivation may be lost.

4. In the *compromise* style, both parties give a little bit in order to reach a resolution to the conflict. This results in both parties kind of winning and may be a satisfactory way of settling the conflict.

5. The *collaborative* style is generally found to be the best of all conflict resolution styles. This will require patience and creativity on the part of the manager. It requires that the manager bring both parties together and gather all facts. Pros and cons of the issues are discussed and solutions brainstormed. The manager and conflicting parties then arrive at mutual conclusions and decisions.

This chapter has discussed some concepts about leadership and management. We hope this gives you some insight into the challenges you might face in a leadership

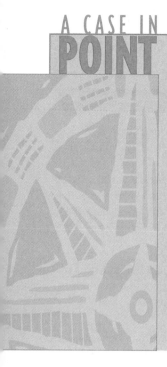

A CASE IN POINT

You are supervising a unit in a long-term care facility. One of your CNAs comes to you to complain that she is sure the CNA she is working with is abusing residents. She says she hears "funny noises" coming from the room where the other CNA is working. When you speak to the other CNA, she denies any problem and states the reporting CNA is just "out to get her" because of personal issues. They each want you to "do something" about the other CNA. Discuss the possible issues here. Decide what additional information you need to make a wise decision. Determine how you will obtain this information. List appropriate solutions and/or actions you might take based on your assessment of the situation. Which conflict resolution style or styles do you think would be the most appropriate and why?

or management role and also food for thought as to how you might handle some common problems.

 ASK YOURSELF

1. How would you prioritize the tasks listed in the case in point?

   _____

   _____

2. Do you think you need to improve your conflict resolution skills? Why or why not? Which skills would you target? How do you plan to make improvements?

   _____

   _____

 CYBERLINKS: FLASH CARDS

Check to see what you now remember by making your own flash cards. Use the CD-ROM that accompanies your textbook to discover how to make flash cards for reviewing and retaining what you have learned.

CONCEPT MAP WORD BANK

LEADERSHIP
MANAGEMENT
Definitions
IMPORTANCE TO NURSE
LEADERSHIP STYLES
CONFLICT RESOLUTION

Refer to Concept Maps and Flash Cards on pages viii–ix for an explanation of how to create and use concept maps. In addition, the CD-ROM guides you through the construction of concept maps by providing a more detailed introduction, more illustrations of examples, and key steps to follow in designing your own maps.

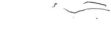

34

The Transition from Student to Graduate Nurse and Beyond

STOP ASK YOURSELF

1. How do you envision yourself professionally five years from graduation? What will you be doing? Where?

_____

_____

2. What will be most important to you in caring for patients?

_____

_____

CYBERLINKS

Interactive Education and career guidance, interactive features, and an online community for nursing students and graduates are available at this site: **www.topsitu.com/world/nursefriendly/topsitu.html**

Supplemental **www.LPNresources.com** can help enhance your learning by leading you to discover other links with more information about the topic you are studying.

Many decisions await the new graduate. There are numerous choices regarding which career path to follow, and more choices continue to emerge. It is important to seek guidance from the people and sources that you trust. But the choice of what to do, where to do it, and all the other related choices must ultimately come from your own reflections and self-examination—must come from within you.

CORE CONCEPTS CHOICES

- Remain an LPN/LVN and seek a position that will allow you to become more competent in your skills while providing quality nursing care for the patients entrusted to your care.

- Remain an LPN/LVN but seek additional education in a specialty area where you may become certified, such as in IV Therapy, and broaden the scope of your practice in patient care.
- Choose to continue your education by entering an ADN or BSN program with the goal of becoming an RN with an even broader scope of practice. Your goals may even be to progress to the role of a nurse practitioner or a nurse educator with a graduate degree.

<table>
<tr><td>CORE CONCEPTS</td><td>TRANSITIONING INTO THE
GRADUATE NURSE ROLE</td></tr>
</table>

What do you foresee as the differences between being a student practical/vocational nurse and being a graduate? When we ask our students that question, the most common answer is "Responsibility." There is no longer an instructor there to answer your questions or guide your thinking until you are able to answer your own questions. Your patient load is greater. You will be going from caring for one to three patients to caring for four or more. You no longer have detailed nursing care plans to hand in and no more drug cards to do. However, you are expected to have those care plans engraved into your brain, and most of the drugs memorized by now. You are assuming a new role, and you might begin to feel uncomfortable and unsure of yourself as you approach it. You are in transition, moving from one role to another.

Another concern is that now superiors will have different expectations of you than they did when you were a student. In some cases, it seems as if health care facilities expect new grads to "hit the floor with both feet running"; in other words, they know you are new but expect that you are bringing 5 years of experience with you.

And if the facility's or its administration's expectations are unrealistic, we find that many graduates have even greater unrealistic expectations of themselves and others. Some new grads enter health care with a set of ideals that are impossible for anyone to live up to. They see all of the changes they think need to be made in nursing, and they want to make them *now*.

Reality shock (Kramer, 1974) is a phrase that has been used over the past 25 years to describe the feelings that new graduates experience when they transition from student to real-life worker. It is common in nursing. New graduates may begin to feel powerless to initiate the changes they feel are necessary in health care and frustrated because they feel they cannot give the kind of nursing care they were taught to deliver in nursing school. Some new nurses allow themselves to be so swept up in this reality shock that they begin to job hop searching for the ideal job; join in the disgruntled troops of nurses already working in their facility; reject their ideals and settle for the mediocre in nursing care; or leave nursing altogether.

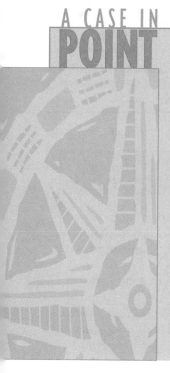

A CASE IN POINT

Judy and Bob are new LPN/LVN graduates. Judy has researched the opportunities and responsibilities related to pediatric nursing. She is definite about her goal to work for three years as a pediatric nurse before exploring other options. Bob hasn't a clue what type of nursing he would like—he just wants to make money in a position he thinks he might enjoy. Six months pass and Judy and Bob run into each other shopping. Judy found a position in pediatric nursing and is happy. Bob has changed jobs twice in 6 months. He started out on a medical–surgical unit but didn't like it. Now he is trying emergency room nursing, but it is not going well. He doesn't like the pace. They say goodbye. Bob is inspired by Judy. She seemed so content. He resolves to find another job, but this time give very serious thought to his choice.

ESSENTIAL SKILLS — GUIDELINES FOR TRANSITIONING INTO THE GRADUATE NURSING ROLE

1. Know your strengths and weaknesses even before you leave school. Ask instructors to help you build on your strengths and work on some of your weaknesses. Use the nursing skills lab to improve your competencies in specific skills. Ask for clinical assignments that will challenge you (e.g., ask for your patient load to be increased; ask to give medications for the whole group of students' patients).

2. Obtain more information on what health care facilities offer new grads. Many have pretty extensive orientation periods; some will assign you a preceptor to guide you through the orientation; some will allow you to go directly into a specialty unit for extensive training.

3. If the hospital does not assign preceptors, see if you can find a more experienced nurse who is willing to take you under his or her wing.

4. Know what expectations your new employer will have of new grads and reconcile that with *your* expectations of a new employer.

5. Work on your organizational and time management skills. You will feel less frustration if you see that you are accomplishing your nursing care in a timely, efficient manner.

6. Be flexible. Not everything in health care is black and white. In nursing school, you may have been taught not to sit on a patient's bed. In reality, that is often the best place for you to be in order to feed a patient without making a total mess and making the patient feel completely dependent. Since infection control is still an issue, place a clean piece of linen on the bed for you to sit on; then put it in the laundry when you are through.

7. Feed your sense of humor! It is difficult to get through nursing school without developing this necessary provider of endorphins for your system. Keep it alive as a nurse. Patients thrive with a nurse who can make them laugh. We even had a doctor one time call a student nurse over to congratulate her for saving the patient several hours' worth of pain medication just by making him laugh!

8. Exercise, eat right, and get plenty of rest. Does this sound like a prescription for good health care? It is. Do it for yourself.

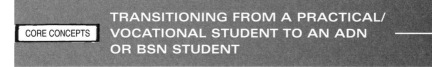

CORE CONCEPTS

TRANSITIONING FROM A PRACTICAL/ VOCATIONAL STUDENT TO AN ADN OR BSN STUDENT

Some of you may decide that you have not had enough of school and want to continue into a more advanced program. This decision might be made immediately after graduation, or it may be made after you have several years experience as an LPN or LVN.

If your state has a nursing articulation model, it will be relatively easy for you to enter an ADN program, as you will be given credit for the education you have already obtained. Other state schools may require that you retake certain courses to meet their criteria. Be sure you research schools and their entrance requirements. Some BSN programs are actually adopting an LPN/LVN to BSN tract to recognize your prior education and experience.

Remember that expectation of a student wanting to become an RN will be more extensive. There will be a stronger emphasis placed on the nursing process and the use of critical thinking skills. You will be taking your previous knowledge to a higher level. There will generally be more reading involved as well as more written assignments. If you have been out of school for a while, it may take a while to adjust to the educational mode again. If you are working, cut back on your hours until you see how time consuming this new role will be. You may need to brush up on certain nursing skills if you have been working in a specialty area and have not used all of your skills recently.

CORE CONCEPTS | **LIFELONG LEARNING**

In our opinion, whether you go on into an ADN or BSN program or whether you choose to remain at the LPN/LVN level either temporarily or permanently, you must continue to learn on a daily basis. Anyone who has been a nurse for any length of time will tell you that what you learned as "true" 6 months ago may no longer be true today. Techniques change; equipment changes; technology changes. We believe that a nurse who thinks there is nothing left to learn is a dangerous nurse. This is also the nurse who can become bored or burned out. So take advantage of facility inservices, attend workshops, present at workshops. Never let your nursing knowledge become stagnant.

Make the most of your nursing career. It is the only career in which your life will become so closely intertwined with the lives of others. You will see people during their finest hours; you will see them during their lowest moments. They may see you the same way. Some days, you will feel good about the nursing care you gave; other days, you will not. You will pick yourself back up dozens of times, dust yourself off, and start again. You will experience a wide range of emotions—some you didn't even know you had. You will make a difference in every life you touch, and you will be touched in return. No other profession offers these kinds of rewards—and heartaches. The nature of nursing is that it is a profession in which the choices are many. You are limited only by the limitations you place on yourself!

STOP | ASK YOURSELF

1. What do you hope to gain from being an LPN/LVN in addition to a salary and stability?

   _____

   _____

2. What plans do you have to continually update your knowledge? Will you participate in nursing organizations, subscribe to journals? If not, why not?

   _____

   _____

CYBERLINKS: FLASH CARDS

Check to see what you now remember by making your own flash cards. Use the CD-ROM that accompanies your textbook to discover how to make flash cards for reviewing and retaining what you have learned.

CONCEPT MAP WORD BANK

CAREER CHOICES

TRANSITION

CONTINUED LEARNING

Refer to Concept Maps and Flash Cards on pages viii–ix for an explanation of how to create and use concept maps. In addition, the CD-ROM guides you through the construction of concept maps by providing a more detailed introduction, more illustrations of examples, and key steps to follow in designing your own maps.

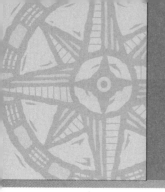

References

ALLEN, C. (1997). *Nursing process in collaborative practice: A problem-solving approach* (2nd ed.). Stamford, CT: Appleton & Lange.

AMERICA ONLINE, INC. (2000). Search engine results showing number of terms and percentages.

ANDREWS, M. M., & BOYLE, J. S. (1996). *Transcultural concepts in nursing care* (2nd ed.). Philadelphia: Lippincott-Raven.

ASK JEEVES, INC. (2001). Questions for an Ask Jeeves Search, Health Care Consumers Will Need Your Assistance.

ATKINSON, W., FURPHY, L., GANTT, J., & MAYFIELD, M. (Eds.). (1995). *Epidemiology and prevention of vaccine preventable diseases* (2nd ed.). Rockville, MD: U.S. Department of Health and Human Services.

BACON, J. (1995). Healing prayer: The risks and rewards. *Journal of Christian Nursing, 15*(3), 14–17.

BALL, J., & BINDLER, R. (1999). *Pediatric nursing: Caring for children* (2nd ed.). Upper Saddle River, NJ: Pearson Education.

BARREN, M. (1995). Take charge of your pain. *Modern Maturity,* 35–37, 80–81.

BERGER, K. J., & WILLIAMS, M. B. (1999). *Fundamentals of nursing: Collaborating for optimal health.* (2nd ed.). Upper Saddle River, NJ: Pearson Education.

BESDINE, R. N. (1990). Introduction. In W. B. Abrams & R. Berkow (Eds.), *The Merck manual of geriatrics.* Rahway, NJ: Merck, Sharp & Dohme Research Laboratories.

BEYEA, S. C. (1996). *Critical pathways for collaborative nursing care.* Menlo Park, CA: Addison-Wesley.

BEYEA, S. C., & NICOLL, L. H. (1997). Research utilization begins with learning to read research reports. *AORN Journal, 68*(3), 402–403.

BEYER, B. K. (1987). *Practical strategies for the teaching of thinking.* Boston: Allyn & Bacon.

BROOKFIELD, S. D. (1987). *Developing critical thinkers: Challenging adults to explore alternative ways of thinking and acting.* San Francisco: Jossey-Bass.

BURGESS, A. W. (1997). *Psychiatric nursing: Promoting mental health.* Stamford, CT: Appleton & Lange.

BURKE, M., & WALSH, M. (1992). *Gerontological nursing care of the frail elderly.* St. Louis, MO: Mosby-Year Book.

BURRELL, L. O., GERLACH, M. M., & PLESS, B. S. (1997). *Adult nursing: Acute and community care* (2nd ed.). Stamford, CT: Appleton & Lange.

BUTLER, R. N. (1969). Ageism: Another form of bigotry. *Gerontologist, 9,* 243–246.

BYRD, R. C., & SHERRILL, J. (1995). The therapeutic effects of intercessory prayer. *Journal of Christian Nursing, 2*(1), 21–23.

CHAFFEE, J. (1985). *Thinking critically.* Boston: Houghton Mifflin.

CLARK, C. C. (1978). *Assertive skills for nurses.* Wakefield, MA: Contemporary Publishing.

COBB, K. (November 2, 1997). A nutria in every pot? *Houston Chronicle,* 10A–11A.

CORBETT, J. V. (1996). *Laboratory tests and diagnostic procedures with nursing diagnoses* (4th ed.). Stamford, CT: Appleton & Lange.

DOSSEY, L. (1994). The science of prayer. *Natural Health,* March/April.

DUNN, H. (1961). *High-level wellness.* Arlington, VA: R. W. Beatty.

ERWIN, B., & DINWIDDIE, E. T. (1983). *Test without trauma.* New York: Grosset & Dunlap.

FARRELL, J. (1990). *Nursing care of the older person.* Philadelphia: Lippincott-Raven.

FITZPATRICK, J. J., & WHALL, A. L. (1996). *Conceptual models of nursing practice* (3rd ed.). Stamford, CT: Appleton & Lange.

FRETWELL, M. D. (1990). Comprehensive functional assessment. In W. B. Abrams, & R. Berkow (Eds.), *The Merck manual of geriatrics.* Rahway, NJ: Merck, Sharp & Dohme Research Laboratories.

GALLUP POLL. (1997, February 1). Religion survey results.

GRANT, E., NEWTON, M., & MOORE, S. (1995). Keeping patients on the right track. *Nursing 95, 27*(8), 57–59.

GRODNER, M., ANDERSON, S., & DEYOUNG, S. (1996). *Foundation and clinical applications of nutrition: A nursing approach.* St. Louis, MO: Mosby-Year Book.

GUIDO, G. W. (2001). *Legal and ethical issues in nursing* (3rd ed.). Upper Sadder River, NJ: Pearson Education.

HABEL, M. (1997). Stroke rehabilitation: What you need to know. *Healthweek-Houston/San Antonio, 2*(16), 18–19.

HAYFLICK, L. (1994). *How and why we age.* New York: Ballantine Books.

HERMAN, S. J. (1978). *Becoming assertive: A guide for nurses.* New York: Van Nostrand.

HINTON, W. D. (1997). Are cookies crumbling our privacy? *PC Novice, 8*(4), 83–85.

HOGAN, R. (1985). *Human sexuality: A nursing perspective.* Upper Saddle River, NJ: Pearson Education.

HUGHES, C. E. (1997). Prayer and healing: A case study. *Journal of Holistic Nursing, 15*(3), 318–324.

HUMPHREY, M. A. (1986). Effects of anticipatory grief for the patient, family member, and caregiver. In T. A. Rando (Ed.), *Loss and anticipatory grief.* Lexington, MA: Lexington Books.

HUMPHRY, D. (1991). *Final exit.* Eugene, OR: Hemlock Society.

KEE, J. L. (1999). *Laboratory & diagnostic tests with nursing implications* (5th ed.). Stamford, CT: Appleton & Lange.

KEITHLEY, J. K., KELLER, A., & VAZQUEZ, M. G. (1996). Promoting good nutrition: Using the food guide pyramid in clinical practice. *Medsurg Nursing, 5*(6), 397–403.

KRAMER, M. (1974). *The reality shock: Why nurses leave nursing.* St. Louis, MO: Mosby.

KÜBLER-ROSS, E. (1969). *On death and dying.* New York: Macmillan.

LEVINE, J. R., & YOUNG, M. L. (1994). *More Internet for dummies.* San Mateo, CA: IDG Books Worldwide.

LYNCH, S. H. (1997). Elder Abuse: What to Look for, How to Intervene, *AJN '97* (1):29.

MAINELLI, T. (1996). Internet search services show the way. *PC Novice, 7*(10), 77–79.

MARRINER-TOMEY, A. (1994). *Nursing theorists and their work.* St. Louis, MO: Mosby.

MASTERS, W. H., & JOHNSON, V. E. (1966). *Human sexual response.* Boston, MA: Little Brown.

MATTESON, M. A., McCONNELL, E. S., & LINTON, A. D. (1997). *Gerontological nursing: Concepts and practice* (2nd ed.). Philadelphia: Saunders.

MELZACK, R. (1992, April). Phantom limbs. *Scientific American,* 120–126.

MELZACK, R. (1998, February). Phantom limbs. *Discovery, 19*(266), 20.

MILTON, K. (1997, June). Real men don't eat deer. *Discover, 18*(6), 46–49.

MURRAY, R., & ZENTNER, J. (1997). *Health assessment & promotion strategies through the life span* (6th ed.). Stamford, CT: Appleton & Lange.

NIESWIADOMY, R. M. (1998). *Foundations of nursing research* (3rd ed.). Stamford, CT: Appleton & Lange.

O'TOOLE, M. T. (Ed.). (1997). *Miller-Keane encyclopedia & dictionary of medicine, nursing, and allied health.* Philadelphia: Saunders.

OREM, D. E. (1991). *Nursing: Concepts and practice.* St. Louis, MO: Mosby.

PARTNERSHIP FOR CARING, INC., 1620 Eye Street, NW, Suite 202, Washington, DC 20006 (800-989-9455).

PAUL, R. W. (1993). *Critical thinking: How to prepare students for a rapidly changing role.* Dillon Beach, CA: Foundation for Critical Thinking.

PERRY, M., & MACKUM, P. (2001, April). *Population change and distribution, Census 2000 brief.* U.S. Census Bureau. U.S. Department of Commerce. Washington, DC: Government Printing Office.

PUBLIC LAW 97-248, Title I, Sec. 122 (c) (3), Sept. 3, 1982, 96 Stat. 359.

RANDO, T. A. (1993). *Treatment of complicated mourning.* Champaign, IL: Research Press.

ROY, C., & ANDREWS, H. (1999). *The Roy adaptation model: The definitive statement* (2nd ed.). Stamford, CT: Appleton & Lange.

SIEGEL, K., MESAGNO, F. P., KARUS, D., CHRIST, G., BANKS, K., & MOYNIHAN, R. (1992). Psychosocial adjustment of children with a terminally ill parent. *Journal of the American Academy of Child Adolescent Psychiatry, 31*(2), 327–333.

SPECTOR, R. E. (2000). *Cultural diversity in health and illness* (5th ed.) Upper Saddle River, NJ: Pearson Education.

SPECTOR, R. E. (2000). *Cultural care guides to heritage assessment and health traditions.* Upper Saddle River, NJ: Pearson Education.

STRAUCH, J. (1997). I spy a good ISP. *Smart Computing, 5*(8), 71–74.

STRAUCH, J. (1998). Search service secrets. *Smart Computing, 5*(9), 81–84.

SULLIVAN, E. J., & DECKER, P. J. (1992). *Effective management in nursing.* Redwood City, CA: Addison-Wesley.

THE ASSOCIATED PRESS. (1998, April 3). Internet world is too wide for software engine to search. Beaumont Enterprise. 8C and 7C.

TOGNO-ARMANASCO, V., HOPKIN, L. A., & HARTER, S. (1995). How case management really works. *American Journal of Nursing, 95*(6), 24I–24J.

U.S. DEPARTMENT OF JUSTICE (1999, July). *Legal immigration, fiscal year 1998.* Immigration and Naturalization Service, Office of Policy and Planning, Statistics Branch. Washington, DC: Government Printing Office.

VARCAROLIS, E. M. (1998, p. 727). *Foundations of psychiatric–mental health nursing* (3rd ed.) Philadelphia, PA: Saunders.

VINCENT, C., YOUNG, M., & PHILLIPS, A. (1994). Why do people sue doctors? A study of patients and relatives taking legal action. *Lancet, 343,* 1609–1613.

WONG, D. L., HOCKENBERRY-EATON, M., WILSON, D., WINKELSTEIN, M. L., SCHWARTZ, P. (2001). *Wong's Essentials of Pediatric Nursing* (6th ed.) (p. 1301). St. Louis, MO: Mosby.

YAHOO!, Search engine.

■ SUGGESTED READING

AGENCY FOR HEALTH CARE POLICY AND RESEARCH (1992). *Clinical practice guidelines: Urinary incontinence in adults* (AHCPR Pub. No. 92-0038). Rockville, MD: U.S. Department of Health and Human Services, Public Health Service.

ALFARO-LEFEVRE, R. (1995). *Critical thinking in nursing.* Philadelphia: Saunders.

ASHBY, D. A. (1997). Medication calculation skills of the medical–surgical nurse. Medsurg Nursing, 6(2), 90–94.

EGBERT, L. A. (1990). The spectrum of suffering, *AJN, 8,* 35–39.

ESCHLEMAN, M. M. (1996). *Introductory nutrition and nutrition therapy.* Philadelphia: Lippincott-Raven.

HILL, S. S., & HOWLETT, H. A. (1993). *Success in practical nursing.* Philadelphia: Saunders.

KIRTZWEIL, P. (1993). "Nutritional facts" to help consumers eat smart. *FDA Consumer, 27*(4), 22–27.

LILLEY, L. L., & GUANCI, R. (1997). Persistent potassium problems. *American Journal of Nursing, 97*(6), 14.

McCLELLAND, C. (October, 1997). Personal communication.

NORNHOLD, P. (1997). Nursing on trial. *Nursing 97, 6*(7), 33.

PLUM, S. D. (1997). Nurses indicted. *Nursing 97, 6*(7), 35–36.

RUBENFELD, M. G., & SCHEFFER, B. K. (1995). *Critical thinking in nursing: An interactive approach.* Philadelphia: Lippincott-Raven.

SHORT, M. S. (1997). Charting by exception on a clinical pathway. *Nursing Management, 28*(8), 45–46.

SIMPSON, R. L. (1997). Point-of-care technology: A new perspective. *Nursing Management, 28*(8), 16.

STEHLIN, D. (1993). A little "lite" reading. *FDA Consumer, 27*(5), 12–16.

TOMKY, D. (1997). Taking a new look at an old adversary: Diabetes. *Nursing 97, 27*(11), 41–45.

VALANIS, B. (1999). *Epidemiology in health care* (3rd ed.). Stamford, CT: Appleton & Lange.

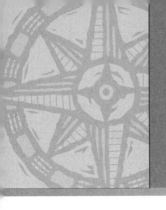

Index

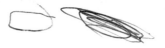

SINGLE PC LICENSE AGREEMENT AND LIMITED WARRANTY

READ THIS LICENSE CAREFULLY BEFORE OPENING THIS PACKAGE. BY OPENING THIS PACKAGE, YOU ARE AGREEING TO THE TERMS AND CONDITIONS OF THIS LICENSE. IF YOU DO NOT AGREE, DO NOT OPEN THE PACKAGE. PROMPTLY RETURN THE UNOPENED PACKAGE AND ALL ACCOMPANYING ITEMS TO THE PLACE YOU OBTAINED THEM. *THESE TERMS APPLY TO ALL LICENSED SOFTWARE ON THE DISK EXCEPT THAT THE TERMS FOR USE OF ANY SHAREWARE OR FREEWARE ON THE DISKETTES ARE AS SET FORTH IN THE ELECTRONIC LICENSE LOCATED ON THE DISK:*

1. GRANT OF LICENSE and OWNERSHIP: The enclosed computer programs and data ("Software") are licensed, not sold, to you by Pearson Education, Inc. ("We" or the "Company") and in consideration of your purchase or adoption of the accompanying Company textbooks and/or other materials, and your agreement to these terms. We reserve any rights not granted to you. You own only the disk(s) but we and/or our licensors own the Software itself. This license allows you to use and display your copy of the Software on a single computer (i.e., with a single CPU) at a single location for academic use only, so long as you comply with the terms of this Agreement. You may make one copy for back up, or transfer your copy to another CPU, provided that the Software is usable on only one computer.

2. RESTRICTIONS: You may not transfer or distribute the Software or documentation to anyone else. Except for backup, you may not copy the documentation or the Software. You may not network the Software or otherwise use it on more than one computer or computer terminal at the same time. You may not reverse engineer, disassemble, decompile, modify, adapt, translate, or create derivative works based on the Software or the Documentation. You may be held legally responsible for any copying or copyright infringement which is caused by your failure to abide by the terms of these restrictions.

3. TERMINATION: This license is effective until terminated. This license will terminate automatically without notice from the Company if you fail to comply with any provisions or limitations of this license. Upon termination, you shall destroy the Documentation and all copies of the Software. All provisions of this Agreement as to limitation and disclaimer of warranties, limitation of liability, remedies or damages, and our ownership rights shall survive termination.

4. LIMITED WARRANTY AND DISCLAIMER OF WARRANTY: Company warrants that for a period of 60 days from the date you purchase this SOFTWARE (or purchase or adopt the accompanying textbook), the Software, when properly installed and used in accordance with the Documentation, will operate in substantial conformity with the description of the Software set forth in the Documentation, and that for a period of 30 days the disk(s) on which the Software is delivered shall be free from defects in materials and workmanship under normal use. The Company does not warrant that the Software will meet your requirements or that the operation of the Software will be uninterrupted or error-free. Your only remedy and the Company's only obligation under these limited warranties is, at the Company's option, return of the disk for a refund of any amounts paid for it by you or replacement of the disk. THIS LIMITED WARRANTY IS THE ONLY WARRANTY PROVIDED BY THE COMPANY AND ITS LICENSORS, AND THE COMPANY AND ITS LICENSORS DISCLAIM ALL OTHER WARRANTIES, EXPRESS OR IMPLIED, INCLUDING WITHOUT LIMITATION, THE IMPLIED WARRANTIES OF MERCHANTABILITY AND FITNESS FOR A PARTICULAR PURPOSE. THE COMPANY DOES NOT WARRANT, GUARANTEE OR MAKE ANY REPRESENTATION REGARDING THE ACCURACY, RELIABILITY, CURRENTNESS, USE, OR RESULTS OF USE, OF THE SOFTWARE.

5. LIMITATION OF REMEDIES AND DAMAGES: IN NO EVENT, SHALL THE COMPANY OR ITS EMPLOYEES, AGENTS, LICENSORS, OR CONTRACTORS BE LIABLE FOR ANY INCIDENTAL, INDIRECT, SPECIAL, OR CONSEQUENTIAL DAMAGES ARISING OUT OF OR IN CONNECTION WITH THIS LICENSE OR THE SOFTWARE, INCLUDING FOR LOSS OF USE, LOSS OF DATA, LOSS OF INCOME OR PROFIT, OR OTHER LOSSES, SUSTAINED AS A RESULT OF INJURY TO ANY PERSON, OR LOSS OF OR DAMAGE TO PROPERTY, OR CLAIMS OF THIRD PARTIES, EVEN IF THE COMPANY OR AN AUTHORIZED REPRESENTATIVE OF THE COMPANY HAS BEEN ADVISED OF THE POSSIBILITY OF SUCH DAMAGES. IN NO EVENT SHALL THE LIABILITY OF THE COMPANY FOR DAMAGES WITH RESPECT TO THE SOFTWARE EXCEED THE AMOUNTS ACTUALLY PAID BY YOU, IF ANY, FOR THE SOFTWARE OR THE ACCOMPANYING TEXTBOOK. BECAUSE SOME JURISDICTIONS DO NOT ALLOW THE LIMITATION OF LIABILITY IN CERTAIN CIRCUMSTANCES, THE ABOVE LIMITATIONS MAY NOT ALWAYS APPLY TO YOU.

6. GENERAL: THIS AGREEMENT SHALL BE CONSTRUED IN ACCORDANCE WITH THE LAWS OF THE UNITED STATES OF AMERICA AND THE STATE OF NEW YORK APPLICABLE TO CONTRACTS MADE IN NEW YORK, AND SHALL BENEFIT THE COMPANY, ITS AFFILIATES AND ASSIGNEES. THIS AGREEMENT IS THE COMPLETE AND EXCLUSIVE STATEMENT OF THE AGREEMENT BETWEEN YOU AND THE COMPANY AND SUPERSEDES ALL PROPOSALS OR PRIOR AGREEMENTS, ORAL, OR WRITTEN AND ANY OTHER COMMUNICATIONS BETWEEN YOU AND THE COMPANY OR ANY REPRESENTATIVE OF THE COMPANY RELATING TO THE SUBJECT MATTER OF THIS AGREEMENT. If you are a U.S. Government user, this Software is licensed with "restricted rights" as set forth in subparagraph (a)–(d) of the Commercial Computer-Restricted Rights clause FAR 52.227-19 or in subparagraphs (c)(1)(ii) of the Rights Technical Data and Computer Software clause at DFARS 252.227-7013, and similar clauses, as applicable.

Should you have any questions concerning this agreement or you wish to contact the Company for any reason, please contact in writing: Prentice-Hall, New Media Department, One Lake Street, Upper Saddle River, NJ 07458.